Forensic Psychology

Drawing on psychological theory and research, this text outlines the core roles of the forensic psychology profession, providing students with a broad overview of the field and bringing to life the work of the forensic psychologists. Written by leading UK practitioners and researchers working in a range of contexts, it invites students to reflect on how psychological literature helps us to understand people in contact with the justice system.

Forensic psychology is continually evolving as a discipline and profession, shaping and responding to changes in legal processes, policies and provision. This book highlights the work of forensic psychologists, which covers a range of areas including assessment and intervention, applied research, consultancy and the training and development of staff working in forensic services such as secure services or community settings. Case studies are used to link psychological theory to practice, showcasing the latest developments in the field, and providing students with insights into best practice. The book further challenges myths in the field, encouraging students to humanise human harm and to apply compassion in their understanding of offending behaviour. Each chapter includes tasks and scenarios to promote critical thinking around theory and practice in what is an exciting time to work in this evolving field.

As a field of study and a profession within the systems for criminal and civil justice, forensic psychology overlaps and interacts with many other areas within and outside of psychology. As such, this volume details the contribution of forensic psychology to a range of presentations and organisational and professional issues, and is an ideal resource for courses in forensic psychology.

Dr Neil Gredecki is a Registered Forensic Psychologist, Chartered Scientist and Chartered Psychologist with over 18 years' experience in the assessment and treatment of forensic clients. He has held posts in HM Prison & Probation Service and in High, Medium and Low Secure Mental Health settings in both the NHS and private sector working with adults and young people, as well as academia.

Dr Polly Turner is a Registered Forensic Psychologist and Chartered Psychologist with over 18 years' experience in the assessment and treatment of forensic clients. She has worked predominantly with assessment and treatment of habitual aggression and personality disorder. She has held posts in High and Low Secure Mental Health settings in both the NHS and private sector and is a Clinical Senior Lecturer at the University of Manchester.

Topics in Applied Psychology Series

Series Editor: Graham Davey,
Professor of Psychology at the University of Sussex,
UK and former president of the British Psychological Society

Topics in Applied Psychology is a series of accessible, integrated textbooks ideal for courses in applied psychology. Written by leading figures in their field, the books provide a comprehensive academic and professional overview of the subject area, bringing the topics to life through a range of features, including personal stories, case studies, ethical debates, and learner activities. Each book addresses a broad range of cutting-edge topics, providing students with both theoretical foundations and real-life applications.

Educational Psychology, Second Edition
Edited by Tony Cline, Anthea Gulliford and Susan Birch

Work and Organizational Psychology, Second Edition
Ian Rothmann and Cary L. Cooper

Sport and Exercise Psychology, Second Edition
Edited by Andy Lane

Health Psychology, Second Edition
Charles Abraham, Mark Conner, Fiona Jones and Daryl O'Connor

Criminal Psychology, Second Edition
David Canter

Counselling Psychology
Edited by Victoria Galbraith

Clinical Psychology, Third Edition
Edited by Graham Davey, Nick Lake and Adrian Whittington

Forensic Psychology
Edited by Neil Gredecki and Polly Turner

Forensic Psychology

**Edited by Neil Gredecki
and Polly Turner**

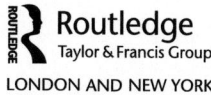

Routledge
Taylor & Francis Group

LONDON AND NEW YORK

Cover image: © Getty Images

First published 2022
by Routledge
2 Park Square, Milton Park, Abingdon, Oxon OX14 4RN

and by Routledge
605 Third Avenue, New York, NY 10158

Routledge is an imprint of the Taylor & Francis Group, an informa business

British Library Cataloguing-in-Publication Data
A catalogue record for this book is available from the British Library

Library of Congress Cataloging-in-Publication Data
Names: Gredecki, Neil, editor. | Turner, Polly, 1980– editor.
Title: Forensic psychology / edited by Dr. Neil Gredecki and Polly Turner.
Description: Milton Park, Abingdon, Oxon ; New York, NY : Routledge, 2022. |
    Series: Topics in applied psychology | Includes bibliographical references and index.
Identifiers: LCCN 2021034667 (print) | LCCN 2021034668 (ebook) |
    ISBN 9780367861322 (paperback) | ISBN 9780367861346 (hardback) |
    ISBN 9781003017103 (ebook)
Subjects: LCSH: Forensic psychology.
Classification: LCC RA1148 .F5567 2022 (print) | LCC RA1148 (ebook) |
    DDC 614/.15—dc23
LC record available at https://lccn.loc.gov/2021034667
LC ebook record available at https://lccn.loc.gov/2021034668

ISBN: 978-0-367-86134-6 (hbk)
ISBN: 978-0-367-86132-2 (pbk)
ISBN: 978-1-003-01710-3 (ebk)

DOI: 10.4324/9781003017103

Typeset in Bembo
by Apex CoVantage, LLC

For Dr Ruth Mann, an inspiring leader in forensic psychology practice and research

Contents

Contributors

Dr Zainab Al-Attar, HMPPS Psychology Service and University of Central Lancashire

Michelle Fletcher, HMPPS Psychology Services

Amy Freel, HM Prison & Probation Service

Dr Emily Glorney, Royal Holloway, University of London

Dr Neil Gredecki, HMPPS Psychology Services & University of Manchester

Dr Kerensa Hocken, HMPPS Psychology Services & Safer Living Foundation

Jude Kelman, HMPPS Psychology Services

Katie Lambert, Coastal Child and Adult Therapeutic Services (CCATS)

Dr Charlotte Lennox, University of Manchester

Karen Lloyd, HMPPS Psychology Services

Dr Caroline Logan, Greater Manchester Mental Health NHS Foundation Trust & University of Manchester

Siobhan Neave, Royal Holloway, University of London

Dr Adrian Needs, University of Portsmouth

Allison Nelson, HMPPS Psychology Services

Rachel Roper, Private Practice and Lead Assessor for Core Role 4, British Psychological Society

Yvonne Shell, Bournemouth University

Dr Jenny Tew, HMPPS Psychology Services

Sally Tilt, HMPPS Psychology Service

Dr Polly Turner, University of Manchester

Dr Jamie S. Walton, HMPPS Psychology Service

Dr Rachael Wheatley, HMPPS Psychology Services

Dr Fiona Wilks-Riley, Private Practice and University of Manchester

Series foreword

Psychology is still one of the most popular subjects for study at undergraduate degree level. As well as providing the student with a range of academic and applied skills that are valued by a broad range of employers, a psychology degree also serves as the basis for subsequent training and a career in professional psychology. A substantial proportion of students entering a degree programme in psychology do so with a subsequent career in applied psychology firmly in mind, and as a result, the number of applied psychology courses available at the undergraduate level has significantly increased over the recent years. In some cases, these courses supplement core academic areas, and in others, they provide the student with a flavour of what they might experience as a professional psychologist.

The *Topics in Applied Psychology Series* consists of eight textbooks designed to provide a comprehensive academic and professional insight into specific areas of professional psychology. The first seven texts cover the areas of clinical psychology, criminal psychology, educational psychology, health psychology, sports and exercise psychology, work and organisational psychology, and counselling psychology, and each text is written and edited by the foremost professional and academic figures in each of these areas.

It is now my pleasure to introduce this eighth book in the series covering forensic psychology. This book maps on to the four core roles in forensic psychology training – assessment and intervention, applied research, consultancy and training others. It seeks to give the reader a broad overview of applied forensic psychology practice in prisons, secure inpatient services and community settings, and all chapters have input from applied forensic psychologists.

Through successive editions, each textbook is based on a similar academic formula that combines a comprehensive review of cutting-edge research and professional knowledge with accessible teaching and learning features. The books are also structured, so they can be used as an integrated teaching support for a one-term or one-semester course in each of their relevant areas of applied psychology. Given the increasing importance of applying psychological knowledge across a growing range of areas of practice, we feel this series is timely and comprehensive. We hope you find each book in the series readable, enlightening, accessible and instructive.

Graham Davey
University of Sussex, Brighton, UK

Please Note: All case studies included within this text are fictional and seek to demonstrate the nature of forensic psychology practice and the characteristics of different offence types.

Part 1

What is forensic psychology?

1   What do forensic psychologists do?

Adrian Needs and Yvonne Shell

Summary

What forensic psychologists do should not be regarded as fixed and unchanging. History certainly demonstrates otherwise. Forensic psychology, as a field of study and as a profession within the systems for criminal and civil justice, overlaps and interacts with many other areas within and outside of psychology. Acceptance of the potential contributions of psychological science within these systems has by no means been automatic. It is unsurprising, particularly given the nature of the range of contexts in which they work, that forensic psychologists as members of a professional group have to be versatile and resilient. Their training reflects this. Practice and the knowledge base of forensic psychology have clearly evolved, and future changes in legal processes, policies and provision alone ensure that this will continue. Yet, there is also scope for self-determination in our use of and contribution to science. These are exciting times to be entering the field.

Introduction

In the words of an early document on their qualification, forensic psychologists form a 'broad church'. The wide range of work and settings encompassed by the profession and selective interest outside it can make it difficult to get a realistic overview. Despite frequent, often misleading, media portrayals, the majority of forensic psychologists are not involved in the profiling of criminals in investigative contexts. Similarly, there are laboratory-based areas of research which tend to figure prominently in undergraduate and MSc courses that are far from typical of the work of qualified practitioners in applied settings. Conversely, there are more representative areas which often receive relatively little exposure.

The impressive trajectory of forensic psychology over the last three decades, in particular, has included refined understanding, innovation and delivery in numerous areas of justice-related policy, procedure and practice. It has been accompanied by a major expansion in the number of people whose work is centred upon the field and by a growth in professional recognition.

It is useful to distinguish between forensic psychology as a field of study and forensic psychology as a profession. The former refers to the academic discipline, sometimes termed the 'knowledge base' of facts, findings and theory. Unsurprisingly, some of this comes from researchers in academic settings. Regarding forensic psychology as a profession, it is important to recognise that in the United Kingdom, the term 'forensic psychologist' is a legally protected title which can now only be used by suitably qualified practitioners who are registered with the Health and Care Professions Council (HCPC);

DOI: 10.4324/9781003017103-2

this is so even if they have achieved the 'gold standard' of chartership in the field by the British Psychological Society (BPS).

It should, however, also be recognised that psychologists from a range of different professional backgrounds sometimes provide direct services within the systems of criminal or civil justice as practitioners, expert witnesses, consultants or action researchers even if these settings are not the usual focus of their work. So, for example, a 2008 survey of psychologists' reports to assist criminal and civil courts found that clinical psychologists formed the largest single professional group engaged in this work.

The early history of the field suggests that acceptance of psychology's potential contributions within the operation of criminal and civil justice has been far from automatic. For example, for many years, the legal profession showed little interest in issues such as the fallibility of memory or the unreliability of confessions. Even several decades after the first attempts at introducing expert testimony on such matters, the Court of Appeal ruled that jurors were perfectly able to judge for themselves issues concerning ordinary human behaviour, without supposed experts complicating things (*R. v Turner, 1975*). Greater integration and influence came largely through demonstrating value and establishing precedents. These were also the hallmark of pioneering work in prisons; some milestones in the history of psychological services in HM Prison Service are depicted in Focus Box 1.1.

The present volume covers a range of activities and issues which are illustrative of forensic psychology as a profession. This chapter reflects its evolution and the competencies that are intrinsic to the work and qualification of forensic psychologists in applied settings. The perspective taken is that components of practice, like development of the field, or psychological phenomena more generally, exist neither in a context-free vacuum nor in isolation from each other.

Focus Box 1.1   The development of prison service psychology in England and Wales through the twentieth century

1925: 'industrial psychologist' asked to conduct research into the vocational interests and aptitudes of 'Borstal boys' (incarcerated male young offenders).

1946: conducting assessments for allocation to training programmes the primary task of the first psychologists to be employed in prisons in England and Wales on a full-time basis.

1952: psychologists employed whose work included assisting in the selection of prison officers.

1950s: psychologists employed to assist medical officers in reports for court.

1960s: development and support of specialist regimes such as group counselling, therapeutic communities, industrial training and the formation of dedicated project groups in headquarters.

1974: review emphasised providing support to management and working with special groups such as lifers.

1980: review highlighted many psychologists engaged in individual as well as group-based work with prisoners along with staff training, research, organisational and operational (e.g. hostage incident) consultancy.

1985: first Control Review Committee special unit for severely disruptive and/or violent prisoners established, with psychological support.

1992: first accredited cognitive-behavioural psychological group work programme (Sex Offender Treatment Programme).

Forensic psychology as a field of study

It would be misleading to assert that forensic psychology is a branch of psychology that is self-contained and separated from other branches. As a discipline, it engages with settings, purposes and issues centred on criminal and civil justice, including the behaviour, usually harmful to others, which triggers the operation of the agencies which then become involved. These facets can be striking, despite interest in them not being exclusive to forensic psychology. It is also not difficult to see that some of forensic psychology's knowledge base has its origins in the adaptation of findings, methods and theory from elsewhere.

So, for example, assessments and interventions have their roots in clinical tradition. Training and consultancy in organisations such as prisons draw upon occupational psychology. The study of offending in young people and the origins of offending in many older ones are enhanced by developmental psychology. Many insights into aggression come from social psychology, and much research relevant to police investigative procedures could be regarded as applied cognitive psychology. Forensic psychology also interfaces with criminology (grounded in sociology), psychiatry (grounded in medicine) and the law whilst shaped and augmented by its own research, developments, settings and contextual influences (including culture, policies and politics).

Finding a summary label for such a broad church was not easy and the title 'forensic' has not met with universal approval. During debates that surrounded its adoption, some insisted that the term should be kept exclusively for work informing the decision-making of the courts, pointing to its Latin origin and sneering at the idea that the meaning of words might change to reflect their emerging usage. Others countered by pointing to examples of how meanings of words often *do* evolve; for example, a once-common definition of 'clinical' was 'of or at the sickbed'. There were already forensic psychiatrists, and the professional body title 'Division of Forensic Psychology' arguably flows better than 'Division of Criminological and Legal Psychology', which it replaced.

Critical evaluation is intrinsic to the development of scientific thinking, and we invite you to consider in your future studies whether forensic psychology's very breadth might be a source of fragmentation or whether apparent successes might sometimes introduce a degree of rigidity and insularity (the orthodoxy of a broad church?). Also, have practitioners and researchers been sufficiently conscious of potential parallels with other sciences? These are often concerned with issues such as the conditions necessary for changes to occur, processes by which new phenomena emerge and patterns and sequences rather than generalisations based on differences in group means.

It is inevitable that forensic psychology is still very much a work in progress. This should be an exciting prospect for those who are drawn to contributing to its development!

Forensic psychology as a profession

Precisely what forensic psychologists do will depend largely on where they work and even ostensibly similar settings can vary widely. For example, prisons vary in aspects such as security category, function and population as well as architecture. It should also be recognised that many forensic psychologists change work settings during the course of their careers. Competencies that forensic psychologists must demonstrate span several areas and client groups. This provides a foundation for versatility and adaptability, qualities which must also serve practitioners in sometimes intense situations with some of the most challenging, complex, disturbed or disadvantaged individuals in society. These sometimes occur in equally unusual environments that involve a heightened awareness of aspects such as security. It is unsurprising, too, that issues of ethics and resilience are rarely far away.

Training as a forensic psychologist

It is usual to start with an honours or joint honours degree in psychology that is accredited to provide Graduate Basis for Chartered Membership (GBC) of the BPS. Conversion courses are available for people who wish to attain GBC (often holders of other degrees, or ones which do not meet BPS criteria). Whilst the BPS relaxed the necessity for GBC to precede stage 1 of qualification (completion of an accredited MSc in Forensic Psychology), lack of GBC can be a disadvantage when applying and studying and still needs to be obtained subsequently (See Figure 1.1).

Although all stage 1 programmes are university based, this is not true of stage 2: the BPS Qualification in Forensic Psychology (QFP) involves practice under supervision and submission of evidence of competence in one or more settings of employment over a minimum of two years. The other options at this stage are to complete a professional doctorate in forensic psychology that leads to eligibility for chartered status with the BPS and registration with the HCPC, or a postgraduate diploma (PgDip) as an HCPC practitioner in forensic psychology that leads to HCPC registration alone; both these options

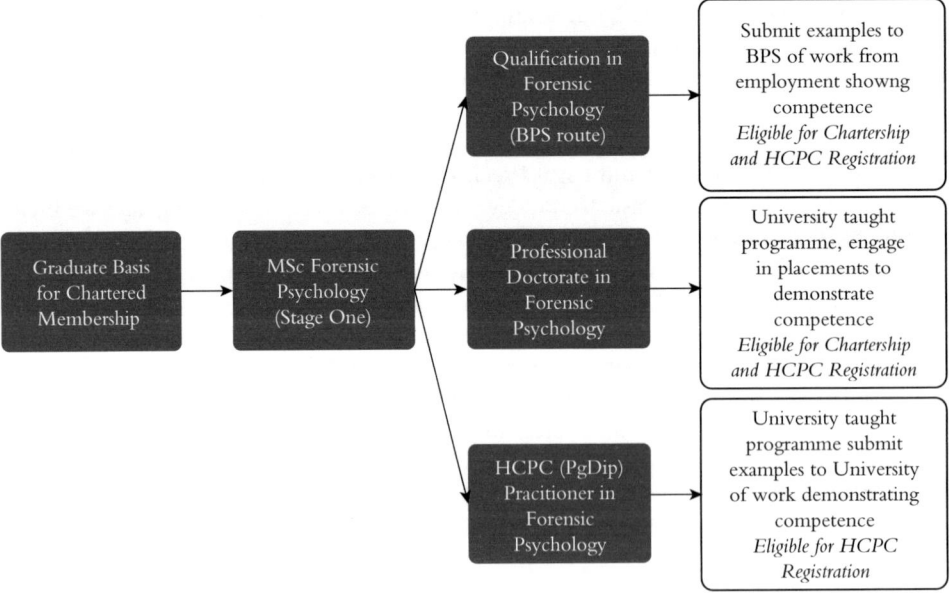

Figure 1.1 Training to become a forensic psychologist

Source: Some Prof Doc programmes incorporate Stage 1 (i.e., an MSc) so the process isn't necessarily as sequential as suggested by the diagram.

are university based. Detailed information on training and qualification is available from the BPS website (www.bps.org.uk).

Competencies articulated as requirements of the BPS route are based on an extended and large-scale project by delegates from across the BPS to identify and represent as standards the work performed by all applied psychologists. The project identified a common core of activities across branches of applied psychology, although of course differences were noted in contexts of practice and specialist knowledge.

> ***Core Role 1***: ***Conducting Psychological Applications and Interventions*** outlines a cycle of identifying, assessing and addressing issues, from initial formulation through planning, implementation and evaluation of effectiveness, with engagement with others including multidisciplinary working as appropriate. This cycle is fundamental to working as a practitioner, whether as a clinician or as a consultant.
>
> ***Core Role 2***: ***Research*** involves designing, conducting, analysing and evaluating an applied, field-based research project.
>
> ***Core Role 3***: ***Communicating Psychological Knowledge and Advice to Other Professionals*** shares an emphasis on problem-solving and making decisions, but directed towards feeding into that undertaken by others; sensitive and appropriate interpersonal engagement with their perspectives is essential, as is awareness of the realities and frameworks of the setting in question.
>
> ***Core Role 4***: ***Training Other Professionals in Psychological Skills and Knowledge***. Analysis of suboptimal job performance involves investigation of a range of factors (including management, feedback and the consequences of desired or undesired behaviour) that are often not reducible to deficits in skills and knowledge alone. Formal training is not always the best solution, and where adopted, active steps must be taken to ensure that gains transfer to and are maintained in the work environment. The specific competencies associated with this Core Role indicate that is not just about what goes on in a classroom.

You may have noted continuities between the core roles in aspects such as formulation, problem-solving and interpersonal engagement. There is also a synergy between them so, for example, experience in delivering training can enhance confidence and skills in consultancy briefings or in conducting groupwork. It can also set the scene for positive working relationships in the demanding multidisciplinary environments of the criminal justice system. Whilst this synergy is an example of the whole being greater than the sum of the parts, there is scope for developing further understanding of the processes which enable competent performance of the outcomes specified in the core roles.

Practitioners must navigate contextual factors including norms, regulations, demands, opportunities, precedents, other professions, management and organisational culture, current policies and the political and ethical climate. In addition, work on what constitutes skilfulness highlights aspects such as sensitivity to situational contexts and creativity in problem-solving. We are also beginning to appreciate the fundamental ramifications of how we make sense 'with' people rather than simply 'of' them (Needs, 2020). To this end, we see the emergence of work on co-constructed/co-produced formulations with those detained in inpatient services (Lewis-Morton et al., 2017). Such skills are much closer to what being a scientist-practitioner entails than template-following and an emphasis on procedures over process which is often insufficient for meeting complex demands (Lane & Corrie, 2006).

It should also be emphasised that forensic psychologists are reflective practitioners. The ability to understand the supervision space and to recognise that supervision is an active process that demands preparation and openness to ongoing learning, professional and personal development is vital. Reflecting on the impact of work and one's responses offers opportunities for learning and insight. Exploring values, beliefs and their influence is a key function of supervision.

Settings in which forensic psychologists work

Prisons

Picking up the narrative from Focus Box 1.1, the embracing of standardised group interventions from the 'What Works' movement (see McGuire, 2013), improved consistency and enabled work with a greater number of prisoners. Its focus on perceived risk and reducing re-offending fitted political imperatives. With financial investment and a management culture increasingly concerned with performance targets and accountability for resources, over the next couple of decades accredited, cognitive behavioural, group-based programmes came to dominate the work of many forensic psychologists in prisons. Although they were largely overtaken by similarly 'risk-need-responsivity' (Andrews & Bonta, 1994)–based assessments of risk, the numbers of psychologists and psychological assistants employed in prisons grew steadily.

This growth broadly followed adoption of the title 'forensic psychologist' and accredited programmes and risk assessment (usually in relation to the Parole Board) came almost to define the contributions of forensic psychologists. This was double edged. Prisoners sometimes saw these activities as policy driven and impersonal, and for several years, opportunities for trainee forensic psychologists to undertake the range of work necessary to complete stage 2 were reduced. Fortunately, in recent years, there has been progress in addressing these issues accompanied by initiatives which once more place how forensic psychologists in prisons are regarded and able to practise on a less restricted footing. These include the establishing of trauma-informed care and applications of the holistic principles associated with 'Enabling Environments' (see Akerman et al., 2018).

In 2020, Her Majesty's Prison and Probation Service (HMPPS) advertised itself as the 'biggest single employer of psychologists in the country' (*The Psychologist*, February 2020), and it is recognised as being a key provider of opportunities for completion of stage 2 for trainee forensic psychologists. There are also other routes for forensic psychologists to work with prisoners, such as working for NHS in-reach services addressing issues relating to mental health or working for 'third sector' organisations offering specialist services in areas such as substance misuse.

Secure psychiatric services

Secure psychiatric services assist individuals who have identified mental health challenges or require assessment. Levels of security ('high', 'medium' and 'low') may influence the nature of practice, and work requires an understanding of mental health presentations and associated assessments and treatments. Once the preserve of clinical psychologists, forensic psychologists now work alongside clinical psychologists or have dual qualification; other colleagues include psychiatrists, psychiatric nurses, occupational therapists and art therapists. Such specialist forensic mental health services offer assessment for the presence of mental disorder, consideration of any indication of risk to others, subsequent treatment of identified disorder and work towards successful reintegration into society. How forensic psychologists contribute within forensic health settings varies depending on the setting. What is common to all, however, is the requirement for a comprehensive understanding of mental health legislation and of the different pathways available for the progression of detained patients through the system.

Probation

Although numbers never quite expanded in the way envisaged 10 years earlier, the National Probation Service is another notable employer of forensic psychologists. (By the time of publication, Community Rehabilitation Companies, introduced in 2014, should be a thing of the past.) Probation services are particularly focused on risk assessment, mitigation and management. Forensic psychologists' roles often concern this area, staff training, consultancy and sometimes research.

Community services

Community Forensic Mental Health Services (CFMHS) provide assessment, specialist treatment and case management of those identified as presenting a risk of harm to others or self. Clients often have complex mental health and social needs, often presenting with vulnerability and their own victim experiences as well as potential for serious risk. Case management includes liaison with other services involved in the management of the individual (e.g. Multi-Agency Public Protection Arrangements or MAPPA). Individuals subject to care and management from CFMHS teams include those on a 'step down' from being detained in secure psychiatric accommodation or subject to Community Treatment Orders. Again, forensic psychologists working in this arena will find themselves working as part of a multidisciplinary team.

Police

In terms of employment of forensic psychologists, this is an area which is at a relatively early stage of development. Some people with a background in psychology work directly as researchers or crime analysts (largely with statistical data), and fewer still work as behavioural investigative advisors. These aside, full-time jobs are rare although there have been precedents in areas such as providing support for stress or training, research and operational support in firearms and hostage incidents. It is more common for psychologists from various (including academic) backgrounds to undertake sessional training or consultancy work in specific areas. Greater details on such roles may be found in Brown et al. (2015).

Courts

As noted earlier, much expert witness is provided by psychologists who would not use the title 'forensic', with clinical psychologists figuring particularly prominently. (When the American Psychological Association recognised forensic psychology as a 'specialty discipline' in 2001, they defined it, rather confusingly for UK readers, as 'the application of clinical psychology to the legal arena'.) The involvement of psychologists from a range of other backgrounds points to engagement with a spectrum of legal concerns. What these psychologists have in common is usually many years of experience in their specialist areas before (accompanied by an appropriate knowledge of legal procedure) assisting the courts with expert testimony. The same applies to the substantial number of forensic psychologists who provide such assistance. For many who have moved into private practice, this may be a core activity. Areas addressed include fitness to plead and stand trial, recommendations for treatment and child custody disputes.

'Other' services

These include non-governmental organisations such as charities concerned with, for example, working with victims of crime or individuals with issues of substance misuse. Each organisation will take a unique approach to how it will utilise its staff group, including forensic psychologists. In such settings, it is possible to find oneself in a position of significant influence, being a key driver of policy and systems change. Senior qualified forensic practitioners may find themselves offered positions of executive roles, moving them away from direct clinical work and practice.

Case study: a week in the life of a forensic psychologist working in a prison

Dan, a forensic psychologist who qualified two years ago with a professional doctorate in forensic psychology, is currently working in a busy remand prison (an establishment where prisoners are held whilst awaiting trial). He meets people with a wide range of psychological presentations and equally varied histories of offending behaviour and contact with the criminal justice system. See Table 1.1 for a typical week for Dan. For most, there are strong emotions associated with their detention including anxiety, shame, anger, frustration, confusion and depression. For some, their psychological response to imprisonment manifests itself in self-harming behaviour or suicide attempts. For others, the expression of anger can be a means by which to try and wrestle some feelings of control of a situation in which they feel powerless. They may feel resentful of the system of which Dan may be perceived to be part. In addition, the research base confirms the high percentage of those in prison with backgrounds of personality disorder, learning difficulties, childhood trauma or mental illness. In his work, Dan must hold in mind prisoners' psychological well-being, their needs and also the offending behaviour that led them to this point in their lives and may recur; a major purpose of working with offenders is of course the prevention of future harm.

Let us consider what a working week for Dan may look like, focusing on a particular referral.

Referral

Much of Dan's work is centred upon mentalisation-based therapy groupwork and conducting risk assessments using the HCR-20 (see Chapter 3). However, the week had hardly begun before he received a referral regarding a young male, Jim, who had been placed in the prison's segregation as a result of setting fire to his cell whilst still inside it. Staff had commenced the Assessment, Care in Custody and Teamwork (ACCT) process

Table 1.1 A typical week from Dan's diary

Monday	Tuesday	Wednesday	Thursday	Friday
8.30–9.00 Check e-mails	8.30–9.00 Read files for MBT★ referrals	8.30–9.30 Continue work on HCR-20 Historical factors	8.30–9.00 Check e-mails	8.30–9.00 Check e-mails
9.00–12.00 Attendance at local training for staff on safety and breakaway techniques	9.00–10.00 Discussion with wing staff about new referral	9.30–11.00 Attend meeting to review prisoners currently subject to an open ACCT	9.00–10.00 Review offender records prior to group	9.00–13.00 Report writing for those who have completed MBT groupwork
12.00–13.00 Referral meeting	10.00–11.00 Assessment with offender referred for fire-setting	11.00–12.00 Psychometric assessment of prisoner for MBT group	10.00–11.00 Scoring of psychometric material for MBT group	
	11.00–12.00 Scoring of psychometric assessment measures for fire-setting incident	12.00–13.00 Psychology Department meeting	11.00–13.00 MBT groupwork prep, group facilitation and debrief	
14.00–16.00 Review of prisoner files for completion of HCR-20	14.00–16.30 MBT groupwork prep, group facilitation and group debrief	13.30–16.00 Groupwork supervision for MBT group	14.00–16.00 Individual supervision to discuss individual cases	14.00–16.00 Completion of functional analysis of a further fire-setting episode, includes meeting with offender and segregation staff
16.00–17.00 Phone discussion with probation officer on offender	16.30–17.00 Complete case notes from assessment and MBT group	16.00–17.00 Case note write up	16.00–17.00 Complete case notes from MBT group	16.00–17.00 Complete case notes

★ Mentalisation-Based Therapy

of care planning for prisoners identified as at risk of suicide or self-harm. The ACCT process requires that particular actions are undertaken by prison personnel and the referral sought clarification as to whether the fire-setting was an attempt to disrupt prison routine in a reckless way or was in fact an attempt at self-harm/suicide.

Dan began by considering available background information including past reports. The nature of offender records can be variable (for example, due to limited previous contact with the criminal justice system), and it can be helpful to speak to a range of professionals to supplement this. Crucially, Dan spoke to wing staff where the prisoner had been located. Wing staff were able to let Dan know that he had been waiting a considerable time for transfer to a prison closer to home, had a history of cutting his arms and legs and that he was perceived as argumentative with prisoners and staff on the wing. He spent considerable periods of time on his own and was described by staff as 'demanding'. Staff also had suspicions that Jim was using drugs, specifically new psychoactive substances, e.g., Spice. Overall, they felt that the fire-setting incident could have been an accidental result of substance misuse, a form of self-harm, or a demonstration of frustration at his situation to precipitate a move from the establishment.

Assessment

Dan was aware that when contact began the first thing to establish was Jim's consent to participate and the beginnings of the professional relationship would be central to the success of the referral. He was mindful of the power imbalance and complexities relating to genuine-informed consent in secure settings. During the assessment, interviewing (see Chapter 5) was supplemented with the use of a number of psychometric assessment tools, their selection depending on presenting issues, training in use or the availability of supervision on their use.

Dan also referred to the evidence base on fire-setting to help him explore hypotheses and derive a framework within which to make sense – with Jim – of the fire-setting behaviour.

Formulation

Dan used several sessions to complete a collaborative formulation (see Chapter 5). He knew that he was fortunate that his role within the prison permitted this, as many of his peers in other establishments would like more time, for example, to conduct their risk assessments and, outside of specialist units, some these days have little opportunity to complete individual interventions.

The understanding reached by Dan and Jim was that the cell fire-setting incident served two purposes. One function of the behaviour served to release feelings of frustration, anger and resentment. Jim was able to articulate that he has minimal ways of dealing with his distress and that historically he had set fires as a means of seeking to regulate his emotional state. However, Jim was able to acknowledge that the fire-setting on this occasion also served a second function, of trying to force his removal from the wing to a prison closer to home.

Recent literature on typologies of fire-setting behaviour and perpetrators (see Chapter 10, this volume), combined with the collateral detail that Jim had been previously diagnosed with emotionally unstable personality disorder (see Chapter 15, this volume), suggested additional hypotheses concerning Jim's problems in managing life's demands and distress.

Communication and confidentiality

The issue of confidentiality is a thorny one in the forensic setting. As made explicit by Dan when gaining consent from Jim for the work to be undertaken, there could only be limited confidentiality. The findings around the dual function of the fire-setting behaviour in Jim's cell needed to be communicated to prison staff. This was despite the potential implications of sharing this information and the possibility that this might lead Jim to withdraw his cooperation from addressing the function of emotional expression of the fire-setting behaviour. Although Jim's response would provide additional evidence about how he responds to perceived unfairness (a possible 'offence-paralleling behaviour'), Dan was aware of the need to help staff to think sensitively about how they could best respond to support Jim and keep him and those around him safe.

Intervention

Jim had repeatedly refused to engage in groups. Given the seemingly pivotal role of distress in Jim's fire setting behaviour, following discussion during supervision with his line manager, Dan drew upon material on distress tolerance from a form of enhanced cognitive behavioural therapy and used it with Jim on an individual basis. However, midway through the treatment and with no prior warning, Dan arrived in the segregation unit to find that Jim had been transferred from the prison the day before. This caused some concern for Dan as he was aware of the evidence that exiting interventions, prior to completion, may elevate risk. Due to this, Dan wrote a closing letter to Jim providing an account of the positive work he had undertaken to date. Dan also wrote to the psychology department in the receiving establishment notifying them that Jim had been midway through a piece of psychological therapy and the focus of that work.

Evaluation

It is critical that forensic clinical work is well evaluated. In this instance, Dan was unable to do this as Jim was transferred prior to completing the intervention. Evaluation may use psychometric measures and other forms of self-report, ideally combined with collection of data from wing staff concerning changes in behaviour. In this case, Jim had set a fire during the second week in segregation. Dan had sat with Jim following this incident and completed a functional analysis of the behaviour to encourage maximum learning from the episode. The subsequent six weeks of treatment were incident-free. It was important that all relevant information was included in Jim's record for future reference, for example, to facilitate future risk assessments.

Conclusion

It is the closeness rather than uniqueness of forensic psychologists' alignment with a range of distinctive settings and demands that is intrinsic to their professional identity. The same applies to the synthesis of knowledge and expertise required to provide an effective service in these settings. Recognition has come from taking opportunities to establish, over time, the relevance, value and integrity of psychological science and its representatives.

We must continue to be responsive and willing to embrace flexibility without compromising standards. Active engagement and reciprocal influence in contexts are as influential in the development of specialist knowledge, activities and services as they are in the development of individual human beings. Taking a lead from other sciences, all can be seen as dynamic systems consisting of 'multiple components that constantly interact with each other and with internal and external processes that change and evolve over time' (Hayes et al., 2015, p. 29).

This possibly unfamiliar perspective is equally relevant to handling what confronts us and what we seek to influence as practitioners, including orienting us to features and dynamics that do not come 'clearly defined and readily packaged' (Lane & Corrie, 2006, p. 23). This extends to reflective understanding of the wider sociopolitical context in which we operate and the service context in which we practice; these are part of the landscape that we jointly inhabit with the individual in front of us. Individuals in criminal justice settings often have long-standing problems with experiencing connectedness (including a sense of 'with') and therefore moving from current positions. It is through our engagement and our facilitating that of others – with the integrity that leads to trust – that we mobilise development in individual offenders and in the criminal justice system itself.

Recommended further activity

You are encouraged to access the HMPPS Forensic Psychology Podcast (https://pod. link/1533101974) and listen to the following episode which explores concepts discussed in this chapter:

Episode 1: An introduction to forensic psychology [15/10/2020]

Learning outcomes

When you have completed this chapter, you should be able to:

1   Suggest reasons why knowledge and practice in forensic psychology are still evolving
2   Describe the range of settings in which forensic psychologists work
3   Outline core roles required for qualification, their rationale and their interrelatedness
4   Understand the role of assessment, formulation, intervention and evaluation

Key concepts and terms

- Contexts
- Scientist-practitioner
- Reflective practice
- Assessment
- Expert witness
- Formulation
- Communication
- Intervention
- Research
- Evaluation
- Consultancy
- Staff training
- Multidisciplinary working
- Accredited programmes
- Problem-solving
- Risk
- Dynamic systems
- Supervision
- Integrity

Sample essay questions

1   To what extent has forensic psychology generated a knowledge base of its own that is effective for its purposes?
2   How have the contexts in which forensic psychology is practised influenced the evolution of this practice?
3   How important is it for forensic psychologists to work with managers and personnel (as well as those suspected or convicted of crimes) in criminal justice settings?

Recommended further reading

Akerman, G., Needs, A., & Bainbridge, C. (Eds.). (2018). *Transforming environments and rehabilitation: A guide for practitioners in forensic settings and criminal justice.* Routledge.

Brown, J., Shell, Y., & Cole, T. (2015). *Forensic psychology: Theory, research, policy and practice.* Sage.

Lane, D. A., & Corrie, S. (2006). *The modern scientist-practitioner: A guide to practice in psychology.* Routledge.

References

Andrews, D. A., & Bonta, J. (1994). *The psychology of criminal conduct.* Anderson Publishing.

Hayes, A. M., Yasinski, C., Barnes, J. B., & Bockting, C. L. H. (2015). Network destabilization and transition in depression: New methods for studying the dynamics of therapeutic change. *Clinical Psychology Review, 41,* 27–39.

Lewis-Morton, R., Harding, S., Lloyd, A., Macleod, A., Burton, S., & James, L. (2017). Co-producing formulation within a forensic setting: A co-author with a service user and the clinical team. *Mental Health and Social Inclusion, 21*(4), 230–239.

McGuire, J. (2013). "What works" to reduce re-offending: 18 years on. In L. A. Craig, L. Dixon, & T. A. Gannon (Eds.), *What works in offender rehabilitation: An evidence-based approach to assessment and treatment* (pp. 20–49). Wiley-Blackwell.

Needs, A. (2020). Veterans, horses and the rediscovery of "with". *The Psychologist, 33,* 56–61.

2 Challenges in developing evidence-based practice in forensic settings

Charlotte Lennox and Polly Turner

Summary

This chapter begins by exploring the terms evidence-based practice and scientist-practitioner and how they relate to forensic psychology. We outline core research methods and how research design is guided by the questions we ask. The chapter highlights the core ethical principles of research, how forensic research can challenge these and provides an overview of the current process for ethical approval. We present a summary of intervention research within forensic settings and a single case of a randomised controlled trial of a complex intervention for prison leavers, where we will discuss the main strengths and limitations of trial methodology within forensic settings. We conclude considering whether we can do more to understand 'how' interventions work.

Introduction

Psychology is a science and psychologists are scientist-practitioners. However, what do we mean by the term scientist-practitioner? The scientist-practitioner model argues that applied psychologists should be trained in both practice *and* science, as the two can never be considered independent. Psychologists must embrace and apply the core principles of their basic scientific training to all aspects of their work including clinical work. Many students of psychology perceive the research components of their degree programmes as unnecessary and irrelevant to real-life psychology practice. Indeed, some psychologists have rejected the notion that 'pure' research is applicable to daily practice. Yet, the essence of the model is that the practicing psychologist should think and act scientifically and be committed to integrating science with practice (see Shapiro, 2002). Indeed, forensic psychologists need to be committed to evaluating and applying the latest scientific evidence to their practice, as well as contributing to that evidence base. The training of forensic psychologists embodies this.

Research and scientific enquiry are central to stages 1 and 2 of applied training in forensic psychology (see Chapter 1 for details on the training routes). MScs in forensic psychology (stage 1) build on the BSc research training with teaching of advanced methods and analysis culminating in an empirical forensic psychology study (i.e. the MSc dissertation). Supervised practice (stage 2) requires candidates to undertake applied forensic psychology research. Core Role 2 of the British Psychological Society (BPS) Qualification in Forensic Psychology (QFP) has this explicit focus on research, requiring candidates to submit applied forensic research for assessment. Yet, Core Role 2 is not the only core role which requires research skills to be evidenced. The

DOI: 10.4324/9781003017103-3

BPS qualification and Health and Care Professions Council (HCPC) training routes expect to see consistent evidence of the scientist-practitioner approach across the period of supervised practice across all core roles (e.g. assessments and interventions, consultancy and training other professionals). In this chapter, we will outline how research is embedded beyond direct research activity and more broadly into forensic psychology practice.

Evidence-based practice

Evidence-based practice (EBP) originated in the field of medicine but is of significance to forensic psychology. EBP means using the *best current available evidence* to help *inform a decision* about the *care and treatment an individual* should receive. The main aims of EBP are to improve the quality of care, to provide accountability to the decision made and to ensure interventions have demonstrable value within the resources available (Spring, 2007). So, let us look at EBP in more detail. EBP's three components are, research evidence, clinical expertise and patient preference. This is often referred to as the 'three legged stool' (Lilienfield et al., 2013; Spring, 2007).

How do forensic psychologists appraise what constitutes the best current available research evidence?

This first leg of the stool focuses on research evidence. This can be divided into examining issues related to (a) therapeutic efficacy (how well an intervention works in controlled settings), (b) therapeutic effectiveness (how well an intervention works in the 'real-world') and (c) the psychological processes at work (e.g. emotion, personality traits, thinking; Lilienfield et al., 2013). Central to EBP is a system for classifying what constitutes the best evidence; the hierarchy of evidence (see Figure 2.1) can help us to appraise this evidence and takes a top-down approach, with research designs ranked on the rigour (strength and precision) of their research methods. However, different hierarchies exist for different research methods (quantitative versus qualitative e.g. Daly et al., 2007), and even within the same method professionals may disagree on the exact rank of information; therefore, many different hierarchies exist. Two commonly used examples are the Oxford Centre for Evidence-Based Medicine Levels of Evidence (OCEBM, 2011) and the National Health and Medical Research Council (NHMRC, 2009).

A well-conducted systematic review is generally considered to provide the best evidence as they are based on the findings of multiple studies, identified using a comprehensive and systematic literature search. However, this position at the top of the evidence hierarchy is not absolute. Systematic reviews can take years to complete and are reliant on there being enough well-conducted primary studies to include in the review. In addition, the systematic review itself may not be well conducted, and therefore, you must still independently appraise the methodological rigor and strength of any findings. Systematic reviews may be quickly superseded by more recent evidence. For example, a large, well-conducted randomised controlled trial (RCT) may provide more convincing evidence than a systematic review of smaller poorer quality RCTs.

If a current, systematic review is not available, then the next step would be to work down the hierarchy of evidence to primary studies to answer their question. However,

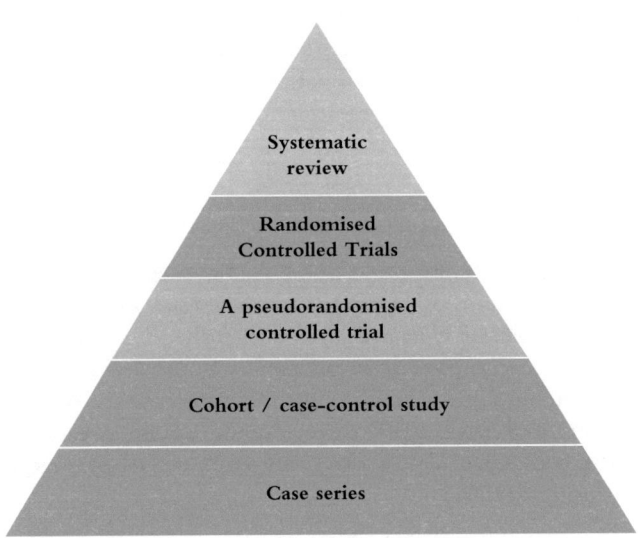

Figure 2.1 Adapted hierarchy of evidence by OCEBM (2011) and NHMRC (2009)

this depends on the question being asked and so an understanding of the different questions and how these correspond to different research designs is needed. For example, if a question is about aetiology or prognosis of mental illness, then the ideal research design is often a longitudinal cohort study. If a question were about the efficacy and effectiveness of a psychological intervention for offending behaviour, then the research design would be an RCT. Figure 2.2 shows research designs that best fit various question types.

One of the core aims of EBP is to improve practice with evidence; however, this evidence has faced a number of critiques and resistance (Hammersley, 2005; Lilienfield et al., 2013; Spring, 2007). The 'evidence' relies heavily upon positivistic designs. Whilst these are objective, scientific and independent, they take a reductionist view, reducing very complex human behaviour and quantifying it down to an effect or outcome. For example, the 'what works' paradigm within offending behaviour interventions (see McGuire, 2013) can be seen to predominantly focus on one outcome, for example, reoffending rates, as evidence of effectiveness. However, doing so ignores insights into the mechanisms involved in the actual behaviour change, arguably, what forensic psychologists are more interested in.

Likewise, EBP with its emphasis on robust designs and outcomes has led to limited description and 'theorising' of the core features of an intervention. All interventions are based on a theory (Pawson & Tilley, 1997), but 'off-the-shelf' theory can narrow the lens to blinker attention away from important mechanisms that lie outside of that framework (Moore & Evans, 2017). Understanding context is vital, what 'works' in one time and place for one person may be ineffective, or even harmful, elsewhere (Pawson & Tilley, 1997). In recent years, there has been an ever-increasing focus on building and testing theory throughout the development and evaluation of interventions (Craig et al., 2008); however, this has mainly been within public health interventions, and to date, forensic psychology has lagged behind. We will return to

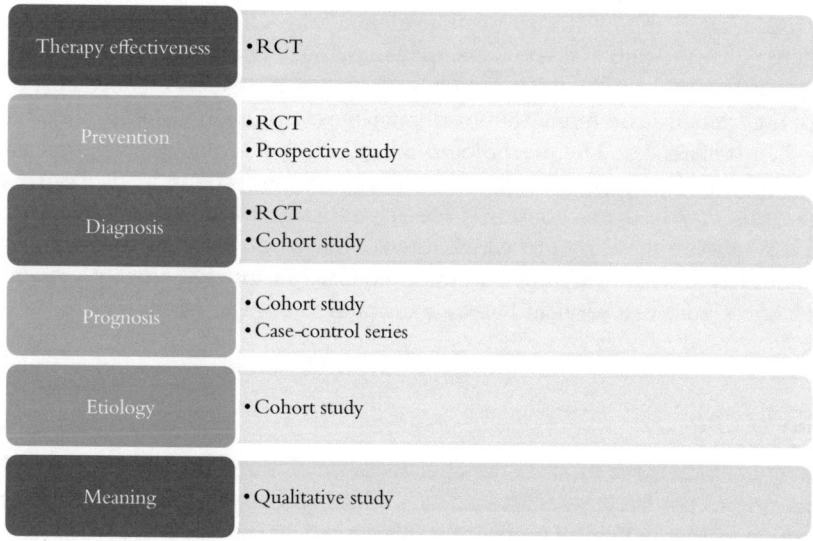

Figure 2.2 Research question type and corresponding research design

intervention theory development, evaluation and its importance for forensic psychology later on in the chapter when we focus on the Engager Research Programme. In summary, as scientist-practitioners, we must systematically evaluate the research evidence. The hierarchy of evidence approach can assist here. We also need to consider the pros and cons of individual research design techniques, in order to critically appraise.

How do forensic psychologists make an informed decision?

This second leg of the EBP stool is clinical judgement and clinical experience (Lilienfield et al., 2013). As scientist-practitioners, forensic psychologists review the evidence base, but they must also rely on their clinical skills and training. To develop a formulation, the psychologist needs to draw on clinical expertise and knowledge as well as relevant theory and research (see Chapter 5 for more on formulation). This enables consideration of the costs and benefits of a range of potential interventions. Indeed, the latest evidence on effective risk assessment demands that the forensic psychologist incorporates clinical expertise with scientific evidence (see Chapter 4 for an overview of structured professional judgement approaches within the assessment of risk).

How do forensic psychologists consider the views of the individual?

The third leg of the EBP stool is client preferences and values (Lilienfield et al., 2013; Spring, 2007). Psychologists must ensure all actions are ethically driven. At the heart of this is ensuring that clients are collaborative partners in all interventions; free to make informed decisions about the care they receive. It is our responsibility to ensure individuals have access to the most accurate information to make informed decisions. The clearest example of this is perhaps in interventions to treat trauma. There are a number of evidenced-based approaches to treating trauma (e.g. CBT, prolonged exposure, eye movement desensitisation and reprocessing therapy). These differ in the extent to which the individual must describe and experience the traumatic event. Clients must be made aware of the strengths and limitations of all available treatment options, so they can freely express their preferences. The psychologist must then choose the most appropriate treatment based on the research evidence, clinical expertise and the individual's preferences. At times, this may lead to choosing a less scientifically robust yet still evidence-based approach. However, the extent to which forensic clients are able to freely express preferences about treatment is a significant ethical concern in forensic settings, where clients do not 'choose' to access services but are mandated to engage. More on this later in this chapter.

Summary of EBP

The forensic psychologist must ensure clear focus on all three components of EBP. They must interrogate the latest research evidence whilst also applying their clinical expertise and accommodating individual preferences. This is not an easy task, and reflective practice is critical to examining decisions carefully. Yet, as we have said, the forensic psychologist must also contribute to the research evidence. We will now consider the history of applied research in secure settings.

Research ethics within forensic settings

Research involving those in secure settings has a dark past. Nazi doctors possibly conducted the most dreadful of all atrocities during World War II. These experiments led to the formulation of the Nuremberg code, the first international code for ethics laying down the guidelines for research on human subjects. This was followed by the Declaration of Helsinki in 1964, which has since had numerous revisions. But the core principles have remained the same: (a) informed consent, (b) minimise the risk of harm, (c) protect anonymity and confidentiality, (d) avoid using deceptive practices and (e) right to withdraw. Whilst these guidelines mainly put a stop to most research involving prisoners in the United Kingdom and other European countries, prison research within the United States thrived and continued until relatively recently. If you are interested to read more on the history of prisoners involvement in research, see Kalmbach and Lyons (2003) and Hornblum (1998).

We need to ask the question; can prison research or that in secure settings ever be ethical? Research within secure settings tests the limits of the core ethical principles of research. Informed consent: can participants ever truly give informed consent when their imprisonment/restrictions undermine their liberty and autonomy? (Christopher et al., 2011). Voluntary: can participation be truly voluntary when the environment is considered 'inherently coercive'? (Charles et al., 2016). Anonymity and confidentiality: Can we afford true anonymity and confidentiality when the closed nature and restrictive movement of secure settings and the safeguarding of participants and researchers means that confidentiality and privacy cannot always be assured? Other factors that may not be considered complex issues in research in other settings are in forensic settings. For example, it can be difficult to distinguish between someone's refusal of care and their denial of care. Also distinguishing compliance and noncompliance, for example, when participants do not turn up for appointments, have they not turned up because they do not want to engage in treatment or have the secure setting not facilitated them being able to turn up, for example, not having the staff to accompany them to an appointment. In addition, people in secure settings are typically more vulnerable due to higher rates of mental illness, learning difficulties and lower levels of literacy, than people in the general population.

All these factors mean that researchers in forensic settings need to consider how they conduct research very carefully. All research has ethical issues, and all ethical review processes will ask the researchers to identify the issues and describe their plan for how they will mitigate these issues. See Activity Box 2.1, which provides you with an opportunity to identify ethical issues and how you might mitigate them for an RCT conducted in a forensic setting.

Activity Box 2.1   Identify the ethical issues relevant to this study

Engager is a randomised controlled trial where 50% of participants are randomised to receive the Engager intervention plus usual care (the intervention group) and 50% to receive usual care alone (the control group). People are included in the study if they are:

- male,
- serving a prison sentence of two years or less and
- have between 4 and 20 weeks remaining in prison until release.

The research team approached those people who met the aforementioned criteria. The research team provided them with an information sheet about the study and obtained consent. After participants had consented, they completed the baseline assessments. The first part of this was to see if participants had a common mental health problem (depression, anxiety and/or trauma). If they did have a common mental health problem, then they continued into the trial and were randomised to one of the two groups. If they did not have a common mental health problem, their participation in the study ended. For those randomised, they were informed of which group they had been allocated to and were all seen again by the researchers to collect data 1 week before they were released from prison and then at 1, 3, 6 and 12 months post-release from prison.

1   Identify the ethical issues in the example given previously.
2   Next, identify how these ethical issues could be overcome.

Ethical review process for prison research

All research should undergo ethical review to ensure that it will be conducted within the core ethical principles of research. At the time of writing, all researchers wanting to conduct research with staff and/or offenders in any prison establishments are required to formally apply for research approval to the HMPPS National Research Committee (NRC). This includes Contracted Prisons, Young Offenders' Institutions (YOIs), Secure Training Centres (STCs), National Probation Service (NPS)/Community Rehabilitation Companies (CRC) regions and their subcontractors or within Her Majesty's Prison and Probation Service (HMPPS) Headquarters. The NRC exists to ensure: (a) that the research applicant, Ministry of Justice (MOJ) and HMPPS attain best value from the research conducted, (b) the resource implications and impact of the research on operational delivery are considered, (c) the robustness and relevance of the research are adequately assessed and (d) matters of data protection/security and research ethics are dealt with in a consistent manner. In addition to HMPPS approval, research within prisons considered to be 'health related' and also requires the approval of the NHS Research Ethics Service (RES).

NHS RES takes a restrictive approach, advising: 'health research involving prisoners or young offenders should relate **directly** to their healthcare and be of such a nature that it could only be conducted in this population'. This has had the impact that it prohibits the involvement of prisoners in research not exclusively relevant to prison populations. Charles et al. (2016) reviewed all applications to NHS RES between 1 April 2010 and 31 March 2012 to examine those who involved prisoners. Of the 14,355 applications to NHS RES, only 0.7% involved prisoners. A wide range of health areas were covered, but the vast majority fell into two main areas: mental health (50%) and infection (11%). Most studies were questionnaire-based studies (53%), and very little research was available to prisoners involving interventions, with only seven studies falling into this category. The authors concluded that most UK research involving prisoners appears to be 'non-beneficial', that is offers no prospect of clinical benefit. This study is now nearly a decade old, and yet, the NHS RES guidance remains the same with little indication that this will change. It is therefore more important than ever that forensic psychologists are committed not only to engaging with but also to producing beneficial research for those residing in forensic services.

So, we have shown the importance of EBP that forensic research can challenge ethical principles and that the current ethical process may constrain research. However, research needs to be and is being conducted; next, we will look in more detail at our evidence base for interventions within forensic settings.

What is our current evidence base?

PROSPERO is an international database of prospectively registered systematic reviews in health and social care www.crd.york.ac.uk/PROSPERO/. There are a number of published prison/secure setting systematic reviews listed, but three of the most relevant will be discussed briefly turn.

Kouyoumdjian et al. (2015) reviewed RCTs of interventions to improve the health of people in prison and in the year after release. They found that most studies were conducted with adult males in the United States and focused mainly on substance abuse and mental health. In most studies, the overall risk of bias was classified as high. Risk of bias was most often the result of a lack of blinding of participants and staff to the intervention and of a subjective outcome assessment (e.g. patient-reported symptoms of mental disorders). They found the number of RCTs was surprisingly small, considering the large size and significant burden of disease in this population. Many studies were conducted as pilot studies but were often not scaled up, which indicated a failure of knowledge translation.

Yoon et al. (2017) reviewed psychological therapies for prisoners with mental health problems. They found a medium effect size for psychological therapies (0.50, 95% confidence interval [0.34, 0.66]), with the most evidence for CBT and mindfulness-based interventions for depression and anxiety symptoms. The authors highlighted that the mechanisms underlying how and why these interventions bring about the outcomes needed further investigation. They also highlighted a number of trial design issues, such as small samples, difficulties with post-treatment follow-up and lack of fidelity measures to check the consistency and quality of the intervention delivery.

Most recently, MacInnes and Masino (2019) reviewed psychological and psychosocial interventions offered to forensic mental health inpatients. The studies were too heterogeneous to allow for a meta-analysis. Therefore, they concluded that currently, there are no consistent significant findings to inform practice in inpatient forensic settings. The authors highlighted that key priorities for future research should be: more trials with larger sample sizes, ensuring participants are representative of the overall forensic inpatient population, using standardised outcomes and clearly describing both treatment arms.

These three systematic reviews demonstrate that RCTs within prison and forensic settings are possible and feasible, but that their unique context can make standard trial procedures more difficult to achieve. These reviews also highlight the real dearth of trial-based evidence to inform practice. Currently, we do not have sufficient evidence of 'what works' within forensic settings, and virtually no evidence at all, about how or why interventions work. The Engager Research Programme https://www.plymouth.ac.uk/research/primarycare/criminal-justice/engager is the first of its kind, a theoretically developed intervention evaluated within an RCT and parallel process evaluation. Engager provides a blueprint for intervention developers and evaluators on how to undertake the process. By following this process, we will, in the future, have a better understanding of how interventions work or don't work, the outcomes they produce and their efficacy and effectiveness. See Case Study for more details on the Engager Research Programme.

Case study: Engager Research Programme

Intervention and trial science development

Engager was a manualised, person-centred intervention aiming to address common mental health needs (anxiety, depression and/or trauma) as well as to support wider needs such as accommodation, education, social relationships and money management. Engager was delivered by support workers and a supervisor who had experience of delivering psychological therapy. A mentalisation-based approach underpinned all elements of the intervention.

The theory of how the intervention would work was developed by bringing together evidence from:

* a realist review of psychosocial care for individuals with complex needs,
* focus groups with individuals from underrepresented groups,
* a series of organisational case studies,
* a rapid realist review of the intervention implementation literature and
* a realist informed formative process evaluation.

In parallel to the theory development of the intervention, trial methodological development included:

- selection of outcome measures through the reviewing of the literature, piloting of measures and obtaining a consensus from a range of stakeholders which outcomes to include;
- developing ways to best describe and quantify usual care and intervention receipt; and
- piloting of trial procedures in a pilot trial.

The delivery of the Engager trial was a significant logistical achievement. A total of 280 individuals were randomised across three prison settings to receive the Engager intervention, plus usual care (n = 140) or usual care only (n = 140). We achieved an impressive follow-up rate of 66% at six months post-release from prison. However, we found no consistent differences between the two groups for any of our outcome measures. This was a huge disappointment to us but our in-depth and detailed mixed method process evaluation was of real importance given the neutral trial finding. It showed us that implementation was suboptimal with only 44% (n = 62/140) receiving the minimum dose of the intervention. Implementation barriers included problems with the recruitment and retention of the practitioners delivering the team, adverse health and criminal justice system context and weaknesses in our intervention theory. However, importantly, it showed that when engagement was positive and was matched with full delivery of the intervention as intended, individual positive changes were achieved, although even these were not always reflected in their quantitative outcome measures.

Strengths and limitations

Our theoretical development work was comprehensive, but we found that there was little prior evidence or theory specific to male offenders for us to build on. Our trial methodological development enabled the efficient running of the first fully powered trial of a mental health intervention for prison leavers with common mental health problems. There were potential weaknesses in our trial methodology in terms of follow-up rates and outcome measures, with the latter not being sufficiently sensitive to small but significant changes for the participants who engaged well with the intervention.

Therefore, what can we learn from the Engager Research Programme? Well it is clear that reducing interventions down to one outcome measure may be problematic. As mentioned, doing so ignores important aspects of behaviour change, limits our theorising of interventions and we may not actually have adequate outcome measures to test such complex interventions. Historically, process evaluations have been seen as small qualitative add-ons to trials and of little importance to the trial. From the outset, the Engager process evaluation was seen as being on par with the trial. Given the neutral finding, the process evaluation became even more important and had it not been planned to be so comprehensive we would not have been able to identify specific areas of theory and/or intervention delivery that were faulty. Therefore, robust process evaluations are vital for all complex intervention (Moore et al., 2015).

Conclusion

EBP has made a significant contribution to our knowledge of intervention effectiveness and influences practice daily. Evidence in forensic practice is constantly evolving.

Forensic psychologists must remain abreast of the latest developments that affect practice to ensure best practice, as well as having a duty to contribute to the evidence base. However, EBP is not without its critics, who have suggested that our current evidence is reductionist, lacking in theory and true understanding of behaviour change. We have also seen that research within forensic settings can be complex and challenging. However, it is exactly this environment that makes this area of research so unique. But, context is key; we must move away from the only outcome of interest being reoffending to one where we try to understand the mechanisms involved in the actual behaviour change. We must also improve the quantity and quality of forensic psychology research, something we must all strive to achieve.

Learning outcomes

When you have completed this chapter, you should be able to:

1   Explain the key features of 'EBP'
2   Understand the relationship between research designs and research questions
3   Identify some of the key challenges to undertaking research within forensic settings
4   Explain the key ethical principles underpinning research and how they apply to forensic research

Key concepts and terms

- Evidence-based practice
- Scientist-practitioner
- Hierarchy of evidence
- Systematic reviews
- Randomised controlled trials
- Evaluation
- Intervention development

Sample essay questions

1   What can EBP offer to the field of forensic psychology?
2   Why should forensic psychologists be trained in both science and practice?
3   Evaluate the application of ethical principles to forensic research.

Recommended further reading

Adshead, G., & Brown, C. (Eds.). (2003). *Ethical issues in forensic mental health research*. Jessica Kingsley Publishers.
Brown, S., & Sleath, E. (2015). *Research methods for forensic psychologists*. Taylor & Francis.
Towl, G. (2006). *Psychological research in prisons*. Blackwell.

References

Charles, A., Rid, A., Davies, H., & Draper, H. (2016). Prisoners as research participants: Current practice and attitudes in the UK. *Journal of Medical Ethics, 42*(4), 246–252.

Christopher, P. P., Candilis, P. J., Rich, J. D., & Lidz, C. W. (2011). An empirical ethics agenda for psychiatric research involving prisoners. *American Journal of Bioethics: Primary Research, 2*(4), 18–25.

Craig, P., Dieppe, P., Macintyre, S., Michie, S., Nazareth, I., & Petticrew, M. (2008). Developing and evaluating complex interventions: The new Medical Research Council guidance. *British Medical Journal, 337.*

Daly, J., Willis, K., Small, R., Green, J., Welch, N., Kealy, M., & Hughes, E. (2007). A hierarchy of evidence for assessing qualitative health research. *Journal of Clinical Epidemiology, 60*(1), 43–49.

Hammersley, M. (2005). Is the evidence-based practice movement doing more good than harm? Reflections on Iain Chalmers' case for research-based policy making and practice. *Evidence & Policy: A Journal of Research, Debate and Practice, 1*(1), 85–100.

Hornblum, A. M. (1998). *Acres of Skin: Human Experiments at Holmesburg Prison.* Routledge.

Kalmbach, K. C., & Lyons, P. M. (2003). Ethical and legal standards for research in prisons. *Behavioral Sciences and the Law, 21*(5), 671–686.

Kouyoumdjian, F. G., McIsaac, K. E., Liauw, J., Green, S., Karachiwalla, F., Siu, W., Burkholder, K., Binswanger, I., Kiefer, L., Kinner, S. A., Korchinski, M., Matheson, F. I., Young, P., & Hwang, S. W. (2015). A systematic review of randomized controlled trials of interventions to improve the health of persons during imprisonment and in the year after release. *American Journal of Public Health, 105*(4), 13–33.

Lilienfeld, S. O., Ritschel, L. A., Lynn, S. J., Cautin, R. L., & Latzman, R. D. (2013). Why many clinical psychologists are resistant to evidence-based practice: Root causes and constructive remedies. *Clinical Psychology Review, 33*(7), 883–900.

MacInnes, D., & Masino, S. (2019). Psychological and psychosocial interventions offered to forensic mental health inpatients: A systematic review. *British Medical Journal Open, 9*(3), e024351.

McGuire, J. (2013). "What works" to reduce re-offending: 18 years on. In L. A. Craig, L. Dixon, & T. A. Gannon (Eds.), *What works in offender rehabilitation: An evidence-based approach to assessment and treatment* (pp. 20–49). Wiley-Blackwell.

Moore, G. F., Audrey, S., Barker, M., Bond, L., Bonell, C., Hardeman, W., Moore, L., O'Cathain, A., Tinati, T., Wright, D., & Baird, J. (2015). Process evaluation of complex interventions: Medical Research Council guidance. *British Medical Journal* (Clinical research ed.), *350,* h1258.

Moore, G. F., & Evans, R. E. (2017). What theory, for whom and in which context? Reflections on the application of theory in the development and evaluation of complex population health interventions. *SSM: Population Health, 3,* 132–135.

National Health and Medical Research Council. (2009). *NHMRC levels of evidence and grades for recommendations for developers of clinical practice guidelines.* Australian Government.

Oxford Centre for Evidence-Based Medicine. (2011). *OCEBM levels of evidence working group: The Oxford 2011 levels of evidence.* Oxford Centre for Evidence-Based Medicine.

Pawson, R., & Tilley, N. (1997). *Realistic evaluation.* Sage.

Sackett, D. L., & Wennberg, J. E. (1997). Choosing the best research design for each question. *British Medical Journal* (Clinical research ed.), *315*(7123), 1636.

Shapiro, D. A. (2002). Renewing the scientist-practitioner model. *The Psychologist, 15*(5), 232–234.

Spring, B. (2007). Evidence-based practice in clinical psychology: What it is, why it matters; what you need to know. *Journal of Clinical Psychology, 63,* 611–631.

Yoon, I. A., Slade, K., & Fazel, S. (2017). Outcomes of psychological therapies for prisoners with mental health problems: A systematic review and meta-analysis. *Journal of Consulting and Clinical Psychology, 85*(8), 783–802.

Part 2

Assessments in forensic contexts

3 Forensic clinical interviewing

Caroline Logan

Summary

Forensic clinical interviewing is an essential part of the professional practice of psychologists working in criminal justice and forensic mental health services. It is largely through purposeful face-to-face encounters with offenders or forensic mental health clients that information is collected about such vital topics as offending behaviour and its motivations, potentially relevant mental health problems and future risk. However, guidance on interviewing skills and their development is sparse. Whilst the substantial forensic and investigative interviewing literatures are relevant, they do not adequately address the professional requirements of forensic psychologists. And the rich literature on clinical interviewing does not satisfactorily account for the practical and ethical challenges of the forensic context. Therefore, this chapter highlights a range of interview skills and techniques, drawn from both the forensic/investigative and clinical interviewing fields, which could be useful to forensic psychologists. The chapter begins by examining what forensic clinical interviewing is and why it needs our attention. It then examines a range of important skills and techniques, using a case example to illustrate their application. The chapter concludes with a discussion of ethical issues raised by being an effective interviewer in a forensic context.

What do we mean by interviewing?

The word 'interview' derives from the French word *entrevue*, which is a combination of the words *entre*, meaning 'between', and *voir*, meaning 'to see'. Therefore, the word 'interview' means, in effect, 'to see each other' (Oxburgh et al., 2016) – it presents an opportunity to see or observe the other person and to understand as well as possible the world, events and experiences from their point of view (Logan, 2018).

An interview suggests a formal encounter with another person – an intentional coming together of at least two people for the purpose of information gathering by one person (the information-seeker, or *interviewer*) from those who are also present (the information-provider, or *interviewee* or indeed, interviewees) and thought likely to have all or some part of the information sought. The term interview also implies an exchange – a question for an answer – and, therefore, the expectation that turns will be taken in that exchange; that is, that one person will speak, and then the other, over and over as the information sought is revealed and the picture it paints builds. Further, the process infers that the interviewer leads, and the interviewee is obliged to respond; the interviewer is the person assumed to have control.

DOI: 10.4324/9781003017103-5

Preparing for an interview

A good interviewer will prepare for the encounter to come, both in terms of collecting and reviewing relevant information about the interviewee and about the topics on which enquiries will be made (Wells & Brandon, 2019). Preparations will help the interviewer maintain control and, therefore, be more likely to obtain the information that is their objective. Preparations will usually be captured in summary notes – like a crib sheet – for the interviewer to use to make sure they keep in mind all that is relevant for the meeting. Such a crib sheet will also list the topics to be enquired about accompanied by possible lead-in questions and follow-up probes. Box 3.1 illustrates a sample interview crib sheet featuring Mr John Smith, to whom we will return throughout the chapter.

Box 3.1   Sample interview crib sheet

Interview on 24 March with John Smith at HMP Grandville for forthcoming Parole Board hearing

Key biographical details

- Age – 52
- Overview – 1st conviction aged 14 (theft); 1st violent crime aged 15 (assault); 1st imprisonment aged 17 (grievous bodily harm – assaulted his father using a brick)
- Index offence – imprisoned 2005, murder of his 3rd wife in front of children
- History of violence – multiple allegations of assault against brother (1980s–1990s), father (1980s), 1st wife (1990s) and deceased 2nd wife (2003, convicted assault plus restraining order); committed murder whilst wife and children were living in a homeless shelter
- Other history – multiple convictions, mainly acquisitive crime including burglaries – mainly homes single females – intent??
- Diagnosis – psychiatric report prepared for 2005 trial identified narcissistic personality disorder; refused to engage in a formal assessment
- Interventions – refused to engage in offending behaviour programmes except Thinking Skills; denies problems
- Parole Board – hearing scheduled for June

Important points from 1st interview on 12 March

- Motivation to engage varied
- Tried to control the interview (talked a lot, spoke over me, directly critical of me e.g. 'You aren't very smart, are you?')
- Noted pattern of minimising violent conduct (victim blaming – e.g. of father, 'He made me who I am, so he deserved a beating'; of 1st wife, 'She had it coming')

- Notable pattern of self-aggrandisement (e.g. 'I am by far the cleverest man in here')

  Key topics for this interview

- Upbringing and family relationships

  - Tell me about your early family life. [*Who raised you? What periods of time did you spend away from your family?*]
  - How did you get on with your parents? Describe them.
  - Did your parents get on well together? [*Did they ever separate?*]
  - How did your parents discipline you? [*How often did they need to? What kinds of things did you do that resulted in punishment?*]

- Note

  - Self-awareness – how does he think he is regarded by others?
  - Role in and perceived responsibility for the difficulties within his family
  - Why was he violent towards father and brother?

- Next session to focus on intimate relationships then his offending behaviour

  Objectives

- Try to stay in control
- Do not be defensive when he is critical

Interviewees may be able to anticipate the nature of the topics about which they will be questioned – for example, Mr Smith should anticipate that a forensic psychologist preparing an assessment report for his forthcoming Parole Board hearing will ask about his past in order to understand something his future needs. However, interviewees will not always be informed in advance of the questions or even the general nature of the enquiries to which they will be invited to respond. Therefore, whilst interviewers are prepared, interviewees are encouraged if not expected to respond in the moment (Shea, 2017). This is to encourage more spontaneous and therefore potentially revealing answers as opposed to ones that are pre-prepared and possibly misleading.

The interview engagement

Interviewee responses to lead-in questions should result in some degree of probing by the interviewer – such as invitations to say more, requests for clarification, reflections on the nature of the response given – in as much of a calm, fluid and conversational exchange as the interviewer can encourage (Shea, 2017). And this is important, interviewers have a responsibility, regardless of the circumstances of the encounter, to try to create a relaxed, thoughtful, curious and reflective exchange with the interviewee. This is because such a context is widely believed to be most conducive both to the flow of information from the interviewee and to the creation of opportunities for the interviewer to observe the nature and pattern of that person's responses (Rogers, 1959).

Interviews are usually conducted face-to-face – that is, with all the participating individuals in the same room as one another at the same time. This is thought to enable the interviewer to perceive the interviewee's responses to questions across several sensory modalities – what they *see* and *feel* in the presence of the interviewee, in addition to what they *hear* the interviewee say. However, interviews can also be carried out remotely using a virtual platform (like video link, Skype or Zoom) or by telephone only.

The interview ends when the questions prepared have all been asked, the responses adequately probed and the sought-after information obtained in whole or in part – or when one or all participants need a break. All interviewers should aim to finish interviews neatly and in good time (i.e. not rushing at the end) and with interviewees feeling fine – and listened to. This means that, if the same interviewer returns to continue the discussion, or when another interviewer comes along for a different purpose, the interviewee will be more likely to engage because the impression they were left with last time was positive.

Reflecting on the interview afterwards

It is good practice for forensic psychologists to pause and reflect on every interview. Did it meet the objectives they had when the interview was planned? Did they get the information they expected? What was the quality of the information obtained and how credible was it? Did the interviewee reveal anything that was odd, novel or unexpected? What went well? What did not go well? What should the interviewer do differently next time, either with this interviewee or the next one? These reflections are an essential element of interview craft, ensuring self-awareness and the potential for skill development and improvement, as well as more mindful interviews with clients (Shepherd, 2019).

Interviews versus other encounters with clients

Interviews may be contrasted with other kinds of meetings, such as for the purpose of enquiries (e.g. *clarifications* in relation to a prison work application), the communication of information (e.g. a *briefing* about the person's work duties during the day ahead), the receipt of information (e.g. a *handover*, or *situation report* or *debriefing* from one team about to go off duty to the next team coming on) or the delivery of interventions (e.g. a *therapy session* or *consultation* between a therapist and a client to help them think about changing their behaviour). However, there are some processes and tasks in all these encounters that are shared with the interview, and it is these that we will explore in more detail in the following sections.

Why must psychologists in forensic settings develop their interview craft?

The interview scenario sketched previously is the ideal. Whilst it outlines the key elements of an interview – planning and preparation, the interview itself, followed by post-interview reflection – the scenario implies that such encounters are a gentle and agreeable to-and-fro between a competent interviewer and an engaged and forthcoming interviewee. Such interviews definitely do occur. However, in forensic settings, it is best to be prepared for more challenging encounters. Mr Smith is an example of an interviewee that a forensic psychologist would do well to prepare for. Why are some interviews more of a challenge and what do more challenging interviews look like?

Psychologists who work in forensic settings work in the main with people who have difficulties that have a bearing on their offending and harmful behaviour. For example, many people in prison have problems with their personalities, which may have resulted directly in conflict with others, leading to arrest, conviction and detention. This is because personality problems, especially if they are severe, impact on a person's relationships with others (McMurran & Howard, 2009). Psychologists work with such people to understand those difficulties and their consequences for the person, both in the past and future. This is with the intention, through interventions and supervision arrangements delivered by the psychologist and others, of reducing the difficulties and weakening their potential association with criminal behaviour. However, those same difficulties will challenge the interviewer's ability to do their job of eliciting information from the client (Ackley et al., 2010). These tensions or challenges may be arranged into three broad types, and they are summarised in Focus Box 3.2.

Focus Box 3.2 Interviewing challenges for the forensic psychologist

1. Motivating interviewees to engage with interviews

The contexts in which a forensic psychologist sees clients for interviews are ones in which the client has limited freedom to choose (Meloy, 2005); in the main, the clients of forensic psychologists do *not* want to be interviewed in detail about their vulnerabilities, their shameful behaviour, their intimate thoughts and feelings and so on. Such clients permit themselves to be interviewed because they can usually see that it is in their interests to cooperate. But they may still be reluctant, ambivalent, anxious or even angry about having to do so.

2. Detecting distorted responding in interviews

A client's responses to interview questions may not marry up with objective facts – or information they have given previously or to others. That is, their responses are distorted, either deliberately because of a desire to deceive or as a result of the problems they experience in their lives. In forensic interviews, a degree of distortion in responses should be assumed to exist *until it is proven otherwise* (Meloy, 2005).

3. Gaining and maintaining a good level of interview craft

Forensic clinical interviewing is a skilled undertaking. It is not just a matter of asking questions and writing down answers. Interviewers need to prepare for each client they interview, anticipate how they will engage and the topics to cover, coax them into a conversation guided by the interviewer's objectives for the encounter whilst managing the client's own, build that conversation over time maximising opportunities for the interviewer to hear and observe information relevant to the reason they are there, take brief notes whilst observing everything, line up the next few questions to ask, maintain a good level of rapport, manage interruptions and bring it all to a tidy conclusion (e.g. Shea, 2017). There is a lot to do!

And there is more. Interviewers will need to adjust their interview technique to suit the needs of clients with different kinds of presentations or in different contexts (e.g. interviewing a man in prison who is on the autism spectrum versus a woman in hospital who has a diagnosis of borderline personality disorder). And in the course of all this, interviewers may need to manage a client's strong responses to questions that could be upsetting (e.g. anger, guilt, shame, distress and ambivalence), as well as their own feelings if they react emotionally to what they are told (e.g. anger, revulsion and dislike). This is no small or insignificant undertaking. Yet, the stakes are high – and interviewers who are not very skilled may be more likely to attribute problems in the interview to the client, leading unfairly to a more critical or judgemental assessment of that person (Gladwell, 2019). For example, an interviewee might be sullenly unforthcoming – and an interviewer may conclude that this is evidence of antisocial attitudes and beliefs. However, the client may simply have held back his responses because the interviewer was mumbling or muddled or dominating or obviously judgemental, or all four, and he was afraid to reply in case he said the wrong thing.

Such challenges, perhaps the third one most of all, mean that the skills and techniques required to undertake and manage interviews with clients in forensic settings – your *interview craft* – should be recognised, developed and maintained throughout your career. What can forensic psychologists do to develop and maintain their interview craft? They can learn from colleagues who specialise in clinical interviewing (e.g. psychologists, psychiatrists and nurses who try to find out from people with severe mental health problems where those problems originated and why they recur, for example, Shea, 2017) *and* from those who specialise in forensic and investigative interviewing (e.g. police officers and social workers who try to find out from suspects and witnesses what they know about specific events or crimes, for example, Oxburgh et al., 2016). And they can put those skills together into the practice of *forensic clinical interviewing*. This term refers to face-to-face meetings with clients (or service users or patients) in order to discuss matters relevant to the reason for their detention in a secure facility or the restrictions legally imposed upon them (Logan, 2018). Forensic clinical interviewing has several important features, which we will now consider.

Essential skills and techniques in forensic clinical interviewing

Essential skills in forensic clinical interviewing are mapped out in Figure 3.1. What are they and how do they work?

Planning and preparation

As in most things in life, interview preparation is essential, most especially when anticipating an interview with a client of a forensic service; fail to prepare, then prepare to fail. What preparations are required?

PLANNING AND PREPARATION	ENGAGING WITH THE INTERVIEWEE	EVALUATION AND REVIEW
clarify your purpose (*your terms of reference*) research the client (*biography & personality*) refine your interview strategy (*to take account of each client's needs*)	initiating an interview with a client (*motivate them to engage*) rapport building detecting and managing distorted and deceptive responding managing and understanding resistance	were my objectives met? how credible was the information I obtained? was anything unexpected? what went well – or not well? (*what will I change next time?*) communicating your findings (*& managing challenges to your observations*)

Figure 3.1 A map of essential skills in forensic clinical interviewing

First, to find out as much as possible about the person to be interviewed and be clear about why such an interview is required. For example, who has commissioned it and for what purpose, how long it is likely to take and what is required of the client and others (e.g. speaking to family members, reading records, discussing matters arising with the clinical team), what is known about the client and the reasons why they are involved with a forensic service and what they are like as a person. This information, especially any information about their personality, will help the psychologist be ready for the interviewee (Ackley et al., 2010).

Think about Mr Smith. He has been described as controlling and self-aggrandising. These characteristics will likely be a feature of most interviews conducted with him – he tries to control interviews in order to minimise the hurt they may cause him and to positively influence their outcome. A psychologist seeing Mr Smith for the first time should anticipate having to work hard to gain his trust, to keep to the agreed agenda, to get beyond his desire to present himself in a good light, to probe him firmly about uncomfortable topics that he may prefer not to talk about and to stay in control of the interview.

Second, based on what has been discovered, prepare a strategy for interviewing each client (Wells & Brandon, 2019). A strategic approach to interviewing helps to maintain focus across each and every interview, and it means simply having a plan for how the interview(s) are likely to pan out. Therefore, the interviewer should prepare what will be discussed and in what order (think about the interview plan in Focus Box 3.1), how they will phrase lead-in questions and follow them up, how they think the person may respond in general and to difficult subjects specifically (e.g. by being controlling) and what kind of resistance they might encounter to (e.g. using strong emotions to discourage probing questions).

In general, interviews should start with less contentious topics (e.g. employment history) building up to more demanding subjects (e.g. offending behaviour) as it progresses. Such an order of play allows the interviewer to *baseline* the interviewee on the easy topics – that is, to gauge their general pattern of responding when relaxed (e.g. eye contact, posture, tone of voice and movement) – before moving on to more demanding matters. This is because a change in any of these characteristics (e.g. reduced eye contact when it was previously good, or folded arms and legs when posture had previously been open) could signify defensive or deceptive responding and trigger more extensive probing on the topic initiating the observed changes. Where deceptive responding is suspected, it is good practice to avoid challenging the person until later in the interview. By that time, the interviewer will have had the chance to build rapport and have a better sense of how to challenge his or her account safely. And at such a late stage, if the client decided to disengage as a result of being challenged – because their efforts to mislead the interviewer had now failed – the interviewer has most of the required information. Therefore, using a strategic approach helps to provide a framework for the interview(s) to come, which will help the interviewer keep their focus, be in a better position to detect avoidant or deceptive responding and maintain control. See Figure 3.2 for an outline of a basic interview strategy.

BASELINE	**INFORMATION GATHERING**	**CONFIRMATION & CHALLENGE**
neutral or low threat questions and queries background subjects	relevant subjects commitment to detail	difficult subjects and relating to earlier responses challenges

Figure 3.2 A basic interview strategy for forensic psychologists

Engaging with the interviewee

As suggested previously, forensic psychologists should aspire to interviews with all their clients who are relaxed, thoughtful, curious and reflective (Shea, 2017). And such an aspiration should be worked on from the very start. Four essential engagement tasks will now be considered (see Figure 3.1).

Initiating a forensic clinical interview

Forensic psychologists generally work with clients whose attendance at an interview is unlikely to be a matter of free choice; 'complete voluntariness should never be assumed' (Meloy, 2005, p. 422). Therefore, the decision to engage is not made unreservedly, and the consequences of participation, for the interviewee's self-esteem and their future prospects, may be significant and enduring. However, the psychologist has a duty to try to understand offending behaviour in order to prevent any future victims of a person known to have been harmful before. Therefore, the approach to a person who may not be very motivated to engage should be made with an awareness of this potential barrier and with a view to encouraging participation by emphasising their contribution.

With Mr Smith in mind, an invitation to him to engage in an interview could go something like this:

INTERVIEWER: *Hello Mr Smith. My name is Jane Doe and I'm a forensic psychologist in this prison. I have been asked to undertake an assessment of you ahead of your Parole Board hearing in June. What have you been told about this assessment?*
[explore expectations and anticipate some reluctance]

INTERVIEWER: *I have read a lot about you in preparation for this assessment. What's been your experience of being assessed in the past?*
[explore his experiences and responses to reports]

INTERVIEWER: *I appreciate that you have been assessed lots before. What worries you about undertaking a fresh assessment with me?*
[encourage discussion and your understanding of his point of view, and be empathic – consider offering to show Mr Smith a draft copy of the report so he can comment on it, which would allow you to correct errors and ensure his views are represented]

Also important at this early stage is a discussion about the limits of confidentiality and consent, which ought to follow directly from the aforementioned opening questions. Such a discussion must be recorded in contemporaneous notes from the session, and ideally, the client should be asked to sign a consent form. This process of easing the person into an interview – a person like Mr Smith, for example – should be regarded as an investment in their motivation to engage with you for the duration.

Rapport-building

Rapport is like oil in the mechanism of any encounter, which makes it an especially important attribute of interviews in which there may be some reluctance by the client to participate (Oxburgh et al., 2016). But what do we mean when we talk about rapport?

The term rapport refers to relating to another person in a harmonious way. Both parties are relaxed, conversation is flowing and there is a good level of mutual understanding if not trust between those present (Shea, 2017). In interviewing terms, the purposeful exercise of rapport-building means the effort of trying to create such an atmosphere, such fluency, by intentionally getting alongside that person and trying to understand something of the world through their eyes.

Rapport building depends on three things (e.g. Rogers, 1959): (i) the interviewer providing the client with unconditional positive regard, irrespective of how they engage with the interviewer; (ii) the interviewer being patient and determined to acquire and to accept an understanding of the world from the client's point of view, that is, an accurate empathic understanding and (iii) the interviewer being genuine, open and sincere. It is the interviewer's responsibility to establish and maintain rapport.

There are many challenges to the achievement of rapport in forensic clinical interviews. For example, a client like Mr Smith may feel threatened by the interviewer's efforts to empathise with him – perhaps because it makes him feel less in control. Therefore, he could try to sabotage what the interviewer does to this end, such as by accusing her of being patronising or using non-verbal communication to indicate his contempt for her efforts. And such responses could make the forensic psychologist falter, lose confidence in what she is doing and ultimately, lose control of this part of the interview – and feel cross with the interviewee for not cooperating. Here's what such an exchange could look like and how the interviewer could more helpfully respond:

INTERVIEWER:	*What age were you when your mother died?*
MR SMITH:	*I was 11 years old.*
INTERVIEWER:	*That must have been tough for you.*
MR SMITH:	*What do you care?! [looks contemptuously at the interviewer]*
INTERVIEWER:	*Sounds like this might be a topic you'd rather not talk about.*
MR SMITH:	*No shit, Sherlock.*
INTERVIEWER:	*In my experience, kids who lose their parents when they are young can have a tough time letting other people know how they feel, which can leave them feeling really lonely and frustrated – and mistrustful of people like me who come along and show an interest. I would understand if that's how you felt. [pause long enough for him to feel that a response is expected, maintain eye contact] Would you like to talk about this time in your life now, or shall we come back to it later?*

In formal interviews, forensic psychologists need to do a lot of thinking on their feet. That quick thinking will be aided by the interviewer being clear about what their interview strategy is and what their objectives are for each and every interview. However, they will nonetheless stumble on occasion and sometimes fail to respond well to sabotaging behaviour on the part of the interviewee (e.g. by showing irritation with Mr Smith's responses in the exchange mentioned previously). Quick thinking will also be aided by the psychologist being alert and attuned to the task. Poor interviews are more likely to follow from interviewers being unclear about what they want, offended when their efforts are rebuffed, as well as feeling tired and sluggish.

Detecting and managing distorted and deceptive responding

The most reliable way to detect deception is to ensure that the interviewee engages in the interview and talks (Vrij et al., 2017). Information from the client can then be compared with what they have said on different occasions, to this interviewer or others, recently and in the past; the devil is always in the detail. Therefore, that investment in good planning and preparation, interview initiation and careful rapport-building will make a big contribution to keeping the conversation going, maximising opportunities to notice anomalous responding and to explore its possible reasons (Shepherd, 2019). Taking a strategic approach to interviewing, a client can also help interviewers to spot the client's efforts to avoid talking about particular topics such as by closing down the flow of conversation on that subject or displaying strong emotions in response to specific questions, which encourage the interviewer to move on to something else. The more resistant the interviewee becomes to reasonable enquiries, the more guarded or sabotaging they are, the fewer opportunities will be presented to detect deception. On such occasions, interviewers should not panic. Instead, they should consider pausing the assessment and trying to re-engage with the client and rebuild rapport whilst reflecting on the reasons for the resistance they encountered.

Managing and understanding resistance

Resistance refers to non-compliance with an invitation or command. It is thought to originate from three sources: (1) when the recipient perceives that their acceptance of the invitation or command would place limitations on their freedom to choose what they do (referred to as *reactance*), (2) when the recipient does not want what the invitation or command will generate (referred to as *scepticism*) and (3) when the recipient does not wish to alter that they are already doing (referred to as *inertia*; Place & Meloy, 2018). For example, a forensic psychologist may invite a client – like Mr Smith – to talk about his offending behaviour. He may evidence resistance to doing so because he would rather talk about things that represent him in a better light (reactance). Alternatively, he could be resistant because he would rather talk about his great hopes for his future than his unhappy past (scepticism). Finally, Mr Smith may be reluctant to talk about his offending behaviour because the previous topic of conversation (how well regarded he is by his peers and the prison staff) was much more interesting (inertia). Interviewers have a key role to play both in the production and in the management of resistance in their interviewees.

Strategies for overcoming resistance amount to either making the invitation or command more attractive than was hitherto realised or by reducing their reluctance to do what has been asked of them. For example, and again thinking about Mr Smith, here are different ways of asking questions that are more – and less – likely to evoke resistance.

Resistance-evoking questions:

INTERVIEWER: *I would like to talk about your mother now. Tell me about her.*
MR SMITH: *I don't want to talk about my mother. [A reactance response]*

INTERVIEWER: *How did your mother's mental illness affect you?*
MR SMITH: *What's that got to do with anything? [A sceptical response]*

INTERVIEWER: *Can we talk about your offending behaviour now?*
MR SMITH: *God, must we? [An inertia response]*

Resistance-reducing questions:

INTERVIEWER: *I am really interested to know more about your family. Can we talk about them now, or would you prefer to talk about the work that you have done in your life so far? [Give the choice of the next topic to him – but you decide the options given]*
MR SMITH: *Let's do my family now, get it over with.*

INTERVIEWER: *It would be really helpful to me to understand how your early life was affected by your mum's mental health problems. Sometimes, when a person grows up with a parent who has got a lot on their mind, that child can be really affected – the parent isn't always there to help and comfort them, and the child can look to other people or activities to substitute for that missing parent. I would really like to know what that time was like for you and whether you think it has any bearing on how you got on with the other women in your life. Can I ask you a bit about that? [A justification is given for the next topic of enquiry]*
MR SMITH: *I don't think her illness has anything to do with anything. It just happened. But ask your questions if you must.*

INTERVIEWER: *I have read a lot about your offending behaviour, so I don't need to go through it with you.*
MR SMITH: *Thank goodness for that!*

INTERVIEWER: *But I did have a couple of questions about some stuff I couldn't understand from the accounts I read. In particular about the burglaries you've been convicted of.*

MR SMITH: *Oh?*

INTERVIEWER: *It would be really helpful if I could ask you a couple of questions just about them. Can I do that? It would really help me to be clear in my report about what support could be useful for you following your release from prison. [That is, it could be in his interest to answer these particular questions]*

MR SMITH: *Oh, okay.*

Evaluating and reviewing your interviews

As suggested previously, interviewers should take the opportunity to reflect on their performance after every single interview. However, forensic psychologists may not be the only professionals reflecting on their interviews with their clients. In forensic settings, the opinions of all practitioners are likely to be scrutinised and challenged, resulting in them having to account for their assessment procedures – including their interview methods – their diagnoses and formulations, and their recommendations (Meloy, 2005). Therefore, psychologists must have a good level of clinical expertise, professional credibility and personal resilience to be able to engage in this kind of work, both with the offenders they are interviewing and the legal bodies and multidisciplinary teams they serve. Practitioners should be prepared to be questioned and criticised. A high level of self-awareness and good quality clinical supervision will help to anticipate from where the criticisms may come and why.

The ethics of good interview craft

Good interviewing practice by psychologists in forensic settings means encouraging an interviewee to either volunteer or reveal information about themselves – what they have done or experienced, their attitudes or beliefs, thoughts and feelings – which they may not wish to reveal or that they may later regret having done so. There are four ethical principles in applied psychology (e.g. British Psychological Society, 2018), all have direct relevance to forensic clinical interviewing. Focus Box 3.3 summarises these principles.

Focus Box 3.3 Ethical principles in forensic clinical interviewing

1. Respect

This principle requires that psychologists recognise the inherent worth of everyone regardless of any actual or perceived differences in gender, age, social status, ethnicity, capacity or any other such group-based characteristics. All human beings are worthy of equal moral consideration and must be treated as such.

Therefore, personal feelings about the client resulting from the way the client treats them (e.g. with disrespect), or because of the nature of their offences (e.g. violent offences towards women or children), must not impact on their evaluation of the individual

2. Competence

This principle requires psychologists to ensure that they have and maintain an adequate level of specialist knowledge, skills and experience in order to provide the services asked of them and to acknowledge and seek to address deficiencies in their skill set when they are brought to their attention.

Therefore, interviewers should recognise, acquire and maintain the skills they need to be competent, seek support through regular training and supervision and accord every client the same high level of professional practice.

3. Responsibility

This principle requires forensic psychologists to understand the considerable power and control they may exercise in their professional role and to use both carefully and with a high level of awareness and consideration. Such awareness is intended to ensure that the trust of others (e.g. interviewees and stakeholders) is not abused.

This principle is exercised in the support psychologists must offer clients to make fully informed choices – about participation, about what they choose to discuss and withhold and about the consequences of engaging in an interview with a forensic psychologist.

4. Integrity

This principle requires psychologists to be accurate, consistent and honest in their professional actions, communications, decision-making, methods and outcomes. Integrity invites forensic psychologists to set aside self-interest and be as objective and open to challenge as possible. Thus, it is beholden upon practitioners to do good for all the people they work with and do no harm.

This latter requirement – non-maleficence – can be a challenge to apply in forensic clinical interviewing when the outcome of such an engagement may be a report that recommends continued detention in prison because risk cannot be safely managed in the community, a recommendation clearly not in the interviewee's interests. However, the greater good may be served by an extended period of detention and possibly treatment, which could be in the client's best interests also.

Conclusion

Much like watching sports on television (e.g. tennis and golf), interviewing looks straightforward until you try it and the challenge of doing so many things at once becomes clear. The task in the application of good and defensible interview craft is the intentional application of the various component parts of a competent interview and maintaining a lightly held control over the dynamic between the interviewer and interviewee, what Shawn Shea refers to as a 'delicate dance' (Shea, 2017). Practice will never make perfect – there is much in a forensic clinical interview that is difficult to anticipate, even by a very experienced and practiced interviewer. But practice and good preparation are critical.

Learning outcomes

When you have completed this chapter, you should be able to:

1 Identify challenges in forensic clinical interviewing
2 Identify the skills necessary to be a competent interviewer in forensic settings
3 Evaluate the interaction between client factors and interviewer characteristics in forensic clinical interviews
4 Understand the importance of rapport in facilitating interviews with forensic clients

Key concepts and terms

- Forensic clinical interviewing
- Interview craft
- Interview strategy
- Rapport-building and maintenance
- Deception and its detection
- Resistance

Sample essay questions

- Discuss how you might prepare to interview a controlling and violent man with a history of domestic abuse (like Mr Smith in Focus Box 3.1) and contrast these preparations with those you might make to interview a distressed and self-harmful man with a history of fire-setting.
- Evaluate the strengths and weaknesses of rapport-building as an essential task in forensic clinical interviewing practice.

Recommended further reading

Gladwell, M. (2019). *Talking to strangers: What we should know about the people we don't know.* Penguin.

Meloy, J. (2005). The forensic interview. In R. J. Craig (Ed.), *Clinical and diagnostic interviewing* (pp. 422–443). Jason Aronson Inc.

Oxburgh, G., Fahsing, I., Haworth, K., & Blair, J. (2016). Interviewing suspected offenders. In G. Oxburgh, T. Myklebust, T. Grant, & R. Milne (Eds.), *Communication in investigative and legal contexts: Integrated approaches from forensic psychology, linguistics and law enforcement* (pp. 135–158). Wiley Blackwell.

Shea, S. (2017). *Psychiatric interviewing: The art of understanding: A practical guide for psychiatrists, psychologists, counsellors, social workers, nurses, and other mental health professionals* (3rd ed.). Elsevier.

References

Ackley, C., Mack, S., Beyer, K., & Erdberg, P. (2010). *Investigative and forensic interviewing: A personality-focused approach.* CRC Press.

British Psychological Society. (2018). *Code of ethics and conduct.* BPS.

Logan, C. (2018). Forensic clinical interviewing: Toward best practice. *International Journal of Forensic Mental Health, 17*(4), 297–309.

McMurran, M., & Howard, R. (Eds.). (2009). *Personality, personality disorder and violence: An evidence-based approach.* John Wiley & Sons.

Place, C., & Meloy, J. (2018). Overcoming resistance in clinical and forensic interviews. *International Journal of Forensic Mental Health*, *17*(4), 362–376.

Rogers, C. (1959). A theory of therapy, personality, and interpersonal relationships as developed in the client-centred framework. In S. Koch (Ed.), *Psychology: The study of a science: Formulations of the person and the social context* (Vol. 3, pp. 184–256). McGraw-Hill.

Shepherd, E. (2019). The hunt for non-barking dogs and other curiosities: Identifying and managing anomaly within forensic interviews. *International Journal of Forensic Mental Health*, *18*(1), 66–84.

Vrij, A., Meissner, C., Fisher, R., Kassin, S., Morgan III, C., & Kleinman, S. (2017). Psychological perspectives on interrogation. *Perspectives on Psychological Science*, *12*(6), 927–955.

Wells, S., & Brandon, S. (2019). Interviewing in criminal and intelligence-gathering contexts: Applying science. *International Journal of Forensic Mental Health*, *18*(1), 50–65.

4 Forensic risk assessments

Michelle Fletcher, Neil Gredecki and Polly Turner

Summary

The completion of risk assessments forms a core component of the work of many forensic psychologists and is a key feature of training routes for forensic psychologists. Although forensic psychologists undertake a range of assessments, the focus in this chapter will be on risk assessments. These assessments are undertaken in a range of settings and for a range of different purposes, including Court (family and criminal), Parole Hearings and Mental Health Review Tribunals. Forensic psychologists undertake risk assessments to ensure that other professionals are able to make well-informed and evidence-based decisions pertaining to forensic clients. In this chapter, we will consider approaches that forensic psychologists take to conducting risk assessments with a specific focus on violence.

Introduction

There may be many reasons for undertaking assessments, but two common referrals relate to understanding why an individual has committed a criminal offence and that of determining an individual's treatment needs to help manage this risk. It is important for the psychologist to develop an understanding of the pathway that an individual takes that leads to their offending behaviour, even if the offender has difficulty understanding this themselves (i.e. has little insight). If the professional can gain an understanding of the offence pathway using the process of offence analysis, then both intervention and risk management recommendations can be made that will enable both the forensic client and the professionals to reduce, or at least manage, any future risk. Within this chapter, we will consider the process of conducting assessments in forensic services and ensuring that the assessments are responsive to the individual client (the forensic client that is being assessed). The focus will be on examining what we know about risk to others rather than risk to self. Part 3 of this book looks at specific forensic populations and assessment issues/ processes with these individual groups.

Forensic risk assessment

Let us start by thinking about some key terms: risk and assessment. *Risk* is a threat or hazard that is incompletely understood and therefore can be forecast only with uncertainty. *Assessment* is the process of gathering information to assist in decision–making. It is not simply providing a diagnosis or prognosis, but an individualised inquiry. Within the forensic context, risk assessment can be defined as '*the systematic collection of information to*

DOI: 10.4324/9781003017103-6

determine the degree to which harm (to self and others) is likely, at some point in time' (O'Rourke, 2008, p. 160).

There are general and specific goals of risk assessment. General goals include preventing risk to self or others and to protect the public, others and/or the individual. Specific goals include formulating risk, guiding risk management and intervention, communicating risk to others, improving consistency and transparency of decisions and protecting the rights of the individual and decision makers from liability. Risk is contextual and risk assessment is complex and has many facets as outlined in Focus Box 4.1.

FOCUS BOX 4.1 **FACETS OF RISK ASSESSMENT**

A thorough risk assessment involves consideration of the following facets:

- Nature – What is the risk?
- Severity – How serious is it?
- Frequency – How often might it occur?
- Imminence – How soon might it occur?
- Likelihood – With what probability?

Fundamentally, the aim of risk assessment is to understand the nature of the risk posed and to then put processes in place to either prevent or decrease the likelihood of future offending. This is achieved by several smaller goals including using the assessment to structure and guide interventions and to devise management and supervision strategies to minimise the risk posed by an individual. It is important that forensic psychologists ensure an evidence-based approach to risk assessment as their assessments can be used to determine an individual's suitability for release into the community or their continued detention. An underestimation of risk could result in the individual being released to the community which could potentially put the public at increased risk. Likewise, an overestimation of risk could result in the individual being detained unnecessarily. Both are equally damaging situations which need to be avoided.

Approaches to risk assessment

There are two main approaches to risk assessment: discretionary and non-discretionary. These terms refer to how information is weighted and combined to reach a final decision, regardless of the information that is considered and how it was collected.

The discretionary approach, also referred to as the clinical or judgemental approach, is that where the evaluator has substantial professional judgement in the decision-making process, including which information to consider and how to gather it, as well as how to weight and combine it. It is sometimes characterised as being informal, subjective and impressionistic. In contrast, the non-discretionary approach, also referred to as the actuarial or statistical approach, is an approach based on the information available to the evaluator. Here, they make an ultimate decision according to fixed and explicit rules, developed *a priori*. Also, non-discretionary approaches tend to rely on empirical research to determine which information to consider, how to gather it and how to weight and combine it. It is very specific in focus, designed to predict certain outcomes over certain time frames and in certain populations. The non-discretionary approach is sometimes characterised as being mechanical and algorithmic.

Approaches to risk assessment have evolved over time. Let us consider the history of risk assessment further in terms of how approaches to risk assessment have developed over time.

ACTIVITY BOX 4.2   IDENTIFYING RISK FACTORS FOR VIOLENCE

Before moving on with this chapter, make a list of factors that you think are risk factors for violence. Once you have your list of proposed risk factors, compare the list to the VRAG-R and HCR-20 (v3) risk factors as outlined in Figures 4.1 and 4.3. Reflect on whether the lists are similar or different and whether the actual risk factors are different to what you may have expected to see in structured risk assessment guides.

First-generation risk assessment consisted mainly of unstructured clinical judgements of the probability of offending behaviour. This approach relies on decision-making that is unguided by tests or professional guidelines. The clinician makes decisions based on their clinical experience alongside other factors they believe to be relevant, perhaps drawing on their past experiences of working with particular client groups. Clinical experience can be helpful in terms of understanding individual cases, especially where there is limited published literature. However, there can be a risk of favouring experience over research findings and the empirically derived evidence base.

Second-generation risk assessments are empirically based instruments which stress static, historical risk factors, such as the number and type of convictions. This approach is referred to as **actuarial risk assessment**, and it involves the use of statistical techniques to provide an assessment of the level of risk an individual poses in terms of reoffending. Examples include the Violence Risk Appraisal Guide (VRAG-R; Quinsey et al., 2006) and the Risk Matrix 2000 (RM2000; Thornton, 2007). Actuarial approaches are commonly used in non-psychology areas such as insurance. For example, when arranging insurance for our cars, we expect to be asked factual questions such as age, where we live and how many accidents we have had in the past. The answers to these questions help to determine one's level of risk by checking our answers against a database of known risks associated with these different categories. In turn, this informs the cost of the insurance premium.

Actuarial assessments to assess risk of reoffending follow a similar process. Drawing on data from offender populations, they are designed to predict a specific risk for a particular population over a specific time period and context. They are highly structured in terms of the evaluation and decision-making process. For example, a basic risk assessment may indicate that being male, single and under the age of 30 increases the risk of an individual committing a violent act. Whilst this is an overly simplistic example, the basic principles of assessing an individual for the presence of factors statistically related to violence or sexual violence remain in all assessments. Actuarial tools such as the VRAG-R provide a probability of the individual committing further specified offending (e.g. violence). In using the VRAG-R, numerically rating a series of 12 items enables the client to be assigned to a category of high, medium or low risk of offending, predicting their level of risk by comparing them to a given population as opposed to considering individual circumstances and differences. The factors used have been shown to be statistically significant in predicting the probability of the specific offending behaviour occurring in the future. Figure 4.1 outlines the items on the VRAG-R.

One main advantage of actuarial approaches is objectivity, as the assessment of the individual cannot be influenced by any bias of the professional. Another advantage is that they are consistent; all individuals assessed using the specific actuarial assessment are assessed in the same way. However, this approach has limitations; they require an element of professional judgement including which scale to use and how to interpret the scores. The results tend to be pseudo-scientific and may be easily misinterpreted with individuals having an over reliance on results due to the assumption that they are always accurate and objective, when in fact actuarial tools differ significantly in their predictive accuracy (Craig et al., 2006).

It is important to remember that actuarial tools are designed in a specific cultural context with a specific population and may not be reliable and valid when used with other populations and cultures. Whilst they can be helpful in producing risk predictions amongst groups of people, they fail to consider the individual client and/or their offence pathway and therefore still require clinical judgement in terms of the client's risk and protective factors in their overall assessment.

Third-generation risk assessments utilise both clinical and actuarial methods. They are considered to be more theoretically informed, and they are objective and systematic as they measure static factors, but can also look at dynamic risk or criminogenic needs factors. This approach is referred to as **structured professional judgement (SPJ).** This approach builds on the strengths of the actuarial approaches (i.e. using scientific evidence to identify those factors relevant to risk) yet allow clinical judgement to be used. Here, the forensic psychologist uses their knowledge of the client to assess the presence and relevance of evidence-based risk factors. This allows them to formulate the case (see Chapter 5 for more information on formulation) and to not only make an assessment but also inform intervention. The SPJ approach, like that of actuarial assessments, imposes

Individual VRAG-R Items
• Lived with both biological parents to age 16
• Elementary school maladjustment (up to age 14)
• History of alcohol or drug problems
• Martial status at tie of index offense
• Criminal non-violent history score
• Age at insdex offense
• Criminal violent history score
• Prior admissions to correctional institutions
• Conduct disorded prior to age 15
• Sex offending history
• Antisociality (Facet 4 of the PCL-R)

Figure 4.1 Items from the VRAG-R (Quinsey et al., 2006)

significant structure on evaluation. For example, at a minimum, a fixed and explicit set of risk factors must be considered. These factors are determined by each individual risk assessment guide, yet the approach also allows for other individual case-specific factors to be considered by the psychologist. These factors include some that are historical and therefore static in nature, as well as factors that are dynamic and therefore more changeable. In each SPJ tool, the risk factors are expressly stated with given definitions that the individual is assessed against, thereby improving consistency in decision-making.

There are a range of SPJ guides available to forensic psychologists to assist them in their assessments of risk. These assessment guides are specifically designed for various risk behaviours, and the forensic psychologist selects the guide that will guide them in their assessment of risk. As such, it is important for the psychologist to be clear as to what area of risk they are seeking to assess. Figure 4.2 outlines key guides used to assess risk within forensic populations; although this is only an indicative list and other guides do exist.

The SPJ process requires the psychologist to consider a minimum number of risk factors that are directly related to the type of offending that is being assessed. As with the actuarial approach, these are factors that have been shown to be statistically significant in predicting the probability of the specific offending behaviour occurring in the future. Using the information available to them, the psychologist is required to assess if the specific risk factors are present *and* relevant to the case in order to develop the risk formulation. Figure 4.3 provides examples of the risk factors that are considered as part of the HCR-20 (v3) assessment.

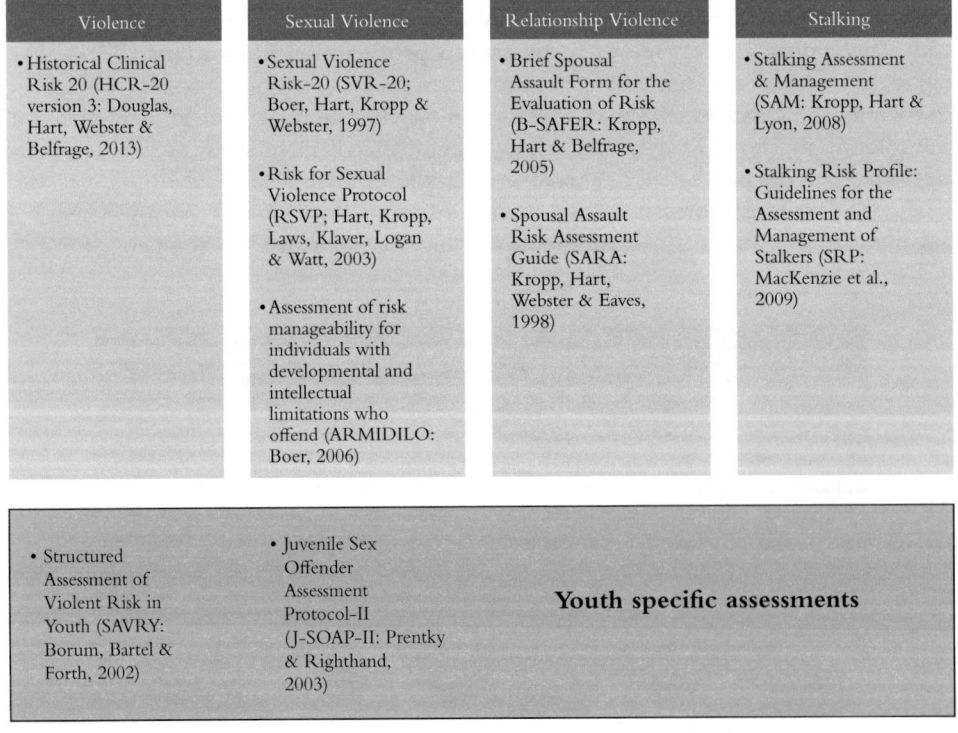

Figure 4.2 Examples of forensic SPJ guides

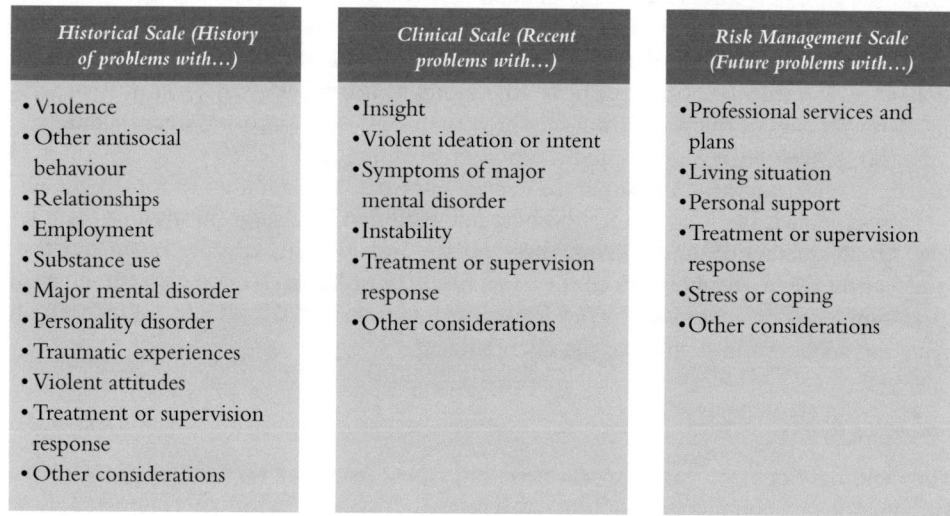

Historical Scale (History of problems with...)	Clinical Scale (Recent problems with...)	Risk Management Scale (Future problems with...)
• Violence • Other antisocial behaviour • Relationships • Employment • Substance use • Major mental disorder • Personality disorder • Traumatic experiences • Violent attitudes • Treatment or supervision response • Other considerations	• Insight • Violent ideation or intent • Symptoms of major mental disorder • Instability • Treatment or supervision response • Other considerations	• Professional services and plans • Living situation • Personal support • Treatment or supervision response • Stress or coping • Other considerations

Figure 4.3 Individual risk factors (items) for the HCR–20 (v3) (Douglas et al., 2013)

In contrast to the actuarial approach, guides such as the HCR–20 (v3) (Douglas et al., 2013) impose structure on decision-making but are considered *guides* rather than psychometric assessments. SPJ guides allow the professional to use their professional judgement in assessing the presence and relevance of each individual risk factor in relation to the offender's risk of reoffending. This allows the psychologist to determine the importance of each risk factor with no 'rules' or scoring regarding how many risk factors should be present to indicate high, medium or low risk. SPJ guides allow for the possibility that only one or two risk factors may be present but may be so significant that they indicate a high level of risk. For example, in a particular case, one single factor such as psychopathy being present may be enough to indicate high risk of reoffending for a client.

One of the main advantages of SPJ guides is that the decisions made using these guides are transparent; it is clear where decisions regarding risk evaluations are made to other professionals and the client. This has the advantages of meeting the aim of open reporting that comes with all psychological assessments as well as providing opportunity to challenge and question the decisions made. This transparency and openness to scrutiny works well with the general aims and methods of psychology as a profession.

A further advantage of the SPJ guides comes in terms of outcome following the assessment. The nature of the risk factors and the process of the assessment of each of these factors encourage the psychologist to consider recommendations for future treatment and intervention to try to minimise the risk that an individual client poses. This action-oriented approach provides the client with an opportunity to change and reduce their risk. Unlike actuarial assessments, there is a clear link between the risk factors rated as relevant and the recommendations made to decrease the impact of the same risk factors, reflecting the concept that risk is a dynamic concept. Actuarial assessments based on risk factors that are static in nature do not measure change over time or acknowledge impact that treatment may have on an individual's risk. Therefore, the aims of the structured

guides are more consistent with the general aims of forensic psychology and the principles of providing clients with the opportunity to change their future behaviour.

A limitation of SPJ is similar to that of actuarial assessments. That is, they still rely on
the assumption that the characteristics of the individual being assessed are consistent with
the characteristics of the population in which the original research was undertaken.

Fourth generation risk assessments promote planning and delivery and are used to
inform case management and supervision arrangements. The addition of fourth generation assessments is the focus on responsivity and readiness to change/motivation. Rather
than simply predicting reoffending, these guides aim to systematically bring together
information about an offender's history and needs in order to develop a treatment plan
and assign levels of supervision. They look at external service factors and are focused on
matching services and support to the client's needs.

Protective factors

The main development during recent years in psychological risk assessments has been the
introduction and consideration of protective factors. Protective factors are considered those
that reduce the likelihood of risk (triggering) factors actually leading to offending; these
factors serve to modify the effects of risk factors and reduce the likelihood of recidivism and
promote abstinence from crime amongst those who previously had engaged in a sustained
pattern of offending (also referred to as desistance). As with risk factors, protective factors
can be the characteristics of the client, their environment or a situation that protects the
individual from relapsing into criminal behaviour. The inclusion of protective factors is
consistent with a strength-based approach (the approach of current treatment programmes
as outlined in Chapter 6) and promotes collaboration with the client within the risk assessment process.

Many clients can feel that the process of risk assessment is overly negative and concerned primarily with past behaviours. Consideration of protective factors and the potential for a scenario where the individual desists from future offending is one way to redress
concerns whilst creating a more hopeful and optimistic outlook where change is possible.
One assessment utilised within forensic services which focuses on protective factors is the
SAPROF (de Vogel et al., 2012). This is arranged into three categories: internal, motivational and external factors (see Figure 4.4).

Specialist populations

When undertaking risk assessments, there is a requirement for the forensic psychologist
to consider specialist populations, recognising that a 'one-size-fits-all approach' is not an
appropriate approach to assessing risk. For example, assessments need to be gender sensitive with consideration being given to the population and any evidence supporting different or additional risk factors. When undertaking violence risk assessments with women,
alongside the HCR-20 (v3) (Douglas et al., 2013), the Female Additional Manual (de
Vogel et al., 2014) may be used. This ensures a gender-sensitive approach to assessment
and consideration of gender-specific risk factors. Further, whilst some guides are gender
neutral, it should not be assumed that all guides are suitable for use with women. This
may include, for example, sexual violence risk assessment guides which have been developed using male only samples. The forensic psychologist is required to identify suitable
guides, and if they do not exist, then they may be required to conduct a theory-informed

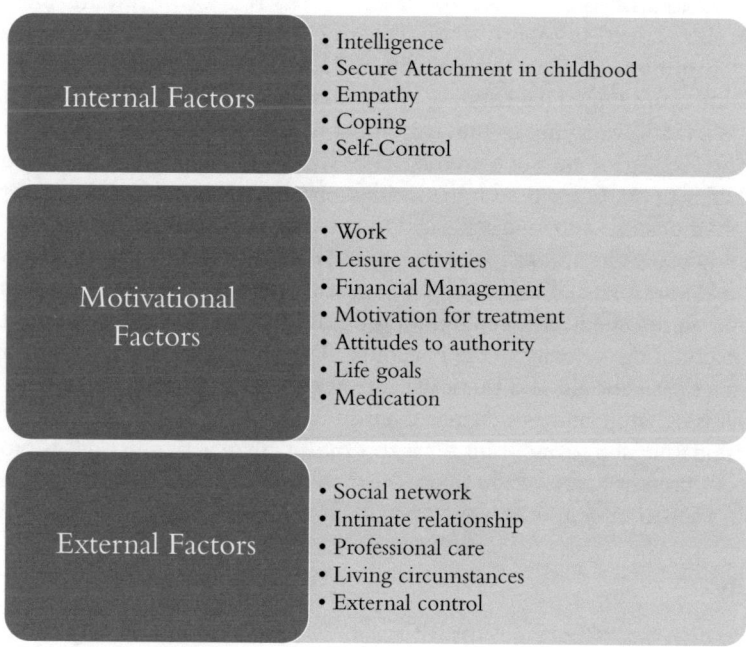

Figure 4.4 Protective factors for violence risk (SAPROF: de Vogel et al., 2012)

formulation of the client's presenting issues/risks. See Chapter 13 for a review of specialist approaches to working with, and assessing, women in prisons.

It is also important to ensure that the assessment guides being used are appropriate to the age of the client. Figure 4.2 also outlines a range of youth-specific risk assessment guides. It is imperative that the forensic psychologist uses guides that are appropriate to the age of the client as the guides are based on research and evidence from specific populations. Likewise, care should be given to the use of assessment guides with clients with intellectual disabilities where specialist guides may be available (e.g. the ARMI-DILO; Boer, 2006). Other considerations include deaf clients and transgender clients, as well as ensuring that assessments are culturally sensitive.

Formulating risk

Risk assessment guides are helpful in drawing the psychologist's attention to various risk and protective factors for the individual client. However, having a list of risk factors is not enough. A comprehensive risk assessment must detail the meaning of the factors and, more importantly, what they mean for the client who is being assessed. One client may present with evidence of two risk factors and present a higher risk of a specific offending behaviour than another client with evidence of 12 risk factors. As such, the forensic psychologist needs to draw together the findings from their assessment, using the evidence from a range of sources in order to form conclusions. This is referred to as a risk statement. Here, the client's risk factors are brought together in order to communicate to other professionals and the client the nature of the risk and the context in which it is likely to be present. In turn, this is used to formulate the client's risk.

Within the field of forensic risk assessment, there is a move towards including risk scenarios in risk assessment reports. Risk scenarios are widely used in business, healthcare and military planning. They are 'possible futures' and used to consider what a person may do in the future and why. Determining risk scenarios involves the process of asking the questions: What are we trying to prevent? What exactly are we worried the person may do? Therefore, scenarios are not a prediction of what will happen but rather a projection of what could happen. Once determined, risk scenarios are useful in aiding the psychologist to consider possible warning signs and future risk management strategies.

As with any psychological assessment, it is important to outline the limitations of any individual risk assessment. This may include factors such as whether the assessment was based heavily on the client's self-report and the extent to which the psychologist has been unable to ascertain the veracity of their account. The absence of key documentation such as victim statements should also be noted. Likewise, it is important to be clear as to the fact that risk is dynamic and can change over time, and that the risk assessment will need reviewing/updating at a given point for it to capture current risk, as well as progress.

Let us now present a case study to see how the findings of a risk assessment may be brought together to inform others as to pertinent risk issues.

Case study

Mr Bryn Ford's index offence was that of Robbery, committed in the city centre at night. He approached the victim who was with their partner and demanded money and his mobile telephone. When the victim refused, Mr Ford produced a knife and later used the weapon to cut the face of the victim before leaving with their wallet and mobile phone. When the victim's partner tried to call for help, Mr Ford punched her in the face and broke her nose. He has previous convictions for violent offences including ABH and GBH against strangers and peers. Whilst he has engaged in criminal activity to fund his use of substances, he has also engaged in reactive aggression, especially when under the influence of substances. He has served several prison sentences and has committed offences whilst on licence.

Having been sentenced to six-year imprisonment, he was transferred to hospital under Section 47/49 of the Mental Health Act (see Chapter 15) when there was a notable change in his mental health. He has a diagnosis of paranoid schizophrenia and antisocial personality disorder. He has not had a formal assessment of psychopathy. Mr Ford was referred to psychology services for a risk assessment as part of his assessment of suitability to transfer to a low-secure forensic mental health hospital. He was assessed by a forensic psychologist who undertook the HCR-20 (v3) with him to help to assess his level of risk and to help guide his formulation.

Excerpt from Mr Ford's risk assessment report

The following is an example of the risk statement section taken from Mr Ford's risk assessment report. In an actual assessment, there would also be a formulation of his violence in order to support professionals in planning his progression and any outstanding treatment needs. Formulation is covered in detail in Chapter 5.

Risk statement *Mr Ford engaged in the current assessment of his general violence. It is important to note that the current assessment is based heavily on Mr Ford's self-report in that*

I have been unable to ascertain the veracity of his account about his past employment and rela-tionships, as well some of his past offences. Therefore, the conclusions reached here may need to be revised should any information become available and this differ from the account given by Mr Ford.

During the assessment Mr Ford was asked about a range of areas relevant to the comple-tion of the structured risk assessment. This was to explore the possible risks posed in rela-tion to his use of violence. The HCR-20 (v3) risk assessment tool was used to guide the assessment.

It is important to emphasise that risk assessment should not be considered static (i.e. fixed). That is, risk should be considered dynamic and contextual (i.e. can change over time). This is important when considering how the factors rated as relevant to risk here should be accommo-dated for within treatment and risk management plans.

General violence: risk statement

The HCR-20 risk assessment conducted in Mr Ford's case highlights a number of risk factors potentially relevant in Mr Ford's use of aggression. The thirteen risk factors rated as present and relevant in his case, and which increase the risk of violence, are:

- *A history of problems with: violence, other antisocial behaviour, substance use, major mental disorder, personality disorder, violent attitudes and treatment or supervision response.*
- *Recent problems with: insight, symptoms of major mental disorder and instability.*
- *Future problems with: personal support, treatment or supervision response and stress or coping.*

The three risk factors rated as possibly present and relevant are:

- *A history of problems with: Employment.*
- *Recent problems with: Treatment or supervision response.*
- *Future problems with: Professional services and plans.*

Based upon the assessment of risk using the HCR-20, the following can be considered potential future risk scenarios:

Future violence would likely involve a physical assault which could be in the commission of a robbery or another offence. It is my opinion that the severity of physical harm from violence would be moderate to high based on his past offending, with the severity of psychological harm being medium to high. Based on Mr Ford's previous use of weapons, it is possible that the violence could escalate to life-threatening levels.

Potential victims of Mr Ford's violence are likely to include adults who are known and unknown to him. It is likely to include both males and females. In the main, Mr Ford's offences have occurred against adult male strangers.

In my opinion, Mr Ford's risk of violence decreases in the context of improved coping and problem-solving skills, improved conflict resolution skills, access to professional support networks and the absence of violence supportive attitudes. It would also decrease in the absence of sub-stance misuse. Protective factors in Mr Ford's case are prosocial coping, leisure activities, medica-tion and professional care.

Limitations to risk assessment

Over recent years, there has been a focus within forensic assessment on structured guides and assessment guides to ensure both reliability and consistency. However, this has potentially led to difficulties as professionals become more proficient in the areas of risk of violence and sexual violence to the possible detriment of other offence types where risk assessment tools are less developed. At times, this has led to psychologists over generalising research findings to make conclusions that, whilst based on valid research, are limited in accuracy.

Another limitation is based on individual differences that can occur within any profession. The danger of a specific risk assessment guide being used is that it encourages the Court (or other formal settings) to believe in a high degree of consistency between professionals. Whilst it is true that all risk guides currently utilised rely on specific instructions that the professional follows, it is also true that some individuals may use different definitions and assumptions to rate both the presence and relevance of an individual risk factor. Therefore, it remains important that the setting in which the risk assessment is being discussed, whether Court or a parole board hearing, continues to assess the level of knowledge and credibility of the professional undertaking the assessment. This should include, as a minimum, the attendance at training events aimed at understanding the risk assessment tool being used and the professional engaging with the wider literature base.

Conclusion

Any assessment undertaken within the forensic psychology field is fundamentally concerned with gathering data to enable a specific question or a set of questions to be answered. This often requires the use of several different assessment methods such as self-report, structured interviews, scrutiny of file information, collection of data from third parties and direct or indirect observation. Today, there are a range of assessment guides that are frequently used and generally accepted as valid guides in all areas of forensic assessment. These include risk assessment guides, assessment measures for personality disorder and cognitive functioning assessments. Within these areas, are a range of psychometric assessments such as self-report questionnaires, actuarial assessments and those that rely on interview schedules. The forensic psychologist needs to determine the most appropriate tool to be used in any given assessment. The psychologist needs: an understanding of the research literature for each assessment tool or approach, an ability to communicate this evidence to other professionals within the criminal justice system, an understanding and communication of the advantages and limitation of each assessment tool used and an ability to effectively communicate findings in a professional non-prejudicial way. Therefore, the role of the forensic psychologist has become crucial not just in predicting the future risk of an individual, and assessing treatment and management options, but also in disseminating an understanding within the wider criminal justice field of risk assessment and management in general.

Learning outcomes

When you have completed this chapter, you should be able to:

1   Outline the various approaches to risk assessment in the forensic context
2   Outline the strengths and limitations of various assessment processes

3 Understand the concept of protective factors
4 Consider the requirement to conduct culturally sensitive assessments

Key concepts and terms

• Risk assessment
• Dynamic risk
• Static risk
• Unstructured professional judgement
• Structured professional judgement
• Actuarial assessment
• Protective factors
• Culturally sensitive risk assessments

Sample essay questions

• Compare and contrast the structured professional judgement approach to risk with the actuarial approach.
• It is important to ensure that assessment guides and risk assessment guides are specific to client groups. Discuss.

Recommended further reading

Otto, R., & Douglas, K. (2011). *Handbook of violence risk assessment*. Taylor and Francis.
Singh, J., Bjørkly, S., Fazel, S., & Leonard, S. (2016). *International perspectives on violence risk assessment*. Oxford University Press.

References

Boer, D. P. (2006). *Assessment of risk manageability for individuals with developmental and intellectual limitations who offend (ARMIDILO)*. Paper presented at the 9th Conference of the International Association for the Treatment of Sexual Offenders (IATSO). Hamburg, Germany, September 2006.
Boer, D. P., Hart, S. D., Kropp, P. R., & Webster, C. D. (1997). *Manual for the sexual violence risk 20 professional guidelines for assessing risk of sexual violence*. Mental Health, Law, and Policy Institute, Simon Frazer University.
Borum, R., Bartel, P., & Forth, A. E. (2002). *Manual for the Structured Assessment of Violent Risk in Youth (SAVRY)*. University of South Florida.
Craig, L. A., Beech, A., & Browne, K. D. (2006). Cross-validation of the Risk Matrix 2000 sexual and violent scales. *Journal of Interpersonal Violence, 21*, 612–633.
de Vogel, V., de Ruiter, C., Bouman, Y., & de Vries Robbe, M. (2012). SAPROF, Guidelines for the assessment of protective factors for violence risk. *Forum Educatief*.
de Vogel, V., de Vries Robbé, M., van Kalmthout, W., & Place, C. (2014). *Female Additional Manual (FAM): Additional guidelines to the HCR-20 for assessing risk for violence in women*. Van der Hoeven Stichting.
Douglas, K. S., Hart, S. D., Webster, C. D., & Belfrage, H. (2013). *HCR-20: Assessing risk for violence* (3th ed.). Mental Health, Law and Policy Institute, Simon Fraser University.
Hart, S. D., Kropp, P. K., Laws, D. R., Klaver, J., Logan, C., & Watt, K. A. (2003). *The risk for sexual violence protocol: Structured professional guidelines for assessing risk of sexual violence*. Mental Health, Law and Policy Institute, Simon Fraser University.

Kropp, P. R., Hart, S. D., & Belfrage, H. (2005). *Brief Spousal Assault Form for the Evaluation of Risk (B-SAFER) user manual*. ProActive ReSolutions.

Kropp, R. P., Hart, S. D., & Lyon, D. R. (2008). *Guidelines for Stalking Assessment and Management (SAM)*. ProActive Resolutions Inc.

Kropp, P. R., Hart, S. D., Webster, C. W., & Eaves, D. (1998). *Spousal assault risk assessment: User's guide*. Multi-Health Systems, Inc.

O'Rourke, M. (2008). Risk assessment. In G. J Towl, D. P. Farrington, D. A. Crighton, & G. Hughes (Eds.), *Dictionary of forensic psychology* (pp. 160–161). Willan.

Prentky, R., & Righthand, S. (2003). *Juvenile sex offender assessment protocol-II (J-SOAP-II) manual*. U.S. Department of Justice, Office of Justice Programs, Office of Juvenile Justice and Delinquency Prevention.

Quinsey, V. L., Harris, G. T., Rice, M. E., & Cormier, C. (2006). *Violent offenders: Appraising and managing risk* (2nd ed.). American Psychological Association.

Thornton, D. (2007). *Scoring guide for the Risk Matrix 2000*. Unpublished manuscript.

5 Formulation

Fiona Wilks-Riley

Case study: Oliver

Thirteen-year-old Oliver returned from school to his care home without any obvious problems. A few minutes later he smashed up the kitchen, pulled doors off cupboards, smashed crockery, repeatedly kicked the fridge, threw the fridge contents all over and he also threw a microwave through a window. Staff expressed there was 'no reason' for Oliver who was usually well behaved to have damaged the kitchen.

Summary

Every year there are media headlines describing behaviour or attacks as being 'for no reason' or motiveless. Although behaviour may appear motiveless to the outside observer, the reality is that it is not. The challenge for forensic psychologists is to help to determine the factors that have caused such behaviour to occur or uncover what purpose it may serve for the person. Then, there may be a chance for effective intervention for the behaviour to not be repeated.

Simply put, the process of understanding the development of an individual's difficulties is known as formulation. After discussing the importance of formulation, this chapter will examine two popular models of formulation in forensic psychology, the SORC (Goldfried & Sprafkin, 1976) and multiperspective model (Weerasekera, 1996), applying these models to the case study of Oliver. The relevance of trauma to forensic populations will then be discussed and a trauma-informed formulation introduced (Greenwald, 2005, 2013) with a structure for sharing it with a client.

The importance of formulation

There are many definitions of formulation within psychology. Bringing together the common elements of these different descriptions Johnstone and Dallos (2014) concluded:

> 'A formulation provides a hypothesis about a person's difficulties, which draws from psychological theory.'

> *(p5)*

Formulation can assist in helping to develop insight into behaviour. It can help foster understanding and empathy into how the individual's difficulties have developed. Accurate formulation will help to inform risk management and indicate relevant treatment targets. Relevant to forensic psychology is that behaviour, including offending

DOI: 10.4324/9781003017103-7

behaviour, inevitably serves some purpose for the individual, that is it possesses a functional value. One approach to formulation is that of functional assessment. Functional assessment aims to determine the functional value or purpose of a behaviour. A commonly used functional assessment framework is SORC (Goldfried & Sprafkin, 1976). SORC has been used to understand problem behaviour in school children (Steege et al., 2019) and applied to the development of personality disorder (Nelson-Gray et al., 2009) as well as offending behaviour.

SORC

The origins of SORC are in the behaviourism movement of psychology where behaviour is viewed as being learned from the environment through the influence of classical or operant conditioning (Lee-Evans, 1994). It might be useful to refresh your understanding of behaviourist principles to assist you with this framework. Radical behaviourists argued behaviour as determined and controlled entirely by the environment. Behaviour theory became more accepting that behaviour is a response not just to the environment, but to what the person brings to it (Nelson & Hayes, 1979). This is the position adopted by SORC. The SORC acronym in its original form stands for:-

Antecedent **Stimuli** – triggers and setting events
Organismic *variables* – personality and physiological factors that a person brings to the situation
Response *behaviour* – the behaviour being analysed
Consequences – things that reinforce or strengthen behaviour

FOCUS BOX 5.1   **EXPLAINS EACH OF THE SORC ELEMENTS.**

Box 5.1   SORC

Antecedent Stimuli – triggers

Triggers are identified as either proximal, occurring just before the behaviour, or distal, occurring historically (Herbert, 1987). In behaviour theory, recent triggers are given more weight. The key point about triggers in this framework is that they are actions or events that are *observable*.

Antecedent Stimuli – setting events

Setting events are the circumstances that increase the likelihood of the response behaviour occurring. These can be *external*, for example, a noisy school environment may be a setting condition for aggression for an individual with autism with sensory issues. Living with a substance using partner may be an external setting condition for a substance user to relapse.

Setting events can also be *internal* for example, a mood state such as feeling stressed or a physical state such as being drunk. They can be linked to behaviour through conditioning such as feeling stressed going into a school playground owing to previous experience of being assaulted there (as consistent with principles of classical conditioning) or learning, that being intoxicated brings more attention (as consistent with operant conditioning).

Organismic Variables

Organismic variables are everything that an individual brings to a situation (Nelson-Gray & Farmer, 1999). They include everything about the individual's physiology and learning experiences that exist before the triggering situation. This includes personality and the beliefs and values a person holds. Cognitive impairments from long-term substance misuse, brain injury, neurodevelopmental disorders, personality disorder and mental illness are other examples of organismic variables.

Response Behaviour

Response behaviour is so called because it is viewed as a response to the individual's environment. Response behaviour must be clearly described in detail with behaviours that can be observed and measured. According to the SORC model behaviour should also be described in terms of its frequency, intensity and duration. Describing behaviour in terms of motor elements (actions), cognitions and physiological experience is also popular. There are several different ways of describing response behaviour (see Lee-Evans, 1994 for review).

Consequences

Key to understanding the consequences of behaviour are the principles of positive and negative reinforcement from operant conditioning. Behaviour that is associated with a gain is positive reinforcement, and behaviour associated with the reduction or removal of something negative is negative reinforcement. Reinforcement leads to behaviour being strengthened and more likely to be repeated. According to learning theory, immediate or short-term reinforcers have more impact on a behaviour being strengthened compared to consequences that occur later (Skinner, 1953). This helps to explain why someone might eat cake but then a minute later starts feeling guilty about breaking his/her diet. The immediate enjoyment of eating the cake being a strong short-term positive reinforcer compared to the guilt experienced later.

Let us now apply SORC to the case study of Oliver.

Case study: background information for SORC

Oliver had a significant history of neglect including deprivation of food. His mother had a heroin addiction and his physical and emotional needs were often overlooked. He and his siblings sometimes fought each other for food. He has cognitive impairment possibly arising from neglect. Oliver has positive relationships with staff in the care home and generally with peers. He worries for his mother and his siblings' well-being.

Core beliefs about himself and others are 'no-one is there for me', 'I can't rely on or trust anyone', 'there's something wrong with me' and 'I don't matter'. His belief relating to aggression is 'it's OK if you need food'.

The night before the incident in the kitchen all the young people in the care home had ordered chocolate bars for the following day. On returning home from school, just prior to the incident, everyone had chocolate bars except for Oliver.

Oliver identified emotions prior to and after the incident and rated the strength of his emotions on a scale of 0–10. See Table 5.1 for more details on each of the factors. He reported feeling guilty after the incident. He was prompted to identify his emotions *immediately after* the incident.

Functions of Oliver's behaviour

SORC assessment helps to identify Oliver's aggression as serving the functions of reducing negative emotional states, as a means of asserting himself in his environment, reminding others of his existence and communicating his need to not be forgotten.

Table 5.1 SORC Oliver

Antecedent stimuli	**Proximal triggers**	Preordered chocolate bar is missing, other people have theirs.
	Distal triggers	Chronic history of not having emotional and physical needs met including a lack of availability of food.
	Setting events – Internal	'They've forgotten me', 'it's not fair' angry (10/10), upset (6/10), humiliated (10/10), left out (10/10), forgotten (10/10).
	Setting events – External	Living with a group of peers with competing needs from caregivers. Limited availability of chocolate in immediate environment.
Organismic variable	**Physiological**	Possible physical and neurocognitive consequences of neglect – cognitive impairment. Possible maternal substance use when pregnant with Oliver.
	Personality and beliefs	Negative self-view and distrust of others. 'No-one is there for me', 'I can't rely on or trust anyone', 'there is something wrong with me' and 'I don't matter'. Aggression 'is OK to get food' and 'food may not be there when I need it'.
Response variable	**Motor elements**	Kicked and threw things. Pulled cupboard doors from their hinges and hit them against the walls. Smashed one window with the microwave. Smashed a lot of crockery from the cupboards.
	Cognitive	Unable to recall thoughts during incident.
	Physiological	Highly emotionally aroused.
Consequences	**Negative reinforcers**	Angry (3/10), upset (4/10), left out (0/10), forgotten (0/10).
	Positive reinforcers	Empowerment (8/10) from showing people, 'they can't mess me about'.

Conclusions of SORC – practice challenges and tips

SORC has strengths in that it draws attention to factors contributing to a behaviour. The consideration of consequences also helps to understand how a behaviour is maintained through reinforcement. The importance of the environment having a critical role in contributing to problem behaviour is clear, and this enables the forensic psychologist to think about ways in which it can be harnessed to help manage problem behaviour.

When SORC is used by new users, it is common for a response behaviour to be referred to as 'substance use' rather than selecting a specific incident of substance using behaviour. As functions of behaviour change over time, this would be a source of confusion. The function of a young person using cannabis with friends for the first time for social acceptance is vastly different to ten years later when he is isolated in his room using heroin in response to withdrawal symptoms. It is helpful to think about a specific incident of a problem behaviour at a specific time and place. It is also common for cognitions not to be recalled during offence when there are high states of emotional arousal.

Another common error in starting to use SORC is to include consequences that are not immediate reinforcers. Clients may identify going to prison or feeling guilty as consequences of behaviour. Oliver has not been aggressive in order to feel guilty. From a learning theory point of view, although a later consequence, his guilt was not an *immediate* response to the incident of aggression and is therefore not a reinforcer. Practitioners need to direct attention to immediate consequences as close to the behaviour as possible.

It can be difficult sometimes to structure information for SORC to 'fit into the right box' which perhaps conceptually do not seem to fit. One example of this is emotions, which can be highly relevant triggers to behaviour being viewed as setting conditions rather than as triggers in their own right. This is because triggers have to be observable and measurable in the tradition of behaviour theory, something which emotions are not.

Historical factors in the SORC model are viewed as less important as they have been seen as less amenable to change compared to recent triggers and indeed not necessarily explored in terms of emotional impact. This is in sharp contrast to the trauma-informed formulation approach (this will be discussed later). SORC places less importance on why problems have developed and more focus on what is maintaining the problem behaviour (Lee-Evans, 1994). This links to the position in SORC that the environment is key to managing behaviour. Whilst the environment is clearly important, the goal in forensic practice is for the client to manage their behaviour rather than it being externally controlled by the environment.

A challenge to adhering faithfully to the SORC model in forensic practice is that 'Response Behaviour', the behaviour being analysed, should be observable and measurable. This is fine when applying SORC to school settings and analysing problem behaviour in the classroom where teachers can observe it. This is more challenging for assessment in forensic practice as the assessor would be in the impossible position of needing to have witnessed the offence as it happened. There may, however, be opportunities for monitoring and observing problem behaviour as it occurs within forensic settings and applying SORC to understanding this.

Sharing formulation with the client, perhaps family members and other professionals, is an important part of the formulation process. This is because it helps to make sense of difficulties, highlights areas that need to be worked on and starts to build therapeutic relationships (Sturmey, 2009). It also enables professionals to develop empathy for the client when problematic histories are shared. The language used in SORC such as antecedent stimuli and organismic variables is jargonistic and complex for clients and other non-psychologists requiring translation into something meaningful. Therefore, SORC can lack simplicity, one of the important elements of effective formulation (see Johnstone & Dallos, 2014 for a review of factors for effective formulation). SORC has, however, been at the forefront of enabling forensic psychologists to understand the function of offending behaviour. Another model of formulation that has become popular in recent years in forensic practice is the multiperspective model (MM) (Weerasekera, 1996), which will now be examined.

Multiperspective model (Weerasekera, 1996)

The MM was originally created to help understand the development of mental disorders, not offending behaviour, and to be used by mental health professionals. It is sometimes referred to as the Four Ps model as it refers to factors that are:

- **Predisposing** – increasing vulnerability to developing the problem
- **Precipitating** – influencing development of problem
- **Perpetuating** – maintaining the problem
- **Protective** – protecting against the development of the problem and building resilience

The MM model requires the formulation of a case from a biological perspective, three different psychological approaches (behavioural, cognitive and psychodynamic) plus four different systemic models (couple, family, occupational and social), a total of eight different perspectives. These should then be integrated into a single formulation (Sturmey, 2008). The model argues more than one approach is needed to explain an individual's difficulties according to Weerasekera (1996). Coping style responses, as in the methods used to respond to stress, are also considered in addition to treatment approaches (see multiperspective grid, Table 5.2). Using the model as it was originally set out therefore involves a lot of information and proficiency in fully formulating a case using these eight perspectives independently.

Commonly, forensic psychologists consider the Four Ps generically and include whichever factors they deem relevant from the approaches with which they are familiar, for example, the cognitive approach, but should consider what is most empirically valid to the case. It appears that there is some drift in how the model is being applied compared to how it was intended to be used. Current use of MM in this way is a very *simplified*

Table 5.2 Multiperspective grid (Weerasekera, 1996)

	Biological	Behavioural	Cognitive	Psychodynamic	Couple	Family	Occupational/ School	Social
Predisposing								
Precipitating								
Perpetuating								
Protective								
Coping style								
Treatment								

version which loosely relates to that set out by Weerasekera (1996). There is also possible drift even in how the model is not referred to as MM, the name designated by its author (Weerasekera, 1996, 2009) but as Four Ps or even Five Ps, in some published papers. The fifth P may be because *Presenting* problems is being included (Johnstone & Dallos, 2014).

The simplified MM may still, however, be a clinically useful framework for formulation in forensic practice. Factors the practitioner selects for inclusion should be guided by research or psychological theories. In this way, the simplified MM may be used as a way of structuring a formulation. This is demonstrated by applying the MM to the case study of Oliver (Table 5.3).

MM conclusions – practice issues and tips

As with SORC, the inclusion of perpetuating factors helps to focus on issues relevant to maintaining the presenting problem. A challenge in practice can be to distinguish between the Four Ps given that factors that are precipitating factors can also be perpetuating. Weerasekera (1996) acknowledged that correctly identifying such factor is not an issue as *'for practical purposes this does not matter'* (p20).

As can be seen from Table 5.2, the two sections for predisposing and precipitating factors in the simplified MM map onto *five* separate sections in SORC. This makes using simplified MM easier than SORC, a strength of this model.

The fact that protective factors feature in simplified MM (and not SORC) is a further strength to this model as it helps to think about the promotion of strength-based factors such as positive engagement with school. Weerasekera (1996) does not, however, provide specific guidance as to what may be protective factors relevant to forensic clients. As we have seen in Chapter 2, it is incumbent on the forensic psychologist to review the latest evidence base for their work. In this case, the forensic psychologist must research what are protective factors for the presenting problem (see Dubow et al., 2016 for review of protective factors for aggression in young people).

Since the original MM was created, there have been many more psychological theories and adaptations of theories than the cognitive, behavioural and psychodynamic in MM. In forensic practice, there may be other theories that identify factors relevant to the development of an offending behaviour. One example of this being that of the Abusive Personality model which requires examination of trauma and insecure attachment when formulating partner abuse (Dutton, 2007; see Chapter 9). The MM, even in its original form, could therefore be potentially restrictive for the clinician and client for constructing

---

Table 5.3 MM: Case study – Oliver

Predisposing	As SORC organismic variables and historical (distal) antecedents (Table 3.1).
Precipitating	As SORC recent triggers and setting conditions (Table 3.1).
Perpetuating	Anxiety over availability of food in environment.
	Sensitivity to feeling excluded and that exclusion means he is forgotten and something is wrong with him.
	In an environment with competing needs of others and where carers have not ensured he had the food he ordered.
Protective	Generally well behaved.
	Felt guilty about aggression indicating desire to behave prosocially.
	Managing to attend school – possibly indicating positive orientation to learning.

a meaningful formulation in forensic practice. Other criticisms of MM include the lack of explanation of the development of the problem, with factors being listed rather than integrated. Indeed, it has been argued this is simply an organising framework as opposed to formulation (Johnstone & Dallos, 2014). The recognition of the meaning or impact of predisposing factors is found in the third approach to be considered, that of trauma-informed formulation (Greenwald, 2005, 2013). Before this, the potential relevance of trauma to offending behaviour will be examined briefly.

Trauma and offending behaviour

Trauma is defined as an '*emotional response to a terrible event like an accident, rape or natural disaster*' (APA, 2020). When we think about trauma, our thoughts may automatically turn to post-traumatic stress disorder (PTSD) as this features in mental health classification systems. PTSD symptoms include reexperiencing and avoidance of the trauma and a current sense of threat and is prevalent in forensic populations (Baranyi et al., 2018). We now understand that exposure to trauma can have impact beyond PTSD in what have been termed complex (Hermann, 1992) and developmental trauma (van der Kolk, 2005). Complex trauma includes emotional dysregulation, negative self-concept and relationship difficulties in addition to PTSD symptoms that can arise from trauma exposure. It has only recently been included in the 11th version of the International Classification of Diseases (World Health Organisation, 2018). Developmental trauma disorder (DTD) equates to complex trauma that occurs in childhood. DTD includes panic, separation anxiety and disruptive behaviour disorders (van Der Kolk et al., 2019) and can arise from exposure to adverse childhood experiences (ACEs).

The potential impact of ACEs on offending behaviour has been a neglected area of research until recent years. Although, not an exhaustive list, ACEs as featured in the 10-item ACE scale (Felitti et al., 1998) includes abuse (emotional, physical and sexual), household dysfunction (violence, substance abuse, mental illness, imprisonment and divorce) and neglect (physical and emotional). Higher ACE scores have been found to relate to a range of offending behaviours (see further reading). In a study of males who had committed sexual offences, experiences of verbal abuse and emotional neglect were thirteen and four times higher, respectively, compared to males in the general population. In fact, half of the individuals who had sexually offended had four or more ACEs compared to 6% of the general population (Levenson et al., 2016). ACEs and their possible links to DTD and complex trauma are therefore relevant and important areas to consider in formulation in forensic practice. The trauma-informed approach was developed to formulate problem behaviour such as aggression in trauma-exposed individuals (Greenwald, 2005).

ACTIVITY BOX 5.1

Identify as many of Oliver's ACEs that you can.

Trauma-informed formulation (TIF) (Greenwald, 2005)

According to the TIF, experiences of trauma (and loss) greatly impact on the development of problem behaviour. Experiences that are traumatic in childhood affect a child's developing view of themselves, others and the world. Such negative experiences also create a host of negative emotions such as shame, sadness, fear, anger, rejection and worthlessness that are stuck and 'piled up' (Greenwald, 2013, p. 79). Reminders of the trauma cause these emotions, thoughts and beliefs to be activated or 'triggered'. In the TIF, the build-up of negative emotions and beliefs is likened to a 'sore spot', as portrayed in Figure 5.1. When a new stressor hits the sore spot, emotions become heightened. This can result in an overreaction in behaviour or a more intense emotional response.

Problem behaviour is therefore 'solution behaviour' as it reduces or provides relief from such negative emotions (Skinner, 1953; Greenwald, 2013). This reduction or relief from negative emotions is the same as the negative reinforcement principle used in SORC.

To complete the TIF, a comprehensive trauma/loss history is needed. Potential traumatic experiences are therefore not confined to the narrow focus of the ACE scale which

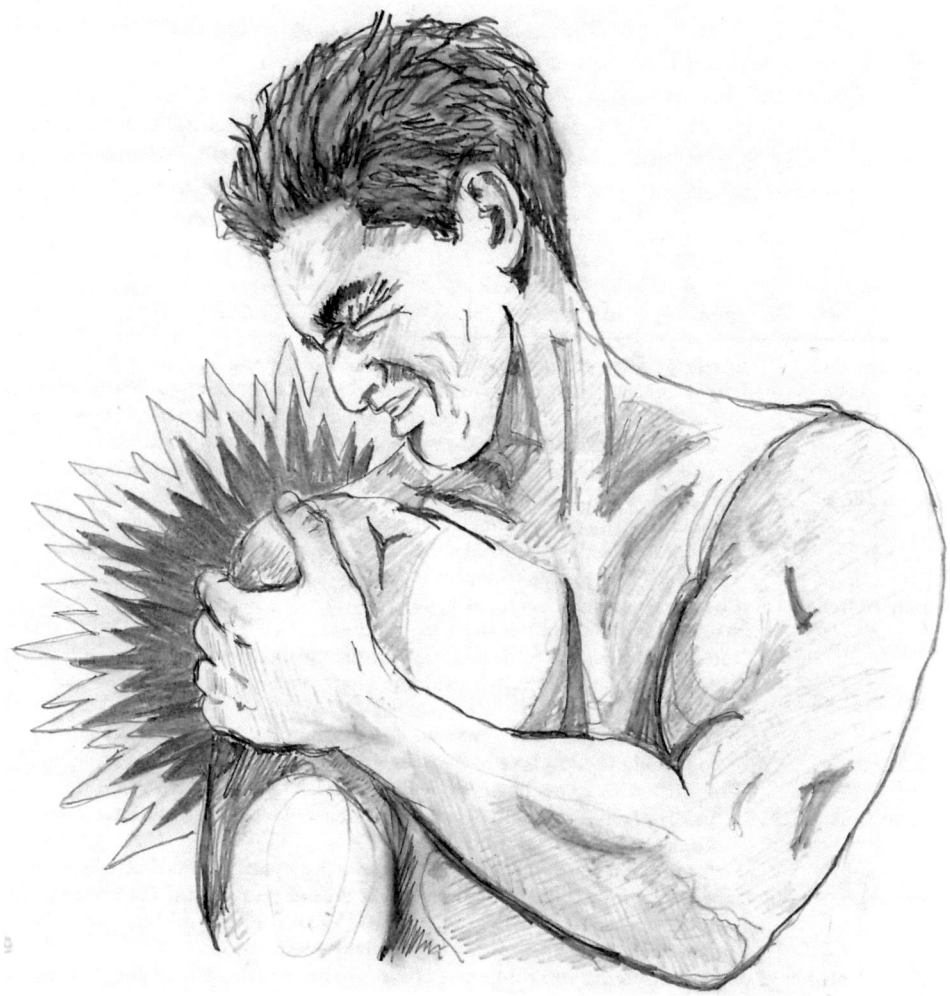

Figure 5.1 Activating the sore spot

omits peer bullying and rejection, bereavement and poverty, for example. Connections between the trauma or loss experiences to the client's associated beliefs and emotions are made. The circumstances of the problem/solution behaviour are then explored, and any trauma-related triggers identified. In this way, the client is not stigmatised, but their behaviour is seen as '*normal and reasonable reactions to unfortunate events*' (Greenwald, 2013, p. 79).

The TIF requires identification of strengths, and resources can be built on in interventions. Strengths and resources are not covered in SORC but are clearly positive aspects of this approach. This is because strengths and resources enable the client to be seen as essentially 'good' and as responding to emotions and beliefs that have been especially challenging. Their problem behaviour is exactly that, a behaviour, and not their whole identity. This explanation is demonstrated in the structure for sharing a TIF as applied to Oliver (Table 5.4). For additional guidance on sharing formulation, see Greenwald (2005, 2013).

Sharing this formulation with staff enabled them to empathise more with Oliver and see his behaviour as emanating from significant neglect experiences. It also helped staff to see the important role they had in being able to help Oliver by trying to ensure his needs were met and he was not forgotten or overlooked.

Strengths to the TIF approach are that it enables drivers to some of the problem behaviour to be identified and provide real meaning for why the problem behaviour develops. Unlike SORC and MM, the emotional impact of historical adverse experiences is given prominence to understanding current behaviour. The sore spot illustration encourages insight into how previous experiences have actively contributed to the

Table 5.4 Trauma-informed formulation – shared (based on Greenwald, 2005, 2013)

Strengths and resources	**Some positive things about you** are that most of the time you get along well with others. You can recognise when you have done wrong and you try do something about it, like, for example, seeing me. You are genuinely caring as I can see from how you worry about your family being OK. You show a sense of responsibility by going to school. You also like things to be fair.
Trauma/loss	**You have had a lot of challenges though,** such as the things we have talked about that you went through when you were growing up. (We purposefully do not repeat these to avoid evoking trauma memories, but these would be included in a written formulation report.)
Negative beliefs	**These experiences seem to have left you with negative beliefs about yourself that aren't really true such as:** 'Other people cannot look after me', 'no-one is there for me', 'I can't rely on or trust anyone', 'there is something wrong with me', 'I am not safe' and 'I don't matter'. You also had learned that sometimes food might not be there for you and that you would need to have to fight for it to survive.
Piled up emotions	**The difficulties you have had seem to have left you with piled up emotions** like feeling forgotten, neglected and worthless **that have become stuck and made a sore spot.**
Triggering situation	**I wonder if** when you did not get the chocolate you ordered **that this could have been hitting that sore spot. It would be difficult for anyone** not getting something they ordered, *but* **I can't help thinking that it is especially hard for you as it has hit the sore spot.**
Solution/problem behaviour	**Most people do anything to get rid of those feelings and for you that involved** smashing things in the kitchen.

development of current difficulties and the approach itself is empathic, which will help to develop the relationship with the client and motivate them to engage in any necessary intervention.

The TIF model is applicable for understanding problem behaviour when it clearly relates to having a function of reducing negative emotional states. It will not be applicable for understanding aggression in all circumstances as in the example of the individual with autism who is aggressive in response to being overwhelmed by the sensory environment.

A criticism of TIF when applied to forensic practice is the view of offending behaviour being '*normal and reasonable reactions to unfortunate events*' (Greenwald, 2013, p. 79). Forensic psychologists do not want to normalise offending behaviour but can still uphold the sentiment of this approach. They can validate how the behaviour was a solution and in this way was effective at the time. The behaviour has been effective in other ways, causing damage to their relationships and in some instances resulting in imprisonment. The idea of needing skills to manage sore spots in different ways feeds in well to a conversation with the client about intervention planning.

Case study: Oliver – intervention

It can be hypothesised that for Oliver to reduce the likelihood of further aggression, he would need intervention to manage negative emotions and communicate his needs effectively. His ACEs have resulted in an anxious, insecure attachment style. The TIF enables understanding of how his environment needs to promote safety and containment with safe and nurturing caregivers to assist him to be able to trust others and develop a positive sense of self. He will also need to address negative core beliefs. There needs to be sufficient food available in his environment in order for him to feel safe and secure that this basic need will be met. There needs to be clear effort to include him in the social group in which he lives. Additional 1:1 time with staff should also assist him to feel valued and that his needs will not be forgotten. The environment thus can have a significant risk management role although it would be unrealistic to expect that Oliver can always be protected by his environment from feeling left out and therefore internal controls need to be developed.

Conclusion

Formulation, although as yet to be endorsed by research, is an important process for understanding behaviour and hence truly relevant to forensic practice. The SORC and MM are popular models in forensic assessment. They both have strengths and weaknesses as models and areas in which they overlap. SORC draws attention to the environmental factors, but at the expense of not embracing the emotional impact of adverse experiences or appreciating emotions as triggers in their own right. The use of the MM has drifted considerably from how it was set out to be used to understanding mental disorder and this needs to be recognised when referencing its use in a more simplified form. Considering MM in its simplified form in will require drawing on models and theories of offending behaviour to identify factors that may be relevant. This could undermine the utility of using MM method of formulation in the first instance. The MM does, however, enable protective factors to be identified. The relatively recent recognition of ACEs as significant to the development of offending behaviour, likely through the mechanisms of developmental and complex trauma, indicates the importance of consideration of such in forensic assessment and intervention. The TIF is a relatively simple approach for formulation. It lends itself well to being shared and is easily understood by clients and professionals. A trauma-informed approach is important given the increased recognition of the association between adverse experiences in offending behaviour.

Learning outcomes

When you have completed this chapter, you should be able to:

1   Identify the core elements of the SORC
2   Identify the core elements of the multiperspective model
3   Identify the core elements of trauma-informed formulation
4   Understand a shared formulation from a trauma-informed perspective
5   Understand why a trauma-informed approach should be considered in formulation in forensic settings

Key concepts and terms

- Positive and negative reinforcement
- SORC
- Adverse childhood experiences
- Learning theory
- Developmental trauma
- Complex trauma
- Multiperspective model
- Formulation
- Function

Sample essay questions

- Compare and contrast two models of formulation to understanding an offending behaviour.
- What does research show about the relevance of trauma to understanding offending behaviour?
- Outline the purpose of formulation in forensic psychology practice.

Recommended further reading

Baglivio, M. T., Wolff, K. T., Piquero, A. R., & Epps, N. (2015). The relationship between Adverse Childhood Experiences (ACE) and juvenile offending trajectories in a juvenile offender sample. *Journal of Criminal Justice, 43*, 229–241.

Crane, C. A., Oberleitner, L. M. S., & Easton, C. (2013). Sub-clinical trauma in the treatment of partner violent offenders with substance dependence. *Advances in Dual Diagnosis, 6*, 5–13.

Levenson, J. S., Willis, G. M., & Prescott, D. S. (2016). Adverse childhood experiences in the lives of male sex offenders: Implications for trauma-informed care. *Sexual Abuse, 28*(4), 340–59.

References

American Psychiatric Association. (2020, 21 September). Retrieved from www.apa.org/topics/trauma/.

Baranyi, G., Cassidy, M., Fazel, S., Priebe, S., & Mundt, A. P. (2018). Prevalence of posttraumatic stress disorder in prisoners. *Epidemiological Review, 40,* 134–145.

Dubow, E., Huesmann, L., Boxer, P., & Smith, C. (2016). Childhood and adolescent risk and protective factors for violence in adulthood. *Journal of Criminal Justice, 45,* 26–31.

Dutton, D. G. (2007). *The abusive personality.* Guilford Press.

Felitti, V. J., Anda, R. F., Nordenberg, D., Williamson, D. F., Spitz, A. M., Edwards, V., & Marks, J. S. (1998). Relationship of childhood abuse and household dysfunction to many of the leading causes of death in adults. *American Journal of Preventative Medicine, 14,* 245–258.

Goldfried, M. R., & Sprafkin, J. N. (1976). Behavioural personality assessment. In J. T. Spence, R. C. Carson, & J. W. Thibaut (Eds.), *Behavioural approaches to therapy* (pp. 295–321). General Learning Press.

Greenwald, R. (2005). *Child trauma handbook: A guide for helping trauma-exposed children and adolescents.* Routledge.

Greenwald, R. (2013). *Progressive counting within a phase model of trauma-informed treatment.* Routledge.

Herbert, M. (1987). *Behavioral treatment of children with problems: A practice manual.* Academic Press.

Herman, J. L. (1992). Complex PTSD: A syndrome in survivors of prolonged and repeated trauma. *Journal of Traumatic Stress, 5,* 377–391.

Johnstone, L., & Dallos, R. (Eds.). (2014). *Formulation in psychology and psychotherapy* (2nd ed.). Routledge.

Lee-Evans, J. M. (1994). Background to behavioural analysis. In M. McMurran & J. Hodge (Eds.), *The assessment of criminal behaviours of clients in secure settings* (pp. 6–33). Jessica Kingsley Publishers.

Nelson-Gray, R., & Farmer, R. (1999). Behavioral assessment of personality disorders. *Behaviour Research and Therapy, 37*(4), 347–368.

Nelson-Gray, R., Lootens, C., Mitchell, J., Robertson, C., Hundt, N., & Kimbrel, N. (2009). Assessment and treatment of personality disorders: A behavioral perspective. *Behavior Analyst Today, 10*(1), 7–46.

Nelson, R. O., & Hayes, S. C. (1979). The nature of behavioural assessment: A commentary. *Journal of Applied Behavioural Analysis, 12*(4), 491–500.

Skinner, B. F. (1953). *Science and human behaviour.* MacMillan.

Steege, M. W., Pratt, J. L., Wickerd, G., Guare, R., & Watson, T. S. (2019). *Conducting school-based functional behavioral assessments: A practitioner's guide* (3rd ed.). Guilford Press.

Sturmey, P. (2008). *Behavioural case formulation and intervention: A functional analytic approach.* John Wiley & Sons Ltd.

Sturmey, P. (Ed.). (2009). *Clinical case formulation: Varieties of approaches.* John Wiley & Sons Ltd.

van der Kolk, B. A. (2005). Developmental trauma disorder: Toward a rational diagnosis for children with complex trauma histories. *Psychiatric Annals, 35*(5), 401–408.

van Der Kolk, B., Ford, J., & Spinazzola, J. (2019). Comorbidity of Developmental Trauma Disorder (DTD) and post-traumatic stress disorder: Findings from the DTD field trial. *European Journal of Psychotraumatology, 10*(1), 1562841.

Weerasekera, P. (1996). *Multiperspective case formulation: A step towards treatment integration.* Krieger Publishing.

Weerasekera, P. (2009). A formulation of the case of Antoinette: A multiperspective approach. In P. Sturmey (Ed.), *Clinical case formulation: Varieties of approaches.* John Wiley & Sons Ltd.

World Health Organization. (2018). *International Classification of Diseases and related health problems* (11th ed.). Retrieved from https://icd.who.int/.

Part 3

Specialist forensic interventions and populations

6 Designing rehabilitative interventions in forensic settings

Jamie S. Walton

Introduction

Providing intervention to people who engage in harmful behaviour is an important role for forensic psychologists. People who repeatedly commit crime often do so against a backdrop of biological vulnerability, personal adversity and socioeconomic deprivation. Words like '*evil*' or '*bad*' are non-scientific. Forensic psychologists stay away from these terms and instead try to understand how behaviour is contextually shaped according to biological factors, learning processes and social conditions – what we might call our 'biopsychosocial circumstances'. To support people in building capacities for leading crime-free lives, forensic psychologists also need to know about the principles of effective rehabilitation. In this chapter, you will learn about a biopsychosocial approach which describes both a humanising perspective of harmful behaviour and organising principles for effective rehabilitation.

A scientific approach to rehabilitative interventions

Just four decades ago, the view in rehabilitation services was that *nothing works* in reducing reoffending. Since then, psychologists and criminologists have gathered evidence about different rehabilitative practices and have determined the mediators of positive effects. These are now known as the 'risk-need-responsivity' (RNR) principles (Andrews & Bonta, 2016). The RNR principles provide an evidence-based framework for designing and implementing rehabilitative interventions. These interventions are often called 'offending behaviour programmes' (OBPs). They are delivered in a group format which involves two clinicians (e.g. psychologist, probation officer and intervention facilitator) supporting eight to ten people learn prosocial skills together.

The *risk principle* has two components. The first component is to assess risk of reoffending with a valid risk assessment. The second is to match level of risk to a proportionate amount of intervention. All things being equal, the most intensive services should be reserved for people assessed as highest risk. The *need principle* specifies that intervention should target characteristics associated with reoffending. These are identified using structured risk assessments and psychometric measures and are called 'criminogenic needs' (Focus Box 6.1). Finally, the *responsivity principle* identifies general and specific procedures for delivery. General responsivity states that intervention should use cognitive-behavioural procedures. These include functional analysis, identifying thinking patterns and teaching cognitive skills. Specific responsivity guides clinicians to attend to the circumstances of individuals such as their culture, learning ability or mental and physical health as a basis

DOI: 10.4324/9781003017103-9

for personalising services. Research continues to find that reductions in reoffending are related to the extent to which intervention conforms to RNR principles (Andrews & Bonta, 2016).

BOX 6.1   CRIMINOGENIC NEEDS

Criminogenic needs are distinguished by their statistically significant association with reoffending. The most common criminogenic needs are outlined in the following. They are called the '*central eight*'. 'Criminal history' is historic and static. The remaining criminogenic needs refer to dynamic risk domains which are changeable, insofar as people can develop new skills, insight, support networks and perspectives.

---

1. Criminal history	2. Antisocial personality pattern
3. Antisocial attitudes	4. Antisocial peer association
5. Family and/or marital	6. School and/or work
7. Leisure and/or recreation	8. Substance use

Despite their validity, the RNR principles are not without criticism. Researchers take issue with the focus of RNR on people's risks at the expense of recognising their strengths. Another issue has to do with criminogenic needs. Whilst they usefully predict *re*offending, the processes underlying them such as biological processes, learning processes and social conditions are not well described. This is important because without this information, it is difficult to know how intervention procedures target mechanisms that mediate change. Identifying the processes underlying criminogenic needs requires a model that is capable of integrating multilevel knowledge about human functioning. Biopsychosocial models are one example of this. Biopsychosocial models are used to integrate information about genes, hormones and brains, learning processes and cognitive systems, and social and cultural factors in order to formulate how individual behaviour is shaped (Figure 6.1). Recently, forensic psychologists have used a biopsychosocial approach to articulate processes underlying criminogenic needs (Walton et al., 2017).

Biopsychosocial processes underlying criminogenic needs

Because of space, it is not possible to describe biopsychosocial processes influencing all criminogenic needs. Instead, I will focus on a few from Focus Box 6.1, specifically, antisocial personality pattern, problematic relationships (family and/or marital) and antisocial peer association. Antisocial personality refers to a pattern of impulsivity, restlessness, rule defiance and aggression. Problematic relationships refer to relationship instability and conflict with partners, and antisocial peer association refers to affiliation with criminal networks. I will first discuss biological processes influencing these criminogenic needs, starting with genes. Genes are a good example of an important point to make about the

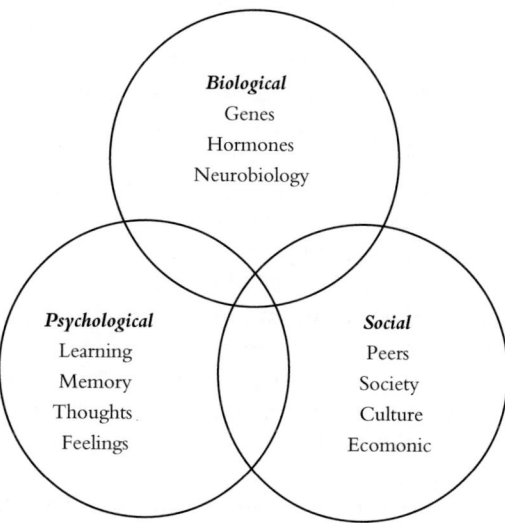

Figure 6.1 Biopsychosocial model

biopsychosocial approach, which is that biological, psychological and social processes are interdependent.

Biological processes

Genes are segments of DNA which instruct how proteins function to build our cells and bodies. They are instructions for life's building blocks. However, genes do not determine our biology, nor for that matter, our behaviour. Genetic influences are environmentally dependent. Two examples relevant to criminogenic needs demonstrate this. The first is a gene called *monoamine-oxidase-A* (MAOA) as a cause for features of antisocial personality such as aggression. The second is a dopamine transporter gene called 'DAT1', as a cause of antisocial peer association. The MAOA gene provides instructions for making an enzyme that breaks down chemicals in the brain which are involved in emotion regulation (e.g. serotonin). In a landmark study, Caspi et al. (2002) found that carrying a low-activity form of the MAOA gene was associated with aggression in adolescents and adults, but only if they had a history of childhood maltreatment. This was not the case for those with the low-activity form of MAOA without a history of childhood maltreatment. In an equally important study, Beaver et al. (2008) found that a particular form of the DAT1 gene was associated with male adolescents befriending antisocial peers, but only if they were from a high-risk family environment marked by absent maternal affection. Such effect of the DAT1 variant was not found for adolescents from families with greater nurturance and emotional closeness. Both sets of findings have been replicated, and they demonstrate an important point, which is that genes are about susceptibility not inevitability. The inheritance of genetic effects depends on inheriting a gene and the environment that regulates it in a particular manner. This is called a '*gene–environment*' interaction. In other words, there is no gene which by itself causes antisocial personality, antisocial peer association or any other criminogenic need.

Hormones are another biological influence. Cortisol and testosterone are well researched for their association with impulsivity and aggression. But again, the picture is complicated. Cortisol is controlled by a group of glands called the 'hypothalamus–pituitary–adrenal' (HPA) axis, which is part of the body's stress response system. It helps ready fight-or-flight behaviour and influences motivation, memory and metabolism. The HPA axis shows a rhythm in humans, where cortisol levels are highest in the morning and then drop throughout the day. Studies tracking daily cortisol report flatter rhythms in male children and adolescents who display impulsive aggression and low cortisol arousal for children and adults who display callous and dispassionate aggression (see Fairchild et al., 2018).

Testosterone is a male sex hormone involved in libido and muscle growth. High testosterone is associated with antisocial personality features such as aggression and rule defiance in men and women. However, these effects are context dependent, for example, on cortisol and personality factors (Carré & Archer, 2018). In fact, testosterone may have less to do with aggression and more to do with increasing *whatever* behaviour maintains status. Evidences come from gaming research which shows how administering testosterone can stimulate prosocial behaviour including generosity when it enhances status in a game (van Honk et al., 2012). Therefore, the problem might be less to do with testosterone increasing aggression and more to do with the way culture rewards aggression with status.

Brain functioning is also important. The frontal lobe of the brain is of particular interest. It supports functions involved in language, memory, reasoning, emotion processing and self-control. The most fore-frontal region is called the 'prefrontal cortex' (PFC; Figure 6.2). The PFC plays a role in higher-order abilities called 'executive functions'. Examples include planning, inhibition and problem-solving. Two subregions of the PFC are the 'dorsolateral prefrontal cortex' (dlPFC) and the 'ventromedial prefrontal cortex' (vmPFC), which are the top side-to-side (i.e. 'dorsal-lateral') and bottom-centre (i.e. 'ventral-medial') areas, respectively. The dlPFC is the cognitive component, involved in working memory, planning and self-regulation. Structural and functional issues in

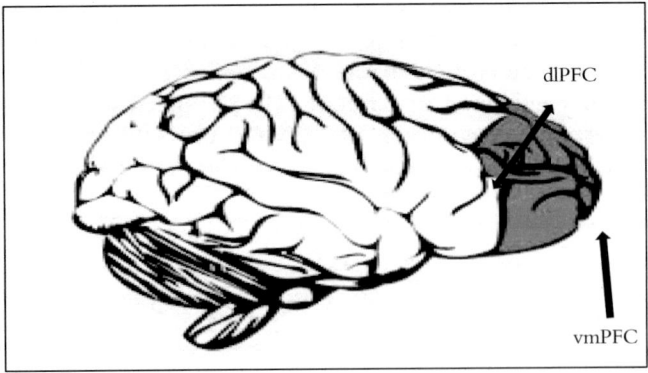

Figure 6.2 Prefrontal cortex

this area are associated with poor self-control, disinhibition and impulsivity and can be found in people displaying antisocial behaviour (Yang & Raine, 2009). The vmPFC is connected to the brain's emotion centre and is involved in representing emotional information for decision-making, including moral decisions. Deficits in this area have distinguished people who persistently engage in crime over their lifetime from those whose crime is restricted to adolescence (Carlisi et al., 2020). The vmPFC is also part of the neurobiological explanation of psychopathy (Blair, 2008), which includes aspects of an antisocial personality pattern including impulsivity and rule defiance/irresponsibility.

Psychological processes

Psychological processes refer to motivational and cognitive systems (e.g. perception and memory) and learning processes, including observational learning such as modelling and imitating and direct behavioural learning such as classical and operant conditioning. The basic motives are those for sex, resources and status, avoiding oppression, forming alliances and giving and receiving care. The attachment system is involved in caring motives especially. Attachment is a biological system as much as anything else, but it includes learning, memory and emotion processes as well as the development of cognitive representations of self, others and the world. Due to space, I will only focus on attachment and behavioural learning processes.

Attachment is the bond that forms between infant and caregiver as the means by which the infant gets their needs met. It then becomes the engine for emotional, social and cognitive development. Optimal development is depended on 'secure attachment'. Secure attachment is characterised by the caregiver(s) being attuned to the child's arousal in order to provide a balance of stimulation, play and soothing. This attuned interaction synchronises the infant and caregiver's biological rhythms, providing the conditions for 'co-regulation'. When co-regulation is occurring, states of positive emotion are being co-created and states of distress are being co-repaired. This begins building the neuro-developmental template for emerging self-regulation, which includes inhibition, self-control, resilience and stable cognitive representations of the world. Childhood adversity such as emotionally deprived parenting or overstimulation and abuse damages this process. When adverse conditions are prolonged, co-regulation is unreliable and the infant's needs are not met. A cascade of changes can occur in the child's brain, shifting the path of neurodevelopment away from prosocial potential, towards illnesses and dysfunctional behaviours during later life. Many of these behaviours are characterised as criminogenic needs, for example, alcohol abuse, aggression and problems in relationships.

Let's consider one effect of childhood abuse from a behavioural learning perspective and in the context of problems in relationships (family and/or marital). The point to remember is that the attachment system responds to *whatever* conditions are available. In nurturing conditions, a child can explore the world knowing that their caregiver(s) will repair it if things become overwhelming. This early secure base promotes abilities for being vulnerable with others and forms a template for intimacy. However, when a caregiver is abusive such that they evoke incompatible states of fear and affection, their closeness becomes a source for distress and a conditioned stimulus for avoidance (Figure 6.3a: classical conditioning). This response can become highly elaborated during adolescence and adulthood through the process of negative reinforcement. This is where attempts at emotional closeness in adult relationships evoke distress and trigger the response of pushing partners away in order to reduce it (Figure 6.3b: operant conditioning). Other responses might include

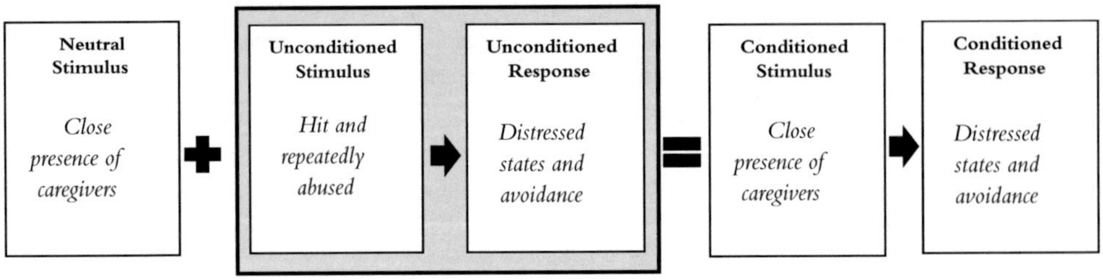

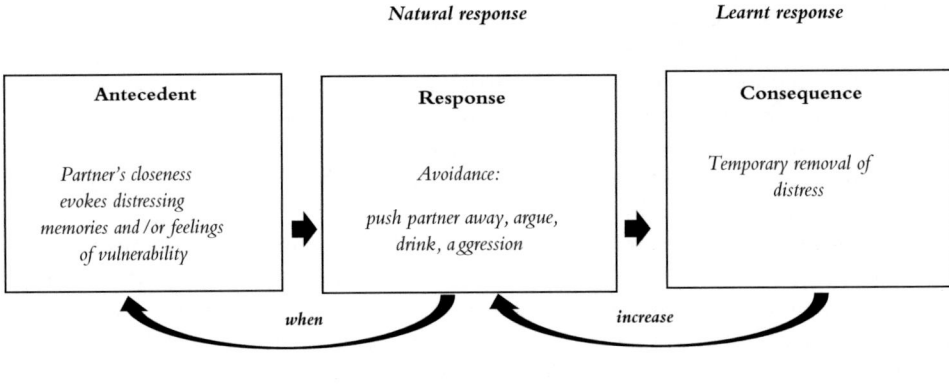

Figure 6.3a Stimulus-Response: closeness becomes a source of fear and a stimulus for avoidance

Figure 6.3b Negative reinforcement: increased frequency and intensity of emotional avoidance

arguing, drinking and aggression. They all serve the same *function* (i.e. consequence) which is to decrease the fear of being close and vulnerable with others. Over time, this avoidance pattern comes at a cost because it erodes scope for connection and reciprocal support which is needed for stability in relationships. In such cases, a confused and frightened child has become a fragmented and insecure adult whose attempts to avoid their own emotional pain increase injury to themselves and others. This brings us to an important issue, which is that beneath criminogenic needs there is often tragedy and hurt.

Social conditions

Social conditions include interpersonal dynamics with peers as well the reverberating influences of contextual factors such as cultural norms and the socioeconomic infrastructure of a community. There is much here that is beyond the scope of this chapter, and so, I will only focus on the effects of living in deprived communities.

Deprived communities have a disproportionately higher prevalence of crime along with a myriad of mental and physical diseases. A clear social influence is that disenfranchised inner-city neighbourhoods with high rates of crime and unemployment, leverage high accessibility to antisocial peers, particularly street socialisation into youth urban gangs.

But the detrimental effects of socioeconomic deprivation run much deeper than this. Poverty gets under the skin. In real terms, it exposes people to numerous disadvantages, including issues to do with household noise that disturbs sleep and rest, malnutrition, reduction of cognitively stimulating experiences including lower home learning resources and higher neighbourhood violence and higher exposure to agricultural toxins. Cumulatively, these disadvantages effect neurodevelopmental trajectories and life expectancy.

Similar to the way the attachment system responds to whatever caregiving conditions are available, personalities and behaviour emerge to fit whatever social niche is provided. In other words, minds, bodies and behaviour are environmentally contextualised. They are adjusted to the cost-benefit pay-offs that are present in the environment and in turn, best-fit strategies will emerge. For example, in a safe cohesive community with good schooling, leisure and healthcare infrastructure, it will prove adaptive to invest in others with trust, sharing, cooperation and care. In such conditions, these prosocial strategies usually develop. However, in a dangerous and deprived neighbourhood, stricken with crime and drugs, such strategies will be less useful or even disadvantageous, and so, they will be down regulated. Instead, high-risk, self-focused and exploitative strategies are more likely to emerge. These may include aggression, excessive risk taking and impulsiveness (*vis-a-vis*, antisocial personality pattern). This is not without consequence. Adaption to adverse conditions simply enables individuals to survive in chronically stressful circumstances, even though the emerging best-fit strategies are often destructive. They are high risk because high risk is what delivers greatest benefit in a high-cost environment. This brings us to another important point, which is that in forensic psychology words like 'risky' and 'maladaptive' are used synonymously. Clearly though, they not the same. What is 'adaptive' is context dependent. Humans adaptively develop best-fit strategies to endure *whatever* social niche they are nested in.

Organising principles for effective rehabilitation

At this point, you are encouraged to think about the processes which influence the emergence of criminogenic needs, and how they are part of a biopsychosocial life lottery. We all play it, and we do not choose our numbers. We do not choose our genes or brains. We do not choose our thoughts or feelings, our caregivers and the learning experiences that shape our neurodevelopment. We also do not choose the environment we grow up in and whether it is safe or deprived and crime ridden. For us all, the reality is that we arbitrarily inherit genes and brains which are choreographed to fit a coincidental environment we happen to find ourselves in. This is not an excuse for harmful behaviour. Rather, it is a way of understanding the harmful side of human potential. The next section discusses six organising principles for intervention. Organising principles are evidence-informed guidelines for designing and implementing OBPs. The first two reflect the risk and responsivity principles of RNR. Principles 3 to 5 build on the need principle of RNR by outlining cognitive-behavioural therapy (CBT) procedures and their links to change processes in biological, psychological and social levels of functioning. The sixth principle focuses on strengthening people's motivation to turn away from crime.

Principle 1: matching intervention to risk of reoffending

Matching the level of risk to intervention intensity is called 'dose-response'. Per risk level, there is an optimum range and a saturation point. For people assessed as high risk, the largest effects on reducing reoffending have been found to occur when intervention moves from 150–200 to 200–250 hours, whereas for people assessed as medium risk, moving from less than 100 to 100–150 hours achieves the largest effects (Makarios et al., 2014). Saturation occurs at about 300 hours for those assessed as high risk, whilst for those assessed as medium risk, it occurs at 200 hours. Beyond these limits, intervention can increase reoffending. Therefore, more is not always better.

Principle 2: intervention should be responsive to people's biopsychosocial circumstances

The biopsychosocial processes underlying criminogenic needs also influence engagement with intervention. A major influence to consider is the effect of childhood adversity on neurocognitive domains such as verbal, attention, memory and executive functions. Using reading and writing to learn, especially with long periods of seated discussion is unlikely to engage many participants. Multimodal approaches that use visual, auditory, reading and kinesthetic methods of presenting information are much more brain-friendly. Modern interventions use body-movement techniques, humour, drawing, gesturing and brain-breaks such as task-switching (Walton et al., 2017). These personalise engagement for different individuals and reset states for learning.

Another responsivity issue is the fact that heightened threat-sensitivity, impulsiveness and aggression, as best-fit strategies for living in hostile environments, make it difficult for people to form trust with intervention staff. When people are presented with interventions, this heightened threat-sensitivity can manifest as a resistance to what is perceived as a pressure to change by authority figures. Coercing people to change is ineffective. Remember, humans develop best-fit strategies to survive in whatever social niche they are nested in. A lot of professional views about what *must* change (e.g. hostility, rigidity, impulsivity and antisocial peers) function to fulfil basic needs such as self-protection, autonomy, status and belonging. The idea of living differently may seem absurd, not least because it looks inconsistent with what is necessary to survive in the harsh environment that a person is accustomed to. So, a person must first have the chance to 'try out' change by learning skills required to achieve it. Modern OBPs therefore set simple terms for safe engagement, where people can come together, explore identity and learn skills to see what works in leading a value-based life (Walton et al., 2017). Staff encourage curiosity about change, rather than demand that people commit to it. A person can choose to engage under the requirement of learning skills, or they can reject the opportunity altogether. In essence, there is an attempt to encourage a recognition that the intervention is not a challenge to autonomy by establishment authority but is instead an opportunity to enhance it through practising alternative behaviour which opens up new choices for living.

Principle 3: intervention procedures that strengthen biological resources

Throughout life, the brain morphs in response to environmental conditions. Brain cells make new connections and the functionality and size of brain regions change. Just as childhood adversity and socioeconomic deprivation can shape neurodevelopmental trajectories, these trajectories can also be reshaped with new learning. This process is called 'neuroplasticity'. CBT procedures that strengthen biological resources include those that produce gains in neurocognition and self-regulation which are at least in part mediated by neuroplastic changes in the PFC and/or biological mechanisms underpinning arousal regulation. The effects of these procedures are also mediated by changes in psychological processes, including metacognition.

Mindfulness is a process of purposefully paying attention to thoughts, feelings, sensations and the environment in the present moment with acceptance. Mindfulness techniques include focused attention, yoga and meditation. These techniques can have positive effects on executive functioning and attention control. The change processes that mediate these effects have been reviewed by Baer (2018) and include reduced cognitive and emotional reactivity and rumination, increased self-compassion and changes in 'metacognition' – a process of being consciously aware of one's thinking. Neurobiological changes seem to occur in prefrontal regions associated with attention and regulating emotion (Hölzel et al., 2011; Siegle & Coan, 2018).

Rhythmic breathing focuses on slowing down breathing and extending exhalation, shifting the breath deeper from the chest to the diaphragm. This technique facilitates physiological soothing through its activation of the bodies 'parasympathetic nervous system' (PSNS) which acts as a counteracting force to the body's stress response system. Rhythmic breathing can improve emotion regulation, metacognition and self-control, and the main neurobiological process mediating these benefits appears to be respiratory stimulation of the vagus nerve (Gerritsen & Band, 2018). The vagus nerve is part of the PSNS and has connections to the voice, heart, lungs and visceral organs. Slow rhythmic breathing can increase vagal activity in a top-down fashion from the executive functioning control network (Gerritsen & Band, 2018). This lowers heart rate, blood pressure and inhibits HPA activity resulting in a decrease in acute stress response. As this happens, the body's slowing and soothing sensations can also influence cognitive perception of stressors in the environment through biofeedback channels facilitating further self-regulation.

Progressive muscle relaxation (PMR) targets the body's stress response system by reducing muscle tension with the successive tensing and relaxing of different muscle groups. Abbreviated PMR scripts instruct several minutes of practice. PMR can reduce psychological distress and improve subjective well-being and is used for reducing anger, tension and aggression. The effects of PMR are in part mediated by a reduction in cortisol (Chellew et al., 2015).

Problem-solving training (PST) aims to apply strategies such as defining problems, generating options, weighing-up costs and benefits, and implementing planned decisions to improve coping with stressors and dilemmas. PST is trained in a structured way to overcome neurocognitive barriers such as cognitive overload, impulsivity and emotion dysregulation. A recent neuroimaging synthesis of PST revealed activation of prefrontal networks involved integrating information and reasoning as potential neurobiological correlates of activation and change (Siegle & Coan, 2018).

Principle 4: procedures that target flexibility in psychological functioning

Intervention procedures targeting self-management, cognitive reappraisal and values form the cornerstone of CBT. They are grouped together based on their goals to enhance flexible forms in psychological functioning.

Self-management refers to analysing and changing the antecedents and consequences of behaviour. This is so behaviour itself can be changed. Antecedents are triggers that come before behaviour. Analysing them provides an indication of *when* a behaviour occurs. A consequence is defined by how it influences behaviour, either increasing or reducing the likelihood of it recurring in the presence of the antecedent. Analysing consequences provides an indication of the function of behaviour, that is, *why* it occurs. The process of analysing what people learn from the consequences of their behaviour in response to antecedents is called '*functional analysis*'. Consider the functional analysis of violence in Figure 6.4. Suppose the individual finds literacy challenging and so this work has been drawn and is simply called '*what happened, what I did, what I got*'.

This individual was violent in a response to a person jumping in front of them in the lunch queue. This evoked a state of feeling undermined. The response of punching this person removed the feeling thereby producing a negative reinforcing effect. It restated their sense of status thereby also producing a positive reinforcing effect. This analysis suggests that the perception of threat is likely to evoke an aggressive response in order to regain status amongst peers and avoid feeling inferior. Self-management suggests several ways of reducing aggression. This could include changing or managing the antecedents, or achieving the consequences in alternative ways. Changing the antecedents could include avoiding the peer or the lunch queue. However, this is a restrictive solution. Managing the antecedents would be a better option. This could include practicing skills to reduce emotional reactivity or respond flexibly to aggressive thoughts (e.g. mindfulness or cognitive reappraisal). To achieve the consequences in alternative ways, new behaviours are needed which can be reinforced to obtain the desired functions (i.e. upholding personal rights and preserving status). This might include practicing interpersonal skills such as assertiveness. Therefore, self-management includes practicing skills to achieve specified goals. What is particular about self-management is the use of behavioural learning processes such as reinforcement to shape people's retention and selection of skills.

Cognitive restructuring involves reappraising thinking and beliefs. This is based on the idea that thinking mediates the association between our experience of things and our emotional and behavioural responses to them. The need to reappraise beliefs is usually because they are problematic (e.g. antisocial) and narrow emotional and behavioural responses. However, some researchers examining interventions that use cognitive restructuring have found that self-report changes in antisocial cognition do *not* predict outcomes in reoffending (Wakeling et al., 2013). That said, in mental health, the effect of cognitive restructuring on conditions such as depression is mediated by changes in problematic thinking (Cristea et al., 2015). Other mediators of change include metacognitive processes, such as *decentring* (Hayes–Skelton & Graham, 2013). This is a process of noticing thoughts and how they change, leading to a non-judging stance towards self.

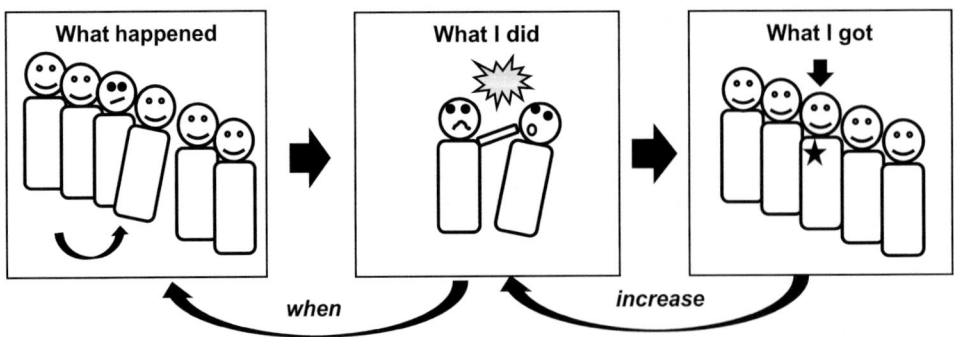

Figure 6.4 Functional analysis of violence: positive and negative reinforcement

Usually, cognitive restructuring involves identifying problematic beliefs through formulation so they can be understood as developing from learnt experience. Using Socratic questions, a psychologist can then help the participant to recognise their learnt biases that shape how they see the world. Socratic questions are non-provocative exploratory questions that evoke metacognitive processes and reasoning. This then paves the ways for more flexible ways for interpreting current situations. This is not about increasing positive ('glass half full') thinking. Rather, it is about achieving a more balanced way of experiencing the world, which is likely to reduce emotional reactivity and increase flexible behaviour.

Values clarification is the process of recognising what makes life meaningful, for example, love, family, security, connection and peace. This process can link personal investment in change to a sense of purpose in life. As is outlined previously, the reality of change for people living in harsh environments can be fraught with uncertainty. Trust, intimacy and being forgiving may be entirely foreign. Putting distance between oneself and antisocial influences may seem completely undesirable. Why would a person choose to do this when those influences are the peers who helped them survive adversity growing up, and with whom they bonded in co-experiencing safety, status and affirmation? They may do it if it was in service of what they deeply cared about in life – perhaps parenthood or their freedom. In short, effort in learning skills for change is likely to be reinforced if it is linked to values. This is because by linking effort to values it becomes energy spent in the service of what matters in life.

Principle 5: procedures that target social resources

Social resources such as interpersonal skills and prosocial networks play an important role in enabling people to contribute responsibly to communities. Group interventions serve as small communities, with live opportunities to practice listening, cooperating and sharing. Prosocial networks can be targeted by analysing a person's social circle and enlisting mentors and professionals which bridge gaps in support. Values clarification can dignify these efforts, but individuals need interpersonal skills to access support. Recognising when interpersonal competency is a barrier to a person's prosocial success and coaching interpersonal skills is a core CBT competency.

Interpersonal competency is the integration of skilful behaviour for appropriately expressing thoughts, feelings and needs, and responding to others. It entails skilfulness of non-verbal communication, choice and tone of words and perspective taking. For those living in threatening environments, hostile social strategies may have a history of reinforcement, whereas prosocial strategies such as listening and compromise may not have been modelled or they may have been punished. Commonly introduced interpersonal skills include assertiveness, negotiation, listening and expressing feelings appropriately. They are taught using a systematic method which involves introducing skill steps, modelling, coaching and giving reinforcing feedback. Interpersonal skills training can have positive effects (Lipsey et al., 2010). However, it remains unclear if these effects are mediated by improved interpersonal skills.

Principle 6: strengthen the intention for prosocial change

Ceasing crime can be difficult. Aggression, impulsivity, emotional avoidance and other developed strategies serve functions in achieving basic needs and avoiding feared realities. These strategies have often gained momentum which creates inertia against investment in change. Procedures already discussed such as values clarification and promoting choice can help. However, they can be further supported with a strength-based approach and motivational interviewing.

A strength-based approach recognises people's discovered and yet-to-be discovered strengths for change. This involves acknowledging the detrimental effects of biological vulnerabilities and adversity, whilst valuing human potential and building personal growth. As mentioned previously, the RNR principles have been criticised on this front, for neglecting people's strengths at the expense of removing criminogenic needs. However, this criticism is misplaced. Targeting criminogenic needs is not about trying to remove strategies or characteristics as if there is a process called 'unlearning'. Nowhere in psychology will you find it. Intervention should be about building repertoires, not restricting them. Targeting criminogenic needs involves using CBT procedures to *expand* an individual's range of behavioural alternatives, thereby empowering them with choices to create healthier conditions. Recognising their aspirations, successes and wisdom is essential to this. In general, a strength-based approach is defined by its emphasis on future-oriented goals, a focus on expanding behavioural repertoires and the effort of a clinician to instil hope and recognise strength.

Motivational interviewing is an approach for promoting a participant–clinician relationship characterised by empathy and attention to the discrepancies between the participant's behaviour and their values. This requires skills in the Socratic method, denoted by the acronym OARS, namely, asking 'open' questions, 'affirming', using 'reflective' listening and 'summarising' information. There is a subtlety to motivational interviewing in the clinician's selective use of the participant's language as direct reinforcers for change. This language is called '*change talk*', and it is language that is suggestive of openness, optimism and ability. Reflecting back change talk, even words like 'can', 'possible' and 'capable', underpins the emphasis of motivational interviewing in promoting self-efficacy. The technique is inherently strength based in recognising that participants have the wisdom and capacities for change and that the clinician serves to help them call them forth.

Conclusion

Preventing harmful behaviour is a challenge. It requires models that can deconstruct human complexity into a manageable number of processes, and procedures that are capable of targeting them. A biopsychosocial approach helps us to do this. It steers the focus beneath criminogenic needs to the processes that constrain neurodevelopmental trajectories, restrict capacities for cooperation and recruit high-risk strategies as a means of adapting to adverse conditions. These processes can then be targeted using evidenced-based CBT procedures as part of working within established principles of effective rehabilitation.

Recommended further activity

You are encouraged to access the HMPPS Forensic Psychology Podcast (https://pod.link/1533101974) and listen to the following episode which explores concepts discussed in this chapter:

Episode 3: How do we help people change? [29/10/2020]

Learning outcomes

When you have completed this chapter, you should be able to:

1   Understand the RNR principles
2   Understand biological processes, learning processes and social conditions that can influence antisocial functioning
3   Have a humanising understanding of harmful behaviour
4   Understand cognitive-behavioural procedures and their links to change processes

Key concepts and terms

* Risk principle
* Need principle
* Responsivity principle
* Organising principles
* Offending behaviour programmes
* Biopsychosocial
* Strength-based approach

Sample essay questions

* If a psychologist designed an intervention that adopted the principles of effective rehabilitation, what would it involve and why?
* Another professional says to you that a person should *'just stop their antisocial activity and start behaving themselves'*. Using a biopsychosocial perspective, explain why change is not always so straightforward.
* How can offending behaviour programmes help a person take responsibility for leading a crime-free life?

Recommended further reading

Walton, J. S., Ramsay, L., Cunningham, C., & Henfrey, S. (2017). New directions: Integrating a biopsychosocial approach in the design and delivery of programs for high risk services users in Her Majesty's Prison and Probation Service. *Advancing Corrections: Journal of the International Corrections and Prison Association, 3,* 21–47.

References

Andrews, D. A., & Bonta, J. (2016). *The psychology of criminal conduct* (6th ed.). Routledge.

Baer, R. (2018). Mindfulness practice. In Hayes, S. C., & Hofmann, S. G. (Eds.), *Process-based CBT: The science and core clinical competencies of cognitive behavioural therapy* (pp. 389–413). New Harbinger.

Beaver, K. M., Wright, J. P., & DeLisi, M. (2008). Delinquent peer group formation: Evidence of a gene x environment correlation. *Journal of Genetic Psychology, 169,* 227–244.

Blair, R. J. R. (2008). The amygdala and ventromedial prefrontal cortex: Functional contributions and dysfunction in psychopathy. *Philosophical Transactions of the Royal Society, 363,* 2557–2565.

Carlisi, C. O., Moffitt, T. E., Knodt, A. R., Harrington, H., Ireland, D., Melzer, T. R., Poulton, R., Ramrakha, S., Caspi, A., Hariri, A. R., & Viding. E. (2020). Associations between life-course persistent antisocial behaviour and brain structure in a population representative longitudinal birth cohort. *Lancet Psychiatry, 7,* 245–253.

Carré, J. M., & Archer, J. (2018). Testosterone and human behavior: The role of individual and contextual variables. *Current Opinion in Psychology, 19,* 149–153.

Caspi, A., McClay, J., Moffitt, T. E., Mill, J., Martin, J., Craig, I. W., Taylor, A., & Poulton, R. (2002). Role of genotype in the cycle of violence in maltreated children. *Science, 297*(5582), 851–854.

Chellew, K., Evans, P., Fornes-Vives, J., Perez, G., & Garcia-Banda, G. (2015). The effect of progressive muscle relaxation on daily cortisol secretion. *Stress, 18*(5), 538–544.

Cristea, I. A., Huibers, M. J., Davprocid, D., Hollon, S. D., Andersson, G., & Cuijpers, P. (2015). The effects of cognitive behavior therapy for adult depression on dysfunctional thinking: A meta-analysis. *Clinical Psychology Review, 42,* 62–71.

Fairchild, G., Baker, E., & Eaton, S. (2018). Hypothalamic-pituitary-adrenal axis function in children and adults with severe antisocial behavior and the impact of early adversity. *Current Psychiatry Reports, 20,* 84.

Gerritsen, R. J. S., & Band, G. P. H. (2018). Breath of life: The respiratory vagal stimulation model of contemplative activity. *Frontiers of Human of Neuroscience, 12,* 397.

Hayes-Skelton, S., & Graham, J. (2013). Decentering as a common link among mindfulness, cognitive reappraisal, and social anxiety. *Behavioural and Cognitive Psychotherapy, 41,* 317–328.

Hölzel, B. K., Lazar, S. W., Gard, T., Schuman-Olivier, Z., Vago, D. R., & Ott, U. (2011). How does mindfulness meditation work? Proposing mechanisms of action from a conceptual and neural perspective. *Perspectives on Psychological Science, 6*(6) 537–559.

Lipsey, M. W., Howell, J. C., Kelly, M. R., Chapman, G., & Carver, D. (2010). *Improving the effectiveness of juvenile justice programs: A new perspective on evidence-based practice.* Center for Juvenile Justice Reform.

Makarios, M. D., Sperber, K. G., & Latessa, E. J. (2014). Treatment dosage and the risk principle: An extension and refinement. *Journal of Offender Rehabilitation, 53*(5), 334–350.

Siegle, G. J., & Coan, J. (2018). Neuroscience relevant to core processes in psychotherapy. In Hayes, S. C., & Hofmann, S. G. (Eds.), *Process-based CBT: The science and core clinical competencies of cognitive behavioural therapy* (pp. 154–178). New Harbinger.

van Honk, J., Montoya, E., Bos, P., van Vugt, M., & Terbug, D. (2012). New evidence on testosterone and cooperation. *Nature, 485,* E4–E5.

Wakeling, H., Beech, A. R., & Freemantle, N. (2013). Investigating treatment change and its relationship to recidivism in a sample of 3773 sex offenders in the UK. *Psychology, Crime & Law, 19*(3), 233–252.

Walton, J. S., Ramsay, L., Cunningham, C., & Henfrey, S. (2017). New directions: Integrating a biopsychosocial approach in the design and delivery of programs for high risk services users in Her Majesty's Prison and Probation Service. *Advancing Corrections: Journal of the International Corrections and Prison Association, 3,* 21–47.

Yang, Y., & Raine, A. (2009). Prefrontal structural and functional brain imaging findings in antisocial, violent, and psychopathic individuals: A meta-analysis. *Psychiatry Research, 174*(2), 81–88.

7 Aggressive and violent offending

Michelle Fletcher, Allison Nelson and Polly Turner

Summary

This chapter will provide an overview of how we define aggression and violence. We will out-line psychological theories that aim to explain aggression and violence, before reviewing therapeutic approaches for working with individuals in prisons, secure forensic hospitals and community settings. The chapter will consider a range of approaches such as traditional cognitive behavioural approaches, as well as third-wave CBT approaches. It will also consider a range of interventions used within prison, secure psychiatric settings and the community.

What is aggression?

The NICE guidelines refer to aggression and violence as 'a range of behaviours or actions that can result in harm, hurt or injury to another person regardless of whether the violence or aggression is physically or verbally expressed, physical harm is sustained or the intention is clear' (NICE, 2015, p. 6). Indeed, it is the intent to harm and not the actual consequences which is argued to determine an act as aggressive (Krahé, 2013). Aggression can achieve many functions and intent to harm may only be one such goal yet it is the *intent* to harm that classifies an act as aggressive. Thus, accidental harm is not aggressive due to the lack of intent. Anderson and Bushman (2002) emphasise that accidental harm because of a helpful action is also not considered aggressive (e.g. pain experienced during a dental procedure).

Aggression is therefore any form of behaviour directed towards the goal of harming or injuring another living being who is motivated to avoid such action (Baron & Richardson, 1994; Berkowitz, 1993; Bushman & Anderson, 2001). The victim should be a living being who is motivated to avoid the harm (Gilbert & Daffern, 2010). Within forensic settings, it is recognised that psychologically harmful behaviour can sometimes be just as damaging to the victim as physically harmful behaviour and therefore behaviours resulting in intentional psychological harm are equally considered aggressive.

We should be clear here that aggression is a behaviour, not an attitude, motivation or emotion (Baron & Richardson, 1994; Novaco, 2011). Cognitions and emotions may underpin aggression but are not in themselves aggressive as they do not necessarily lead to harm. For example, anger (emotion) and hostility (cognition) may increase the likeli-hood of aggression but not in all situations and in some circumstances may actually lead to behaviour that results in positive change. Therefore, if we were to explore anger and/ or hostility to understand aggression, we may include factors not truly related to the use

DOI: 10.4324/9781003017103-10

of aggression. That is not to say that affect and cognition should be ignored, rather they should be viewed as contributing factors.

The literature makes an important distinction between aggression and violence, with the latter representing an act with the intent to inflict extreme harm or severe consequences (see Archer, 1994; Bushman & Huesmann, 2010). Violence is sometimes used to refer to both aggression and violence (McMurran & Howard, 2009). DeWall and Anderson (2011) clarify that all acts of violence are captured by the definition of aggression noted previously; however, not all acts of aggression are judged violent. But why does it matter? As forensic psychologists, we are tasked with providing effective treatment to reduce aggression. If we focus on violent behaviour (i.e. the most extreme acts), then we might miss 'low level aggression'. Goldstein (1999) argues that treatment must target all forms of aggression as lower forms can escalate if unchecked and may be underpinned by similar motivations. Therefore, treatment interventions aiming to reduce violent behaviour must also target behaviours within the aggression framework.

In addition to considering definitions of aggression and violence, it is also important that we consider categories or types of aggressive behaviour as these can often impact on understanding an individual's behaviour as well as ensuring appropriate treatment interventions to address the behaviour. The literature makes a distinction between 'Provoked' and 'Unprovoked' aggression. Provoked aggression has its roots in the frustration–aggression model which was defined by Dollard et al. (1939). This model considers aggressive behaviour that is emotionally driven and often proceeded by strong emotions. This type of aggression is often considered an impulsive act motivated as a defensive strategy. In treatment interventions, this is often referred to 'Reactive aggression' and is viewed as a behavioural strategy that occurs as a direct reaction to a situation or circumstances the individual encounters. In contrast, unprovoked aggression is considered a proactive strategy as opposed to a response. Rather than being motivated by emotion, it is often described as more predatory in and strategic in nature. In treatment, this form of aggression is referred to as 'Instrumental aggression'.

The distinction between instrumental and reactive has, however, proven harder to distinguish in practice, with professionals struggling to differentiate between the two forms (Daffern et al., 2007). Indeed, individuals often may have different motivations within one act of aggression. As a result, there is an acknowledgement of the mixed-motive aggressor (Anderson & Bushman, 2002). Chambers et al. (2008) suggested that many individuals who have committed violent acts can display both proactive and reactive forms of violence. Therefore, treatment programmes aimed at individuals assessed as high risk of committing future violence are likely to be more effective if they consider factors related to both reactive and instrumentally driven aggression.

Why are people aggressive?

Research into aggressive behaviour tells us that there is not one cause of aggression but rather it is the result of several factors interacting with each other (Gilbert & Daffern, 2010). There are a number of psychological theories of aggression that aim to explain why people might act aggressively. Let us review some of the important contributions from these approaches.

Biological theories

Evolutionary theory

Fessler (2010) argues that aggression has an evolutionary component as it can act as a motivator to challenge, prevent and deter transgressions within social networks. Evolutionary theories suggest that individuals are predisposed to violence and aggression and therefore have an innate disposition as described by the 'fight/flight/freeze' response to a perceived threat. Individuals who are at higher risk of becoming aggressive are likely to have a preference for the fight aspect of this response.

Learning theories

Social learning theory (SLT)

SLT (Bandura, 1978) is based on theories of classical and operant conditioning where violence is viewed as a learnt behaviour. 'Instrumental aggression' is positively reinforced by gains and rewards, whereas 'reactive aggression' is negatively reinforced by removing aversive experiences. Bandura developed these learning concepts suggesting that aggressive behaviour is acquired and maintained through directly experiencing or observing behaviour and its positive and negative consequences. Therefore, SLT emphasises the role of the family, peers, childhood experiences and authority figures (Ferns, 2007).

Social cognitive theories

Social cognition involves the study of the mental processes people use to make sense of their social world (Kunda, 2002). Research in this area is based on two factors; first that cognitive processes ought to be central to analyses of personality and second that cognition develops in social context, whereby people acquire thoughts about themselves and the world through social interaction (Augoustinos et al., 2006). The social cognition approach explores the interaction between motives and feelings alongside cognitive processes (Gilbert & Daffern, 2010).

Social cognitive theory of aggression

This model (Bandura, 1989) expands on SLT and proposes that individuals will not only learn behaviours that are similar to those they observe in others but also learn behaviours that are only abstractly similar, as individuals will construct an abstract cognitive representation of the style of behaviour that they observe. This cognitive information is then constructed into symbolic behavioural rules, which are encoded into memory and used to enact future behaviours. Bandura proposes that individuals make judgements about how the behavioural options open to us might meet our personal standards. Options that give us a sense of self-satisfaction and pride are more likely to be chosen over those which give us a sense of self-dissatisfaction or self-criticism. Therefore, aggression is likely to occur due to cognitive distortions linking violence to sense of self-satisfaction, for example, individuals in prison will often state that violence leads to being treated with 'respect' by others and therefore leads to self-satisfaction and further cognitive distortions regarding the value of aggression. Longer term, they might develop beliefs that violence is the best strategy for gaining social status.

Social information processing theory

This model (Crick & Dodge, 1994) describes the way in which an individual actively interprets and appraises social information to select and enact the most appropriate behavioural response. It is hypothesised that this process is comprised of a sequence of stages, social cues are encoded and interpreted, goals are selected, possible responses are then generated and evaluated and the chosen behavioural response is then enacted. It is suggested from this model that habitually aggressive people will interpret social cues as hostile more often than non-aggressive people, otherwise known as a hostile attribution bias. This is particularly the case if the social interaction is ambiguous (Anderson & Graham, 2007). Habitually, aggressive people are said to have limited response repertoires, having typically over relied on aggression to meet their needs. Thus, aggression is accessed more readily as an appropriate behavioural response and is evaluated as effective to meet their goal. Over time, this behavioural appraisal is likely to strengthen hostile attributions and schema supporting an aggressive response (i.e. offence is the best defence).

Biopsychosocial models

It is recognised in forensic psychology that there are often several factors that lead to an individual behaving aggressively and therefore models such as the **General Aggression Model** proposed by Anderson and Bushman (2002) bring together contributions of preceding models and theory into one integrated model. It is based on the principle that behaviour is the result of a complex interaction between the person and the situation. The main assumption being that each individual carries a unique set of learning experiences, biological predispositions and personality factors which shape their cognitive, affective and arousal responses to a given situation and therefore determine the individual's behaviour in response to the situation. Aggressive acts result from a convergence of individual and situational variables. Biopsychosocial models have the advantage of explaining aggression based on multiple motives and encourages a move away from looking at the nature of the aggression and more towards the underlying motivation.

Summary of psychological theories

Several psychological approaches have sought to explain why people act aggressively. Some theories focus on one particular concept that underpins aggressive behaviour such as innate drive, personality types from genetic inheritance or learned behaviour. Social cognitive theories combine social information processing, learned behaviour and the development of schemas and beliefs. Biopsychosocial models combine several factors and therefore are more useful to forensic practice in terms of assessing the risk of an individual acting aggressively and then understanding the treatment needs of individuals who commit violent acts.

ACTIVITY BOX 7.1

Psychological theories of aggression would indicate that aggressive behaviour is something all humans are motivated to enact at times. Take a moment to reflect on a time when you have acted or been motivated to act aggressively. What were the underlying emotions, cognitions and motivations for this behaviour? Consider the different psychological theories of aggression and think about how your behaviour might be understood by the theories.

Let us now explore how theory has been applied by forensic psychologists to support people reducing aggressive and violent behaviour.

Treatment for aggression and violence

As with psychological theories of aggression, there are several different approaches to the treatment of aggression utilised in forensic psychology. Treatment approaches depend on the theoretical model utilised in the design of the treatment and therefore as theoretical models have developed so has the understanding of different treatment approaches.

Group-based interventions specifically designed to address aggression

As with other areas of offending, interventions designed to address aggression and violence are based on the Risk-Need-Responsivity principles as outlined in Chapter 6. Most programmes adopt a CBT approach. Following the risk principle interventions, programmes are divided into high and moderate intensity which correspond to levels of risk as determined by both static and dynamic risk assessments, see chapter 4. Moderate-intensity interventions include programmes such as alcohol-related violence (ARV), controlling violence in angry, impulsive drinkers (COVAID) and the resolve programme.

ARV and COVAID are primarily focused on reactive aggression, where aggression is the result of poor emotional control. The aim of the intervention is to consider violence-related factors such as alcohol and aggression and the interaction between such factors with the focus primarily on reducing aggressive behaviour. Resolve is underpinned by research that suggests individuals with violent convictions often display difficulties relating to emotional management, self-control and possess attitudes supportive of violence. Therefore, sessions are divided into six modules addressing knowledge and skills to manage impulsivity, improve emotional management, challenge attitudes supporting violence and improve conflict management.

Research concerning moderate-intensity interventions indicate some positive impact of the interventions. McMurran and Cusens (2003) demonstrated the effectiveness of COVAID although there remains a need for a wider ranging evaluation study. Robinson et al. (2021) demonstrated that for general offending, individuals who took part in resolve were less likely to reoffend, reoffended less frequently and took longer to reoffend during a one- or two-year follow-up period, compared to matched comparison group. In terms of violent reoffending, although findings indicated a reduction in measures following resolve attendance, these figures were not statistically significant and therefore further research is required.

Kaizen (see Walton et al., 2017) is delivered in Her Majesty's Prison Service as a high-intensity intervention designed to meet the criminogenic needs of adult males who are high or very high risk, typically those with convictions for sexual offences, generally violent offences or intimate partner violence offences. The organising principles (see Chapter 6) are related to biological, psychological and social factors identified as related to aggression and violence. Therefore, as with integrated theories of aggression, Kaizen aims to provide an integrated model of treatment. Kaizen explores both reactive and instrumentally motivated forms of aggression. It is focused on several treatment targets such as building positive relationships, developing skills to manage life problems, creating a sense of purpose and addressing attitudes that promote or condone violence. This programme was introduced in 2017, and thus, research examining the outcomes from this programme is underway. Watch this space!

Life minus violence – enhanced (LMV-E) is a high-intensity programme delivered in secure psychiatric services. It consists of seven modules that cover motivation to change, early influences, emotional management, interpersonal skills, offence/behaviour analysis, consequences and relapse prevention. Each module aims to address the elements identified to facilitate aggression in the aforementioned psychological theories and models (e.g. biological, learning, social cognition and biopsychosocial theories). Daffern et al. (2018) demonstrated that, when compared to a wait list control group, individuals who had completed LMV-E showed reduced risk levels and aggressive behaviour. Yet positive changes were also noted in the comparison group. The treatment group showed statistically significant improvements only in relation to sensitivity to provocation, social problem solving and anger regulation. This highlights the additional influence of the therapeutic milieu in secure services.

Although there are some limitations regarding research into group programmes, there is evidence to indicate that interventions which target emotional management, attitudes supporting violent behaviour, develop interpersonal and conflict resolution skills are effective in reducing future violent and offending behaviour. However, more research into this area is required.

General therapeutic approaches to reduce aggression

In addition to the treatment programmes outlined previously which are specifically designed to address violence and aggression, general therapeutic models can assist in the management of aggression. In secure psychiatric settings, there are a range of therapeutic approaches designed primarily to address personality traits or mental health conditions that also target criminogenic needs relating to aggressive behaviour; these include dialectical behaviour therapy (Linehan, 1993) and schema-focused therapy (Young et al., 2003). Both therapies would view aggression as a maladaptive strategy to meet core human needs. Both view strategies such as aggression as stemming from early experiences and beliefs arising to make sense of these experiences. Whilst there are subtle differences between the mechanisms judged to be most important, both therapies utilise various cognitive, behavioural and psychoanalytic techniques to assist the person to understand the origins of unhelpful strategies in order to develop alternative ways to meet their needs.

More recent research has begun to explore the impact of third-wave CBT therapeutic approaches which build on traditional CBT by having a primary focus on compassion and acceptance as a way of developing understanding and flexibility of thinking. In third-wave approaches, behaviour is viewed in context, and thoughts are considered a form of behaviour and therefore amenable to change. Behaviour, thoughts and feelings coexist rather than having the causal relationship assumed in second-wave CBT. Therefore, the treatment focus is to change the context and relationship between thoughts, feelings and behaviour not to change the thoughts themselves. Third-wave approaches include Compassion Focused Therapy (CFT; Gilbert, 2009) and Acceptance and Commitment Therapy (ACT; Hayes, 2009). Both are being effectively applied within offending behaviour treatment. Although new emerging research indicates some positive aspects to third-wave approaches, they have been applied within criminal justice settings relatively recently and therefore further research is required in this area. Watch this space here too!

ACTIVITY BOX 7.2

Now you have read about the different treatment approaches, return to your aggressive example. Think about what skills or areas addressed in the treatment programmes and consider which approach might have been most useful for you.

Let us now look at how the theory and therapeutic approaches might be applied in real-life practice.

Case study

Daryl grew up in a large family and was one of four brothers. His parents worked but struggled to provide for their family and there were times when Daryl and his siblings were left unsupervised. He was never a victim of violence from his parents but witnessed his parents arguing and his father drinking heavily. Daryl described a chaotic childhood and that he would physically fight with his brothers when they argued.

Daryl struggled to concentrate at school, he found the lessons boring and would get into trouble for not paying attention. In secondary school, he found the work difficult and so interrupted sessions and set off fire alarms. He was suspended for fighting with other pupils. He described this as occurring when he felt embarrassed or disrespected, aiming to send a message that he couldn't be picked on and, thus, people would stay away from him. He was proud of his reputation for being able to fight viewing this as living up to his family's reputation.

Daryl begun to spend time with his older brother's friends and truant from school resulting in expulsion at 15 years old without qualifications. He spent more time with his friends, feeling accepted and protected by them and enjoyed spending time with them. Daryl would drink and take drugs and not think about the consequences of his behaviour. He began to work on a building site and would drink throughout the week and would often drink, take drugs and stay up all weekend attending parties. Daryl found it hard to maintain his employment due to his impulsive behaviour and substance use.

In order to fund his lifestyle, Daryl began to commit robberies with his friends and began to carry a knife in order to threaten victims and coerce them into giving him what he wanted quicker, without the use of physical violence. On the day of the index offence, Daryl had been using substances when he got into an argument with someone and stabbed him.

ACTIVITY BOX 7.3

Before moving on, review Daryl's case study and identify factors that may be relevant to assessment and intervention in his case.

Assessment and intervention

Daryl was assessed for the risk of future violent offending using a structured professional judgement approach which identified he was a high risk of future violence. The risk formulation identified intervention needs relating to impulsiveness, substance misuse, negative peer associations, financial difficulties and attitudes and beliefs that led to the use of aggression to resolve conflict, or to get what he wanted. He did have a good relationship with his mother who he spoke to regularly and she visited him once a month. He had also been attending education to achieve his Level 2 in English and Maths. Daryl had expressed an interest completing a building course and applying for a certificate that would allow him to work on building sites in the future but was not able to do this until nearer his release.

Daryl was referred to the programmes team where he took part in a programme need assessment, and he was found suitable for the Kaizen programme. The Kaizen team developed an individual treatment plan where exercises were planned to address areas highlighted by the assessment which included managing life's problems, positive relationships and healthy thinking.

Daryl attended the programme three times a week for six months. During his sessions, he was introduced to the skill of self-monitoring, which enabled him to identify his triggers, thoughts and behaviour when he was tempted to, or did use aggression or violence. Daryl was able to complete the self-monitoring diaries and would often bring them to session to reflect with the group on times he was tempted to use aggression and/or violence with staff and other residents and how he responded.

Daryl participated well in group sessions exploring his internal behaviour (thoughts, feelings and personal rules) that led to the use of aggression and/or violence in the past. At times, he would get bored with the session and frustrated with other group members, which would result in him acting impulsively and on occasion walking out of group. However, these were useful opportunities to reflect on how emotions and impulsivity could cloud his choices. He engaged in supported learning sessions to think about his behaviour and his application of skills. He stated that he wanted to make changes and not come back to prison, so he needed to know where he had gone wrong and what he needed to do instead.

During the programme, Daryl reviewed his self-monitoring and past use of violence to see if there were any patterns or themes in his behaviour that he could address through the programme. Individual exercises were then introduced which included emotion management, mindfulness, problem-solving, conflict resolution and assertive communication. He then created relapse preventions plans to manage situations that might trigger the use of aggression and/or violence in the future such as being embarrassed in front of his peer group, or in response to a perceived threat.

An important part of the intervention includes the participant learning skills and practicing them to increase their self-efficacy, so they choose to use the skills in the future. Daryl was given the opportunity practice the skills through role play and to receive feedback on his ability to apply the skills.

Once Daryl had finished the main phase the programme his prison offender manager met with him monthly to complete 'New Me MOT'. In these sessions, self-monitoring was reviewed and they discussed how he was applying the skills from the programme. These discussions helped to develop robust release plans and at his parole hearing the year after he graduated from the programme, it was recommended that he progress to open conditions.

Concluding comments

Violence continues to be a concern for society and particularly for those who manage individuals in forensic, secure and community settings. Research informs theories and interventions in order to develop the most effective and efficient way of managing the risk of future violence. Yet as with all our work, we must remain committed to continued research examining the effectiveness of interventions. We need to ensure we are always evaluating the best methods of engaging, supporting and developing individuals to identify alternative thoughts feelings and behaviours that lead them away from using aggression and violence.

Learning outcomes

When you have completed this chapter, you should be able to:

1   Outline theories that aim to explain the use of aggression and violence
2   Outline how theories have influenced interventions to address aggression and violence

Key concepts and terms

- Aggression
- Violence
- Reactive aggression
- Instrumental aggression
- Motivation or function
- Learning theory
- Social cognitive theory
- Biopsychosocial theory

Sample essay questions

- How has psychology influenced the development of interventions designed to address attitudes that support aggression and violence?
- Is it an individual's genetic makeup (nature) that leads to the use of aggression and violence or is it the environment in which they are raised (nurture) that determines behaviour?

Recommended further reading

Anderson, C., & Bushman, B. (2002). Human aggression. *Annual Review of Psychology*, *53*, 27–51.
Ireland, J., & Ireland, C. (2019). Therapeutic treatment approaches for violence: Some essential components. In J. Ireland, C. Ireland, & P. Birch (Eds.), *Violent and sexual offenders : Assessment, treatment, and management* (2nd ed., pp. 319–341). Routledge Taylor & Francis Group.

References

Anderson, C., & Bushman, B. (2002). Human aggression. *Annual Review of Psychology*, *53*, 27–51.
Anderson, K. B., & Graham, L. M. (2007). Hostile attribution bias. In R. Baumeister & K. Vohs (Eds.), *Encyclopaedia of social psychology* (pp. 446–448). SAGE Publications.
Archer, J. (1994). *Male violence*. Routledge.
Augoustinos, M., Walker, I., & Donaghue, N. (2006). *Social cognition: An integrated introduction* (2nd ed.). Sage.
Bandura, A. (1978). Social learning theory of aggression. *Journal of Communication*, *28*(3), 12–29.
Bandura, A. (1989). Social cognitive theory. In R. Vasta (Ed.), *Annals of child development: Six theories of child development* (Vol. 6, pp. 1–60). JAI Press.
Baron, R. A., & Richardson, D. R. (1994). *Human aggression*. Plenum Press.
Berkowitz, L. (1993). *Aggression: Its causes, consequences and control*. Temple University Press.
Bushman, B., & Anderson, C. (2001). Is it time to pull the plug on the hostile versus instrumental aggression dichotomy? *Psychological Review*, *108*, 273–279.
Bushman, B. J., & Huesmann, R. (2010). Aggression. In S. T. Fiske, D. L. Gilbert, & G. Lindzey (Eds.), *Handbook of Social Psychology* (5th ed., pp. 833–863). Wiley.
Chambers, J. C., Eccleston, L., Day, A., Ward, T., & Howells, K. (2008). Treatment readiness in violent offenders: The influence of cognitive factors on engagement in violence programs. *Aggression and Violent Behavior*, *13*(4), 276–284.
Crick, N., & Dodge, K. (1994). A review and reformulation of social information processing mechanisms in children's social adjustment. *Psychological Bulletin*, *115*, 74–101.
Daffern, M., Howells, K., & Ogloff, J. (2007). What's the point? Towards a methodology for assessing the function of psychiatric inpatient aggression. *Behaviour Research and Therapy*, *45*, 101–111.
Daffern, M., Simpson, K., Ainslie, H., & Chu, S. (2018). The impact of an intensive inpatient violent offender treatment programme on intermediary treatment targets, violence risk and aggressive behaviour in a sample of mentally disordered offenders, *The Journal of Forensic Psychiatry & Psychology*, *29*(2), 163–188.
DeWall, C. N., & Anderson, C. A. (2011). The general aggression model. In P. R. Shaver & M. Mikulincer (Eds.), *Herzilya series on personality and social psychology: Human aggression and violence: Causes, manifestations, and consequences* (pp. 15–33). American Psychological Association.
Dollard, J., Miller, N. E., Doob, L. W., Mowrer, O. H., & Sears, R. R. (1939). *Frustration and aggression*. Yale University Press.
Ferns, T. (2007). Factors that influence aggressive behaviour in acute care settings. *Nursing Standard*, *21*(33), 41–45.
Fessler, D. M. T. (2010). Madmen: An evolutionary perspective on anger and men's violent responses to transgression. In M. Potegal, G. Stemmler, & C. Spielberger (Eds.), *International handbook of anger: Constituent and concomitant biological, psychological, and social processes* (pp. 361–381). Springer Science + Business Media.
Gilbert, F., & Daffern, M. (2010). Integrating contemporary aggression theory with violent offender treatment: How thoroughly do interventions target violent behaviour? *Aggression and Violent Behavior*, *15*, 167–180.
Gilbert, P. (2009). *The compassionate mind*. Robinson.
Goldstein, A. P. (1999). Aggression reduction strategies: Effective and ineffective. *School Psychology Quarterly*, *14*(1), 40–58.

Hayes, S. C. (2004). Acceptance and commitment therapy and the new behavior therapies: Mindfulness, acceptance, and relationship. In S. C. Hayes, V. M. Follette, & M. M. Linehan (Eds.), *Mindfulness and acceptance: Expanding the cognitive-behavioral tradition* (pp. 1–29). Guilford Press.

Krahé, B. (2013). *The social psychology of aggression* (2nd ed.). Psychology Press.

Kunda, Z. (2002). *Social cognition: Making sense of people* (5th ed.). MIT Press.

Linehan, M. M. (1993). *Cognitive behavioral treatment of borderline personality disorder.* Guilford Press.

McMurran, M., & Cusens, B. (2003). Controlling alcohol-related violence: A treatment programme. *Criminal Behaviour and Mental Health, 13,* 59–76.

McMurran, M., & Howard, R. C. (Eds.). (2009). *Personality, personality disorder and violence.* Wiley.

NICE. (2015). Violence and aggression. Short-term management in mental health, health and community settings. *NICE.* Retrieved from https://www.nice.org.uk/guidance/ng10/ifp/chapter/About-this-information

Novaco, R. W. (2011). Anger dysregulation: Driver of violent offending. *The Journal of Forensic Psychiatry and Psychology, 22,* 650–668.

Robinson, C., Sorbie, A., Huber, J., Teasdale, J., Scott, K., Purver, M., & Elliott, I. (2021). Reoffending impact evaluation of the prison based RESOLVE Offending Behaviour Programme. *Ministry of Justice.* Retrieved from https://assets.publishing.service.gov.uk/government/uploads/system/uploads/attachment_data/file/957855/RESOLVE_report.pdf

Walton, J. S., Ramsay, L., Cunningham, C., & Henfrey, S. (2017). New directions: Integrating a biopsychosocial approach in the design and delivery of programs for high risk services users in Her Majesty's Prison and Probation Service. *Advancing Corrections: Journal of the International Corrections and Prison Association, 3,* 21–47.

Young, J., Klosko, J., & Weishaar, M. (2003). *Schema therapy: A practitioner's guide.* The Guilford Press.

8 Sexual offending

Neil Gredecki and Kerensa Hocken

Summary

Sexual offending often brings about strong emotional reactions amongst the public as well as clinicians working in forensic settings. Many people ask 'how could they do that?' and attach labels such as 'monster' and 'pervert' when referring to those with a conviction for sexual offending. People can struggle to comprehend both how and why individuals may commit a sexual offence; this can be the case for those who commit the offences too as they struggle to make sense of their behaviour. There a number of assumptions about sexual offending not supported by the statistics and research. For example, the public are more likely to be at risk of being a victim of a violent or general offence (e.g. burglary) than they are of being a victim of a sexual offence, and rates of recidivism are lower than other serious offence types. The stigma and assumptions attached to sexual offending can also be a barrier to addressing offending and reintegrating back into the community for those with convictions for sexual offences. However, this is not to undermine the seriousness of sexual offending. The harm caused clearly warrants the need for evidence-based assessments and interventions. Forensic psychologists play an important role in conducting assessments and providing effective interventions to this client group. This chapter will outline the processes of assessment and intervention with men convicted of sexual offences (MCOSOs) and the importance of conducting these with a focus on the evidence base. It will tackle some of the myths associated with sexual offending behaviour and risks.

Men convicted of sexual offences

This chapter will focus on male clients. It is true that men, women and young people engage in sexual offending or sexually harmful behaviour. However, the reason for focusing on men is that the evidence base for sexual offending assessment and intervention is much more developed for men. You may have also noticed at this point that we use the term *'men convicted of sexual offences'* rather than *'sexual offender'*. As clinicians, we are very mindful of the language and terminology we use as this can have implications for our clients and our work (see Focus Box 8.1).

BOX 8.1 TERMINOLOGY

Social psychology has long shown us that our view of self is shaped by our perceptions of how others views us (referred to as The Looking-Glass Self: Cooley, 1902). One key way we infer what others think of us is through their use of language about

---

DOI: 10.4324/9781003017103-11

us. If we experience people describing us in critical ways, such as 'incompetent' or 'failure', this will likely influence our view of self to incorporate these features and create an inner self-critic. If someone describes us as 'successful' and 'intelligent', we are more likely to have confidence in ourselves. This is why we want to gravitate towards people who make us feel good about ourselves. The way we talk about, and describe, MCOSOs is equally important and influential on their self-identity. If they are perpetually described by the worst thing they have ever done, for example, 'offender', 'sex offender' and 'ex-offender', then the offending identity becomes part of how they see themselves. Research on desistance tells us that having a non-offending identity is important in desisting from offending. Therefore, we need to be aware of the language we use to ensure it is not labelling.

Assessing men convicted of sexual offences

It is important that as forensic psychologists we undertake evidence-based assessments as these assessments inform decisions about the management of clients as well as the interventions they can access. Whilst there are ongoing debates in both forensic psychology and psychiatry about the most effective ways of assessing the risk of future sexual offending (e.g. see Boer & Hart, 2012; Hanson, 2014), what is important is that we undertake thorough assessments based on the research evidence. If we overestimate risk, then individuals could be held in secure conditions for longer than required to manage their risk. Conversely, should we underestimate risk, this can result in clients being released too early with implications for public safety. We therefore have a moral and ethical obligation to provide thorough assessments of risk and need for intervention. But what do we mean by risk assessment in the context of sexual offending?

The concept of risk assessments is discussed in detail in Chapter 4. In relation to MCOSOs, we are referring to an assessment of the likelihood that the individual will engage in sexual offending behaviour in the future. These assessments are also helpful in determining outstanding treatment needs linked to the risk factors in the case. Thus, the assessments assist with the planning of psychological interventions to address individual risk factors linked to risk. We shall now consider risk factors that have been empirically linked to sexual offending risk before considering various approaches to risk assessment.

ACTIVITY BOX 8.2

Before reading this section, write a list of what you think are risk factors for sexual offending. Having read this chapter, review your list and consider how and where you developed these beliefs around risk and the impact of this on how you see MCOSOs.

Risk factors for men convicted of sexual offences

A number of recidivism studies have assisted us in understanding the risk factors of MCOSOs. Figure 8.1 draws on the work of Hanson and Bussière (1998) and Mann et al. (2010), bringing together an overview of risk factors predictive of sexual offending. These risk factors fall into six broad domains.

BOX 8.3 RISK FACTORS

Forensic psychologists often use the term 'Risk Factor'. Here, we are referring to the factors linked to a particular problematic behaviour such as sexual offending. Risk factors can be static (i.e. something that cannot change such as the number of past offences), whilst others are dynamic and can be targeted through intervention (e.g. increasing skills in social intimacy). It is important to ensure that the factors we focus on are generated from the evidence base and large-scale studies rather than what clinicians *feel* are relevant. If we do not focus on risk factors linked to the evidence base then it is likely that our assessments will focus on incorrect or irrelevant factors which can undermine the assessment.

The first two domains are linked specifically to sexual offending history and sexual interests. First, a client's history of committing sexual offences is linked to risk. This is not only about the number of previous convictions but also the types of sexual offences they have committed. For example, whether they have committed offences against diverse groups including other males, as well as committing non-contact offences (e.g. indecent exposure). The second domain is linked to sexual deviance, namely a sexual interest in an area which if acted upon would cause harm. This would include an individual having a sexual preference for children rather than adults or an arousal to rape and sexual violence over consenting sex. Attitudes that support such sexual behaviours are linked to risk, as is sexual preoccupation where individuals think about sex a lot and oversexualise non-sexual matters. Despite common beliefs, not all men who commit sexual offences against children or who engage in rape necessarily have a sexual preference in these areas. The next two domains are linked to general lifestyle instability and criminality, followed by social problems and intimacy deficits. The latter are often important considerations in the MCOSO population.

The penultimate set of risk factors is linked to a client's engagement with professionals. Where clients drop out of interventions or do not comply with the requirements of their prison sentence, probation or license conditions in the community, this is likely to be an indicator of increased risk. Having poor cognitive problem-solving skills and being young are also risk factors.

You may notice from Figure 8.1 that there are factors missing that seem intuitively to be risk factors for sexual offending (e.g. denial and poor victim empathy). For many years, practitioners thought such areas were relevant to sexual offending and they have historically formed the basis of assessments of risk and interventions for MCOSOs. Subsequent research has shown there is little or no relationship between such factors and a risk of sexual recidivism (see Mann et al., 2010). This highlights the importance of always being up to date with the latest research and the evolving nature of the field in order to ensure our practice is evidence based.

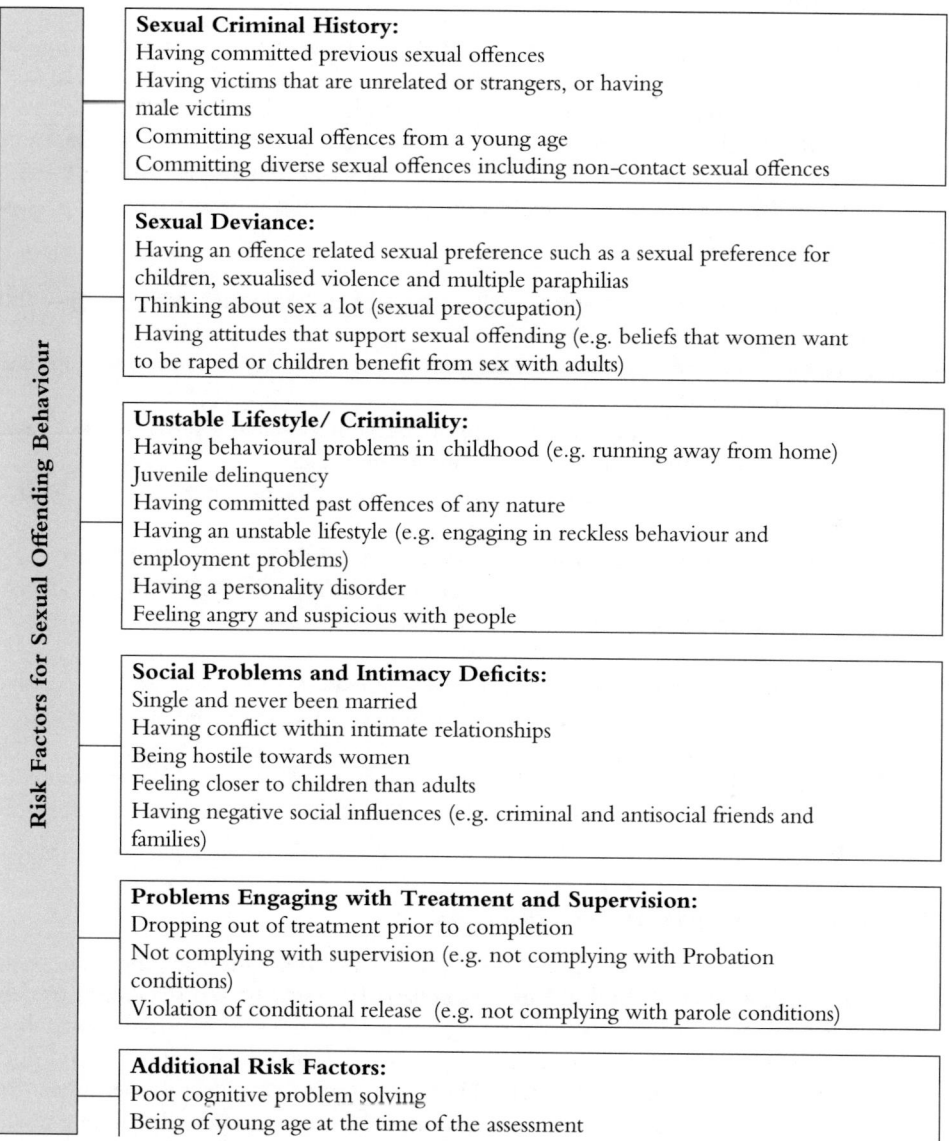

Figure 8.1 Risk factors for sexual recidivism

Some of the risk factors outlined previously are static in nature and the client is unable to change these (e.g. past convictions and employment history). However, there are a number of dynamic risk factors that we, as forensic psychologists, are interested in when we are considering interventions and opportunities for risk reduction. For example, we can work with clients to address their relationship skills, sexual interests, attitudes around employment and their social networks to build in protective factors to help manage risk factors as outlined in the description of self-management strategies in Chapter 6. These dynamic risk factors are the focus of our interventions.

Protective factors

As outlined in Chapter 4, it is fundamental that we consider protective factors in our assessments. Given that the study of protective factors for sexual offending is relatively new, there is not a robust evidence base compared to that of risk factors, and any protective factors identified in the literature must be considered provisional. Perhaps, the most comprehensive account of the protective factors for sexual offending is that by de Vries Robbé et al. (2015). They propose eight domains that could promote desistance from sexual offending. These are:

- Healthy sexual interests – being sexually interested in consenting relationships with adults
- Capacity for emotional intimacy – being able to establish and maintain close intimate relationships with others
- Constructive social and professional support networks – having prosocial peers and being able to work in productive ways with professionals
- Goal-directed living – being able to set and work towards goals in order to live purposefully
- Good problem-solving – the ability to manage life's daily problems prosocially
- Busy with employment or constructive leisure activities – having rewarding, satisfying and constructive activities
- Sobriety – the absence of substance abuse
- Hopeful, optimistic and motivated attitude to desistance – the ability to find positive outcome from life's challenges and being willing to develop oneself.

de Vries Robbé et al. (2015) suggest that any assessment of risk should incorporate an assessment of protective factors, and interventions should aim to build capacities for protective factors.

Approaches to assessing the risk of sexual offending

Recapping on Chapter 4, we know that forensic psychologists can draw on three approaches: unstructured clinical judgement, actuarial assessment and structured professional judgement (SPJ). Unstructured clinical judgement is the least favoured approach as it relies on decision-making that is unguided by tests or professional guidelines and does not provide an evidence-based approach. There are a range of actuarial assessments for use with MCOSOs, yet they differ significantly in their predictive accuracy (Craig et al., 2008). They also offer little in terms of formulation and an understanding of what takes an individual closer towards an offence. SPJ is often the preferred approach. Here, the forensic psychologist uses their knowledge of the client to assess the presence and relevance of evidence-based risk factors; this in turn allows them to formulate the case and to make an assessment and inform intervention. Specific tools used with MCOSOs include the Sexual Violence Risk-20 (SVR-20; Boer et al., 1997), the Risk for Sexual Violence Protocol (RSVP; Hart et al., 2003) and the ARMIDILO-S (Assessment of Risk and Manageability of Intellectually Disabled Individuals who Offend – Sexually: Boer et al., 2004).

Practical considerations for assessments

As we noted in the introduction, many MCOSOs experience feelings of shame and guilt regarding their offending and their own experiences of trauma, and many clients have difficulty articulating how they came to be in the position that they offended. As such, it is necessary to remember the importance of planning our clinical interviews as outlined in Chapter 3. This is particularly important when working with MCOSOs where we must be sensitive to likely levels of shame and guilt when undertaking an assessment. An assessment is the interaction between the client and the assessor, and it is important to develop this relationship in order to understand risk and to help focus the individual needs in relation to intervention and management.

We have offered a broad overview of approaches to assessment with MCOSOs here, and there will be many individual responsivity factors that should be considered when undertaking assessments. Further, there will be individual client and offence characteristics which should be considered. Refer to Gredecki and Hocken (2018) for a fuller discussion of specialist populations and the various approaches to assessment when working with MCOSOs.

Interventions for men convicted of sexual offences

The previous section has outlined the risk factors that predict sexual offending as well as a number of protective factors that may help to reduce offending. Assessing the presence, persistence and severity of these is essential to making judgements about the risk of reoffending and informing risk management plans. Once risk and protective factors are known, it becomes possible to set about finding ways to minimise the risk factors and strengthen the protective factors. This is what offending behaviour interventions aim to do. Interventions for offending are described by different labels, such as 'treatment' or 'programme', but they are referring to the same process; intervening via psychological means to reduce the likelihood of reoffending.

The most popular therapeutic approach used in interventions to reduce sexual offending has been cognitive behaviour therapy (CBT) (see Schaffer et al., 2010). CBT is based on two schools of psychology: behaviourism and cognitive psychology. The basic assumption of CBT is that human distress and problematic behaviours are caused by errors in thinking and problems in managing feelings and behaviour. The therapeutic aim is symptom reduction, primarily via reducing thinking errors and increasing emotional regulation which should lead to improvements in thinking and behaviour. This can take the form of helping participants to restructure their faulty beliefs (e.g. beliefs about sex with children), improve self-monitoring, teach skills for healthy relationships, improve problem-solving abilities and develop healthy alternative behaviour patterns. More recently, interventions for sexual offending have begun to expand the approaches they use to include techniques like mindfulness. This can help participants become more aware of their thoughts and feelings (to improve self-monitoring) and to accept but not act on these (Walton, in press). Research is divided about the extent to which sexual interests can be changed, but a developing consensus is that for those who have a lifelong interest in children and no interest in adults, change may be unlikely (Cantor, 2018); therefore, acceptance methods might be the best approach. An important element of all interventions is that skills are practiced so they become more automatic. This happens both in the therapy session and also in their daily life so the skills are generalised beyond intervention.

Adopting a theoretical basis for interventions

An important aspect of any intervention is to have a theoretical basis from which to base decisions about the intervention such as how long it should be, who should have access to it, what it should target and what format it should take. Models applied to interventions include the risk-need-responsivity (RNR) framework (Andrews & Bonta, 1998) and the Good Lives Model (GLM: Ward, 2002).

The RNR model is the ubiquitous theoretical basis for interventions for offending. The RNR framework (see Chapter 6) sets out guiding principles that, if followed, should lead to the most successful interventions. In the framework, the risk principle refers to the expectation that most effective interventions will target those who are at higher risk. This expectation has reasonable support, since the empirical consensus is that interventions for lower risk individuals are not effective at risk reduction and in some cases may have the opposite effect and increase risk (see Wakeling et al., 2012). The need principle specifies that interventions must target the factors that research has established are the causes of sexual offending (i.e. risk factors). Finally, the responsivity principle sets out that success-ful interventions will have the flexibility to adapt to, and respond to, the individual needs of the participants, in order to make the intervention relevant and accessible to all. The RNR framework has empirical support as interventions adhering to two or more prin-ciples have better outcomes for reducing reoffending (Hanson et al., 2009).

The RNR model is not free from limitations, a prominent one being that it exclusively focuses on reducing risk (symptom reduction), and in doing so excludes attention to participant-specific factors, and in particular, the life experiences that have given rise to the development of the risk factor. Similarly, it does not aim to increase strengths (pro-tective factors) and has been criticised for lacking humanity for its conceptualisation of behaviour as criminogenic rather than being understood as an (understandable) outcome from adverse experiences (Taylor et al., 2020).

The Good Lives Model is a more recent framework to base interventions upon which addresses some of the concerns of the RNR model. Here, the fundamental conceptuali-sation of offending is rooted in understanding all behaviour as being motivated to achieve basic human needs. Therefore, it is not the aim of the behaviour that is unwanted but the means of achieving it. For example, a man engages in an offence of rape because he wants sexual satisfaction and because he wants to feel intimacy. Sexual satisfaction and intimacy are basic human needs, and we are designed to seek them out (Popovic, 2005). Therefore, within the GLM, change can come about by helping individuals to meet their needs in safe ways. This proposal can feel counterproductive because there is a ten-dency to pathologise natural human behaviour when it is observed amongst MCOSOs, for example, seeing the pursuit of sexual satisfaction and intimacy as inherently wrong. Subsequently, the inclination is to want to change or eradicate the desire for those needs (see Focus Box 8.4).

BOX 8.4   PATHOLOGISING OFFENDING

Pathology means the science of disease, so when we use the term 'pathological', we are suggesting that it is caused by disease, so to 'pathologise' someone or some-thing, we are inferring that it is abnormal or 'diseased'. Humans have a tendency to pathologise everyday behaviours when they are viewed in a different context. For example, Rosenhan (1973) demonstrated that keeping a diary as a patient in a psychiatric hospital was described as 'writing behaviour'. In this way, pathologising a behaviour dehumanises, inferring it as abnormal. We see the same phenomenon in forensic psychology, whereby everyday behaviours demonstrated by people who offend can be construed as 'deviant', and this is especially true for people who commit sexual offences. For example, any kind of sexual behaviour and thinking can be construed as wrong or risky. Similarly, the term 'treatment' suggests a problem that needs to be cured. As practitioners, it is important that we are aware of our own human tendency to pathologise and take steps to minimise this.

Ultimately, adopting an integrated approach is favoured in the design of interventions for MCOSOs. Although seemingly diametrically opposed, RNR and GLM are used together in interventions that follow both frameworks (Willis et al., 2013). Carter and Mann (2016) argue that neither should be seen as a substitute for the other and should be used in conjunction. Consequently, most of the interventions for sexual offending that have been in operation since 2000 have drawn on both these models.

A model of delivery for interventions

In an effort to define a novel way forward to design effective interventions, Carter and Mann (2016) offer a two-part model for intervention. The first part is a biopsychosocial (BPS) explanation for the dynamic risk factors for sexual offending. The detail of this is discussed in Chapter 6 of this book. The second aspect sets out six broad principles that they argue should organise interventions for sexual offending. These principles bring together but expand the features of the RNR and GLM models based on empirical evidence about what seems to work to reduce sexual offending. They are:

- Principle 1: Interventions should be designed and delivered in a way that is proportionate to the risk of each participant.
- Principle 2: Interventions will be delivered in a way that makes it accessible and appealing to participants whatever their biological, psychological and social circumstances.
- Principle 3: In addressing criminogenic need, interventions will strengthen biological resources such as neurocognitive functioning.
- Principle 4: In addressing criminogenic need, interventions will strengthen psychological resources, such as cognitive and emotional flexibility and empathic relating.
- Principle 5: Interventions will strengthen social resources such as social capital.
- Principle 6: Interventions will strengthen the intention to desist from offending.

The first two of these principles have clear overlaps with the RNR principles of risk and responsivity. Principles 3, 4 and 5 link to the Need principle of RNR in that interventions should not only address criminogenic need and reduce risk, but they should also strengthen biological, psychological and social resources. The final principle highlights the need to address protective factors. These principles have been adopted by Her Majesty's Prison and Probation Service (HMPPS) in the design of their new suite of interventions for those considered high risk of reoffending (Walton et al., 2017). These interventions recognise the BPS explanation for dynamic risk factors and in particular, that adverse life events (e.g. trauma) can lead to biological vulnerability to offending by, for example, reduced frontal lobe and attentional functions. We draw attention to this here because it is a relatively novel acknowledgment in intervention design. The HMPPS interventions use concepts and exercises that target the biological, psychological and social features of dynamic risk factors and aim to build strengths in each. These interventions have been gradually implemented since 2017. Consequently, it is too early to judge their effectiveness since participants need to be followed up for ideally eight to ten years after intervention to robustly measure reoffending trends.

The effectiveness of interventions with MCOSOs

A critical aspect of intervention science is to know whether the intervention yields the intended outcomes, and in sexual offending interventions, that is held as a reduction in sexual reoffending as measured by reconviction data.

There are a few key studies that bring together data from lots of smaller studies to pool together the results. As discussed in Chapter 2, this is called a meta-analysis and is the gold standard methodology for establishing intervention effectiveness, within social sciences and the medical field (Hariton & Locascio, 2018; The Campbell Collaboration). Overall, these studies show a small positive effect for interventions to reduce sexual reoffending (Schmucker & Lösel, 2017; Gannon et al., 2019). However, this is not a universal finding as some studies within these meta-analyses show a *higher* level of reconviction in the intervention samples (e.g. Mews et al., 2017). This led Carter and Mann (2016) to conclude that intervention effectiveness to reduce sexual reoffending remains controversial. In light of the varied findings, it is important to establish the commonalities amongst those interventions that do best, so they can be replicated. Schmucker and Lösel (2017) and Gannon et al. (2019) are the most recent two meta-analyses to look to here. They conclude that interventions that use CBT, are led by a psychologists and delivered in a group-based format but have individualised intervention targets for participants, are the features of the most effective interventions.

Let's think about how what we have outlined in this chapter might apply in practice.

Case study

Lester's dad was in the army, and they moved around a lot. He was bullied throughout school and found it hard to make friends. As a teenager, he wanted a girlfriend but was not confident to approach females. At 21, he indecently exposed himself to a woman in a pub hoping that she would be interested in him. He later commenced a stable relationship lasting several years, but the relationship ended when she had an affair. Lester had a successful career as a tree surgeon and several hobbies. In his mid-30s, he injured himself through an accident at work and following a period of time off work was made redundant. He described feeling 'useless'. Unable to afford to live alone, he moved in with his sister and niece. His offending occurred against his niece between the ages of 10 and 14 and would occur in her bedroom. The offences started with Lester touching his niece over her clothes progressing to penetration when she was aged twelve.

Assessing Lester

Lester found it hard to talk about his conviction, and it was clear that he experienced shame and guilt around his offending and as such, building a relationship with him was an important consideration when planning and conducting the interview. Based on the assessment, his offending occurred against a backdrop of poor coping linked to his belief that he was useless having lost his job. He would use alcohol to cope with the distress caused by his feelings. He felt emotionally lonely having few friends and no intimate relationship. He self-soothed by masturbating five or six times per week following his relationship ending. He described feeling anxious at the thought of having another relationship due to fear they would cheat on him. He found it easier to relate to his niece and began to confuse their closeness with sexual intimacy.

ACTIVITY BOX 8.5

What thoughts and feelings arise for you when reading this offence account? What is it about your values that lead to this response and what may you need to be mindful of if assessing or working therapeutically with this client group?

Lester's risk factors were poor problem-solving, lack of intimate relationships, sexual preoccupation and possible emotional congruence with his niece. His protective factors were he has capacity for healthy relationships and healthy sexual interests, as well as being busy with employment and hobbies.

Intervention plan

Lester's intervention aimed to reduce the severity of his risk factors and strengthen his protective factors. Given the presence of shame, it should be delivered in a supportive and empathic way, encouraging rather than challenging. An important aim is for Lester to recognise the risk and protective factors identified previously and how they operated in his life. It will not be necessary for Lester to give an account of his offending to do this, and it can be achieved by Lester doing a life history review to spot where the risk factors started to emerge and his protective factors weakened. He will need to develop skills for managing problems to help him cope with difficult life events as well as his own feelings, reducing the need for alcohol and masturbation. Lester will be supported to address his fear about relationships and teach him skills for achieving and maintaining these. This will also help him understand how he came to sexualise his relationship with his niece so that he can learn appropriate boundaries.

Conclusion

We have outlined current approaches to assessment and interventions with MCOSOs. What we have seen is that practice has changed over time and what we once thought were important factors for this population do not have a persuasive evidence base for their inclusion in assessment and intervention. It is always necessary for forensic psychologists to look towards emerging evidence that is starting to influence practice in the field. Our challenge to you is to seek out this evidence giving further consideration as to understanding the circumstances that give rise to the development of risk factors (e.g. Adverse Childhood Events).

Learning outcomes

When you have completed this chapter, you should be able to:

1   Outline the evidence-based risk factors for sexual offending
2   Outline different approaches to undertaking assessments with MCOSOs
3   Outline the aims and methods of interventions to reduce sexual offending
4   Challenge myths around the functions of sexual offences

Key concepts and terms

- Sexual offending
- Static risk factors
- Dynamic risk factors
- Protective factors
- Offending behaviour interventions
- Risk assessment
- Men convicted of sexual offending (MCOSOs)

Sample essay questions

- Men who commit offences against children prefer sex with children than sex with adults. Discuss this in relation to the evidence around sexual offending risk factors.
- Interventions for sexual offending are effective at reducing sexual offending behaviour. Discuss.

Recommended further reading

Gredecki, N., & Hocken, K. (2018). Thinking outside of the box: The assessment of sexual offending recidivism and specialist populations. In J. L. Ireland, C. A. Ireland, & P. Birch (Eds.), *Violent and sexual offenders: Assessment, treatment and management* (2nd ed.). Routledge.

Hocken, K., & Gredecki, N. (2018). Thinking outside of the box: Advancements in theory, practice & evaluation in sexual offending interventions. In J. L. Ireland, P. Birch, & C. A. Ireland (Eds.), *International handbook on human aggression: Current issues and perspectives*. Routledge.

References

Andrews, D. A., & Bonta, J. (1998). *The psychology of criminal conduct* (2nd ed.). Anderson.

Boer, D. P., & Hart, S. D. (2012). Sex offender risk assessment: Research, evaluation, "best-practice" recommendations, and future directions. In J. L. Ireland, C. A. Ireland, & P. Birch (Eds.), *Violent and sexual offenders: Assessment, treatment & management* (pp. 27–41). Routledge.

Boer, D. P., Hart, S. D., Kropp, P. R., & Webster, C. D. (1997). *Manual for the sexual violence risk 20 professional guidelines for assessing risk of sexual violence*. Simon Frazer University.

Boer, D. P., Tough, S., & Haaven, J. (2004). Assessment of risk manageability of intellectually disabled sex offenders. *Journal of Applied Research in Intellectual Disabilities, 17,* 275–283.

The Campbell Collaboration. Retrieved from www.campbellcollaboration.org.

Cantor, J. M. (2018). Can pedophiles change? *Current Sexual Health Reports, 10*(4), 203–206.

Carter, A. J., & Mann, R. E. (2016). Organizing principles for an integrated model of change for the treatment of sexual offending. In D. Boer (Ed.), *The Wiley handbook on the theories, assessment and treatment of sexual offending* (pp. 359–381). Wiley Blackwell.

Cooley, C. H. (1902). *Human nature and social order.* Scribner's.

Craig, L. A., Browne, K. D., & Beech, A. R. (2008). *Assessing risk in sex offenders: A practitioner's guide.* Wiley.

de Vries Robbé, M., Mann, R. E., Maruna, S., & Thornton, D. (2015). An exploration of protective factors supporting desistance from sexual offending. *Sexual Abuse: Journal of Research and Treatment, 27*(1), 16–33.

Gannon, T., Olver, M., Mallion, J. S., & James, M. (2019). Does specialized psychological treatment for offending reduce recidivism? A meta-analysis examining staff and program variables as predictors of treatment effectiveness. *Clinical Psychology Review, 73,* 101752.

Hanson, K. (2014). Sex offenders. In C. Webster, Q. Haque, & S. Hucker (Eds.), *Violence risk: Assessment and management* (2nd ed., pp. 148–158). Wiley Blackwell.

Hanson, R. K., Bourgon, G., Helmus, L., & Hodgson, S. (2009). The principles of effective correctional treatment also apply to sexual offenders: A meta-analysis. *Criminal Justice and Behavior, 36,* 865–891.

Hanson, R. K., & Bussière, M. T. (1998). Predicting relapse: A meta-analysis of sexual offender recidivism studies. *Journal of Consulting and Clinical Psychology, 66*(2), 348–362.

Hariton, E., & Locascio, J. J. (2018). Randomised controlled trials: The gold standard for effectiveness research: Study design: Randomised controlled trials. *BJOG; an International Journal of Obstetrics and Gynaecology, 125*(13), 1716.

Hart, S. D., Kropp, P. K., Laws, D. R., Klaver, J., Logan, C., & Watt, K. A. (2003). *The risk for sexual violence protocol: Structured professional guidelines for assessing risk of sexual violence.* Simon Fraser University.

Mann, R. E., Hanson, R. K., & Thornton, D. (2010). Assessing risk for sexual recidivism: Some proposals on the nature of psychologically meaningful risk factors. *Sexual Abuse: A Journal of Research and Treatment, 22,* 191–217.

Mews, A., Di Bella, L., & Purver, M. (2017). *Impact evaluation of the prison-based core sex offender treatment programme.* Ministry of Justice Analytical Series.

Popovic, M. (2005). Intimacy and its relevance in human functioning. *Sexual and Relationship Therapy, 20*(1), 31–49.

Rosenhan, D. (1973). On being sane in insane places. *Science, 179*(4070), 250–258.

Schaffer, M., Jeglic, E. L., Moster, A., & Wnuk, D. (2010). Cognitive-behavioral therapy in the treatment and management of sex offenders. *Journal of Cognitive Psychotherapy, 24*(2), 92–103.

Schmucker, M., & Lösel, F. (2017). Sexual offender treatment for reducing recidivism among convicted sex offenders: A systematic review and meta-analysis. *Campbell Systematic Reviews, 13*(1), 1–75.

Taylor, J., Akerman, G., & Hocken, K. (2020). Cultivating compassion focussed practice for those who have committed sexual offences. In Elliott, H., Lievesley, R., Blagden, N., Winder, B., Hocken, K., Banyard, P. (Eds.), *Sexual Crime and Trauma.* Palgrave Macmillan.

Wakeling, H. C., Ruth, E. M., & Adam, J. C. (2012). Do low-risk sexual offenders need treatment? *The Howard Journal, 51*(3), 286–299.

Walton, J. (in press). Rehabilitation of sexual deviancy in prisons. In Winder, B., Blagden, N., & Hamilton, L. (Eds.), *Forensic interventions for therapy and rehabilitation: Case studies and analysis.* Taylor and Francis.

Walton, J. S., Ramsay, L., Cunningham, C., & Henfrey, S. (2017). New directions: Integrating a biopsychosocial approach in the design and delivery of programs for high risk services users in Her Majesty's

Prison and Probation Service. *Advancing Corrections: Journal of the International Corrections and Prison Association, 3,* 21–47.

Ward, T. (2002). Good lives and the rehabilitation of sexual offenders: Promises and problems. *Aggression and Violent Behavior, 7,* 513–528.

Willis, G. M., Prescott, D. S., & Yates, P. (2013). The Good Lives Model (GLM) in theory and practice. *Sexual Abuse in Australia and New Zealand, 5,* 3–9.

9 Intimate partner abuse

Fiona Wilks Riley

Summary

Headline reports of homicides by intimate partners are all too familiar. In England and Wales alone every week on average, two women are killed. This is not just a crime that happens to women as on average, one man is killed by an intimate partner every 17 days (National Office of Statistics [NOS], 2019). Homicide represents the extreme form of intimate partner abuse (IPA), which is defined as physical aggression, sexual coercion, psychological abuse and controlling behaviour towards a current or former intimate partner (WHO, 2017). The high prevalence and long-term effects of victimisation show that IPA can be recognised as a significant public health issue (Cranley et al., 2000). Further, the costs of IPA reach far beyond the immediate impact of a victim's physical injury and emotional suffering. They include, but are not limited to costs to police, the criminal justice system, social services, long-term mental health, housing, social care and lost economic output (Home Office, 2019). Children are particularly vulnerable to psychological and occasionally physical harm from exposure to IPA, sometimes leading to their removal into local authority care. This chapter will critically explore key theories of IPA followed by the application of theory to the work of forensic psychologists in psychological formulation, and intervention of IPA with clients.

Models for understanding IPA

The question of how IPA can be understood will be addressed by examining a number of key theories. First, we will consider the Duluth Model, a feminist approach that has dominated the field of interventions aimed to reduce IPA. We will then consider a contrasting theory for the development of IPA, namely that of the Abusive Personality (AP) (Dutton, 2007). This theory includes a focus on borderline personality (BP) traits being key to the development of IPA with the aspects of insecure attachment and trauma being of significance.

Duluth Model

Developed in Duluth, Minnesota, in 1981, the philosophical core of the model is the belief that men may use physical and sexual violence and other abusive tactics to control their partners. Advocates of the Duluth Model view men's violence to women as stemming from a socially reinforced sense of entitlement. Within the model, men are noted to use violence towards women to stop arguments, to stop their partners from doing something and to punish them for noncompliance (Paymer & Barnes, 2007). According to the model, insofar as women are violent at all, it is with rare exception in

DOI: 10.4324/9781003017103-12

self-defence. Emotions such as frustration or anger that a man may experience before committing acts of IPA are considered to be excuses to justify his behaviour (Dobash & Dobash, 1977).

Based on the premise that men act out of a socially reinforced sense of entitlement, the Duluth approach aims to hold men to account for their actions (see www.duluthmodel. org). The 'Power and Control Wheel' is used to demonstrate how behaviour such as threats, intimidation and coercion serve to exert power and control over a victim. Programmes seeking to address emotions or personality disorders as relating to IPA are accused of collusion and of not helping to change men's beliefs and attitudes about women, men and marriage (Paymer & Barnes, 2007). From a scientific perspective, a positive aspect of the Duluth Model is that its core tenet, that male patriarchal beliefs drive intimate partner violence (IPA), can be tested.

What has research into the Duluth Model shown?

In response to increased awareness of violence towards women and children, the first step for researchers was to measure the extent of the problem. A population survey commissioned for the United States in 1975 showed that contrary to expectations, it was females rather than males who were responsible for a greater amount of assaults (Straus & Gelles, 1986). These results were replicated in a 1985 population survey. Both studies showed that IPA perpetrated by women was an issue that needed to be recognised. This conclusion produced strong reactions, with researchers subjected to jeering, hostility, menacing phone calls and even a bomb threat at a venue where the results were presented (Straus, 1992). Despite this opposition, the finding has continued to be supported by research, including Archer's (2000) meta-analysis of 82 studies.

Moreover, the evidence also shows high levels of violence instigated by women. When the argument that women exercise violence only or almost exclusively in self-defence has been investigated, results have shown that women are more likely to be the first to initiate violence and strike the first blow (Stets & Straus, 1990; Capaldi et al., 2007). Studies based on women's self-reports also concur with this (Whitaker et al., 2007). However, the risk of serious injury and of homicide is higher for women victims than for men because men are generally stronger than women and a punch or a kick from a man can cause more serious damage (Straus, 1992).

The idea that patriarchal beliefs fuel and justify IPA has also been investigated. Studies have demonstrated greater approval for women hitting men than of men hitting women (Straus et al., 1997; Simon et al., 2001). Consistent with this, Eckhardt and Dye (2000) concluded in their review that men who were violent towards their wives had no more patriarchal belief than controls. Further, studies examining same-sex relationships have shown that IPA features at a similar level in gay male and heterosexual relationships and that partner violence is highest of all in lesbian relationships (Waterman et al., 1989; Lie et al., 1991). This indicates that IPA exists in same-sex relationships, which cannot by their nature involve roles of male dominance over women.

Understanding the effectiveness of Duluth-based interventions

Vigurs et al. (2016) conducted a review of ten systematic reviews examining the effectiveness of interventions to address IPA. Nine of the systematic reviews included Duluth-based approaches. Vigurs et al. (2016, p. 27) concluded 'the reviews were unable to identify a clear impact of domestic violence perpetrator programmes on criminal justice or victim-related outcomes'. For an intervention to be effective, it needs to address criminogenic needs, the factors that underpin the development and maintenance of offending behaviour (Andrews & Bonta, 2010). Central to the Duluth Model are patriarchy and gender, factors that research has not indicated to be criminogenic needs relevant to IPA. Failing to target criminogenic needs may help to explain why Duluth approaches have struggled to show effectiveness.

Interventions using the Duluth Model continue to be the predominant approach to work with perpetrators of IPA. But the Duluth approach raises ethical issues for psychologists and other practitioners whose organisations expect them to deliver such interventions as part of their job role. This is because there is an ethical obligation for practitioners to provide interventions that are effective and indeed clients, courts and victims expect this (Corvo et al., 2009).

BOX 9.1   PUTTING ETHICS INTO PRACTICE

Identify what may be the ethical implications for a forensic psychologist delivering an intervention based solely on the Duluth Model.

The Abusive Personality

The AP theory provides an alternative approach to understanding IPA (Dutton, 2007). In this theory, IPA has its roots in exposure to traumatic childhood events, which include abuse, neglect, shaming and exposure to IPA. Consequent to these experiences, the child develops attachment insecurity which underpins the development of BP traits in adulthood. Individuals with BP traits are prone to difficulties in regulating affective states such as anger and jealousy that can contribute to aggression in relationships.

Attachment

Attachment is a biological-based system which supports a deep emotional bond between a child and their caregiver who provides security, safety and protection (Howe, 2011; Bowlby, 1969). During exposure to IPA, neither of the child's parents/caregivers is able to demonstrate their ability to protect the child from the fear or distress of the immediate situation. Partner abuse can represent a threat not just to a child's safety but to the attachment bond as it renders the child unable to rely on either of its parents/caregivers for security and support.

Attachment insecurity in childhood has been found to continue into adulthood where such is manifested in patterns of relating to others (Hazan & Shaver, 1987). Brennan et al. (1998) found differences in attachment styles that could be represented by variations in two underpinning dimensions: anxiety (being worried about abandonment and whether someone cares) and avoidance (lack of ability to be close, open and rely on others). Investigating attachment styles in men, Dutton et al. (1994) found that a fearful attachment style, which features both high anxiety and high avoidance, was significant to IPA and partners' accounts of physical and psychological abuse. A similar pattern of results has been found in women with diagnosed BP disorder, whose anxious attachment style was also found to be strongly associated with anger and reactive aggression (Critchfield et al., 2008).

Velotti et al. (2018) found insecure attachment styles featuring high avoidance and/or high anxiety were significantly associated with psychological, physical and sexual IPA perpetration, although the associations were weak. The authors criticised the methods used to assess attachment as these often relied on self-report rather than more sensitive measures such as the Adult Attachment Interview (George et al., 1985). The review, however, contained only a small number of studies involving participants with police records of IPA and this may be why the associations were weak. Those with more serious IPA thus could have more severe attachment difficulties.

Childhood experiences of abuse, shaming, interparental abuse and parental substance abuse not only increase the risk of attachment insecurity but can also be inherently traumatic in their own right. This has led Dutton to explore the relevance of psychological trauma to IPA (Dutton, 2008).

Trauma

Howell et al. (2016) reviewed the impact of IPA exposure on children at all developmental stages in a multi-country study. IPA exposure was associated with increased anxiety, depression, emotional dysregulation and post-traumatic stress. Exposure to IPA has also been found to affect physical health and causes social functioning problems in relationships as well as impacting cognitive and neurodevelopmental functioning (Hambrick et al., 2019). A recent systematic review of 21 studies found that IPA exposure as a child was associated with a four times higher likelihood of engaging in IPA in adulthood (Kimber et al., 2018). The association between witnessing IPA and perpetrating it has influenced social learning perspectives of IPA, identifying it is a learned behaviour. However, most children exposed to IPA do not use IPA in adulthood and this limits understanding of IPA though a social learning approach (Dutton, 2008).

More recently, Gardner et al. (2014) explored the links between violence and childhood maltreatment by looking at the potential mediating variables of anger and emotional dysregulation. The study included 88 individuals on probation with court-ordered intervention for either intimate partner violence (IPV) (n = 48, mean age = 38) or general violence (n = 40, mean age = 34.5). The IPV group were all men, and the non-IPV group were male (77%) and female (23%). Rates of childhood experiences of abuse were high in both the IPV and the, generally, violent group. Physical abuse and neglect were associated with anger in the non-IPV group, but the combination of physical abuse and neglect with emotional abuse related to anger expression in the IPV group. Difficulties in emotional regulation and anger were significantly higher in the IPV group. This research shows that potentially traumatic abusive experiences contribute to the development of violence with emotional abuse experiences being significant to IPV. This highlights the need for forensic psychologists to consider the importance of trauma to the development of IPV (see chapter on working with women for more details on trauma-informed formulation and approaches).

Borderline personality traits

Dutton (2007) originally developed the theory of the abusive personality by highlighting the difficulties in the regulation of anger, fear and jealousy being of particular importance in IPA. Dutton argued that anger and jealousy are borne from a fear of relationship separation and culminate in 'pathological reactions' which can include violent behaviour (Dutton et al., 1996, p. 421). The origin of the fear of abandonment is argued to lie in early attachment experiences.

Anger has been found to be significantly associated with IPA (Norlander & Eckhardt, 2005). Indeed, anger problems were found to be related to more severe and frequent IPA (Holtzworth-Munroe & Stuart, 1994). Foran and O'Leary (2008) found jealousy to be associated with IPA providing further support for the emotions associated with BP as being significant to IPA.

Anger and jealousy are recognised to be characteristics of BP. BP has been studied in its own right in connection with its relationship with IPA. Hines (2008) investigated the dating relationships of 14,154 students (4,054 men and 10,100 women) at 67 universities across the world. Hines found BP to be strongly predictive of physical, psychological and sexual IPA perpetration. BP was measured on a four-point scale, and Hines found that each additional point on the BP scale was associated with the doubling of physical abuse perpetration rates. This signifies the importance of BP to IPV. There were no gender differences with the presence of BP increasing IPV in both men and women in a similar way. This adds further support to there being no gender difference in BP as a risk factor for IPV. It also shows that forensic psychologists need to be alert to the presence of emotions such as anger and jealousy and how these may constitute BP traits. This demonstrates that such emotions are not simply transitory states but are likely underpinned by problems relating to attachment and trauma.

Comments on the abusive personality

The AP theory helps to explain why relationships are challenging and unstable for people with BP traits. This is because there is emotional dysregulation and a fear that the attachment bond will be broken (fear of abandonment) which contributes to anger and aggression. The need to preserve the attachment relationship is paramount. This theory also explains IPA as serving an affect (emotion) regulating function, something which has also been observed in the wider literature on general aggression (Bushman & Anderson, 2001).

The strengths of this theory are that it has been informed by psychological research. It explains IPA in terms of its developmental experiences and the trajectory that these have taken. This is important for forensic psychologists when assessing individuals who have engaged in IPA. The theory provides clear targets for psychological intervention that relate to criminogenic needs namely trauma, attachment and emotional dysregulation. It underlines the need for a trauma-informed approach for assessment, intervention and prevention. Protective factors need to be further explored as adverse childhood experiences (ACEs) do not always predict aggression in adulthood.

The AP theory has implications for forensic psychologists, social care and educational services for the prevention of IPA. Those exposed to abuse, neglect and other adversity in childhood are at increased risk of using IPA in adulthood and should be the focus of attention in an effective approach to prevention. Prevention should proactively support children and those vulnerable in adulthood from a trauma-informed perspective and recognise their attachment needs for safety and security. Trauma-informed interventions to develop emotional management skills and resilience are also needed.

The AP theory is consistent with developments in neuroscience. Blair et al. (2005) developed the neurocognitive model of reactive aggression, sometimes referred to as affective (emotionally driven) or impulsive aggression (Bushman & Anderson, 2001). The neurocognitive model explains how the trauma of childhood abuse can impact emotional regulation systems influencing individuals to operate at a higher baseline level of threat. Individuals with a high baseline threat level are more easily activated to reactive aggression. The AP theory would highlight that the threat could be psychological in the form of a perceived attack to the attachment bond and not solely physical threat.

Assessment

Implications for forensic psychologists from the AP theory are that it is imperative to explore clients' early attachment experiences. This can be done by directly asking how the client was treated by their parents or other care givers and exploring the quality of these relationships. Other adverse experiences in childhood that have had the potential to be traumatic also need to be discussed, albeit not in depth lest traumatic memories should be reactivated and become distressing. A trauma/loss history list may be conducted to assist to contain emotions in this process. The emotional impact from adverse experiences needs to be identified with the forensic psychologist being alert to the potential significance of experiences of threat, rejection and abandonment. The impact on the client's view of themselves/others and the world from their developmental experiences also needs to be elicited on interview. Collateral information from professional reports can be helpful for gathering information about the client's developmental history. A detailed exploration of relationship history is needed to examine patterns of relating to others and how the client has responded to relationship breakdown. The client's level of emotional reactivity should be explored on interview, and a simple scale of 0–10 to gauge the intensity of emotions can be helpful.

The forensic psychologist should also be familiar with the range of BP traits that may be manifest, for example, suicidal ideation/self-harm. Assessment using a personality disorder screen or a full assessment of BP disorder may be helpful. There are the usual caveats though of not relying solely on self-reported information when conducting assessments of personality disorder. There is no requirement, however, to be diagnosed formally with BP for its traits to be clinically significant to IPA. The use of substances should be explored as it is likely that such also relates to dealing with negative emotions associated with potentially traumatic experiences in childhood.

An analysis of the antecedents leading to an incident/offence of IPA needs to focus on how emotions and core beliefs significant to developmental trauma may have been triggered. Structured risk assessments of risk for general violence and even of partner violence arguably do not emphasise the specific significance of negative attachment experiences. These include abandonment and rejection, developmental trauma, emotional dysregulation and BP traits with sensitivity to rejection, abandonment, and perceived threat. Although these are included in a new risk assessment measure currently being piloted for domestic violence risk assessment, the 'PARTNR scale' Partner Abuse Risk and Treatment Need and Responsivity (Wilks-Riley & Graham-Kevan, 2017).

Intervention

Intervention approaches need to address the assessed needs of a client on an individual basis. As stated previously, interventions need to adhere to the principles of risk, need and responsivity and to address criminogenic needs. The empirical evidence indicates support for the AP theory and that attachment, trauma and BP traits are criminogenic needs generally for this client group. The BP traits of emotional dysregulation, abandonment sensitivity, rejection sensitivity, jealousy and anger would need to be targets for intervention.

Effective intervention for BP disorder is dialectical behaviour therapy as recommended by the National Institute for Health and Care Excellence. This has a key focus on emotional regulation. DBT is, however, a 12-month intervention programme which can be difficult to access. The fact that IPA is a community and/or forensic issue indicates that interventions should not solely lie in services provided by prisons or mental health services which are already recognised to be under significant pressure. The Inner Strength Programme (Graham-Kevan & Wilks-Riley, 2012) integrates techniques from DBT and other psychological approaches in an intervention programme to address IPA (this has been redeveloped into the Positive Futures: Relationships Programme (Wilks-Riley, 2021)). This programme has been delivered in prison and community settings. Independent evaluation of its delivery in a community setting (Schrader-McMillan & Raynes, 2020) of 34 participants (M = 31, F= 3) showed an 81% reduction in records of convictions for any form of DVA and a 72% reduction in other offending (e.g. theft, affray). The follow-up period for evaluation was between 6 and 38 months. Of the 66 children who were subject to child protection plans (CPPs) when their parent was referred to the Inner Strength Programme, 23 were on CPPs post-intervention, a reduction of 64%. The number of children in local authority care reduced from 19 to 9, a reduction of 53%. The estimated financial saving to social care was in the region of £56,000 per year per child no longer in LAC. The results of this evaluation are promising, and further evaluation is necessary to include a control group comparison. The results do suggest that successful outcomes may be possible when criminogenic needs are targeted effectively.

Attachment issues and BP traits also need to be borne in mind for the forensic psychologist to ensure that the space for intervention is safe, containing and emotionally validating. Forensic psychologists need to be reliable, dependable and empathic in their approach, and any changes to the delivery team should be avoided in order to foster the development of therapeutic relationships and predictability of the environment. The client may also need additional therapeutic support for post-traumatic symptoms from developmental trauma and insecure attachment. In terms of the intervention pathway, this more specialised therapy would usually follow the emotional management phase. Emotional management training should improve emotional stabilisation, an important early phase of working with trauma (Greenwald, 2013) and personality disorder (Livesley, 2003). The following case study, involving Shelley, is presented to illustrate a psychological formulation and intervention approach in practice.

Case study: Shelley

Shelley grew up living with her mother and did not know her biological father. She felt her mother had no interest in her when she became involved with her stepfather and recalled feeling 'pushed out'. She described her mother as 'emotionally cold with a short fuse' and as 'liking her drink'. Shelley said she has missed out on having a bond with her mother and felt that she did not matter.

Shelley overheard arguments between her mother and stepfather but did not observe any violence. She was bullied at school and felt she did not fit in.

Shelley moved in with her boyfriend, Ben, a day after meeting him. She said that the relationship was unstable and they got into physical fights. She was feeling stressed and having problems at work because of poor attendance. Ben had forgotten they were going to stay in and watch a film one night and told her he was going out with friends. She grabbed some tablets to overdose, 'so he could see how he was making me feel'. He told her to leave. She refused and recalled, 'I felt so angry I could have done anything'. She then started kicking him and screaming hysterically. She described feeling angry, upset and stressed. On exploration, she stated that she had felt 'pushed out' on being told to leave and 'on my own'. She reflected that she had felt 'left out and a bit jealous' over Ben's intention to go out. She recalled thinking, 'I do not matter' and 'he needs to listen to me'.

Shelley's formulation using the AP theory

Applying the AP theory, Shelley's lack of a secure attachment is evident from experiences of emotional abuse and neglect and of witnessing interparental abuse. These experiences can also be viewed as traumatic. Shelley recognised her lack of a positive attachment experience expressing that she had no bond with her mother. BP characteristics of rejection, abandonment, jealousy, anger and emotional dysregulation are evident and have arisen as a consequence of her traumatic experiences and insecure attachment. Ben having forgotten the plan to watch a film, intending to go out with friends and asking her to leave represented further threats to the security of the attachment bond of her intimate relationship. These events triggered feelings of rejection and abandonment to which she was already vulnerable. These feelings fuelled both her desire to self-harm and her aggression.

Shelley's traumatic experiences as a child have influenced her to be emotionally reactive at a biological level, consistent with BP traits and developmental trauma. She is more likely to be highly distressed by relationship conflict and vulnerable to aggression and self-harm at times when she is feeling rejected and abandoned.

Social learning theory may hold some appeal for explaining Shelley's IPA as arising from exposure to interparental abuse. It does not account for the significance of abandonment and rejection as key triggers to Shelley's aggression and her emotional reactivity, as explained in the AP theory.

Shelley's intervention plan based on AP theory

The first phase of work is to help Shelley to understand her behaviour which is aided by the assessment a process. This provides a rationale for the intervention approach. Shelley needs to develop emotional regulation skills through a DBT-informed approach. This also enables a therapeutic relationship to be forged where her attachment needs to feel safe, supported and to develop trust are met.

Shelley would appear to need to recognise her emotional triggers, prepare for managing these better and identify situations in which her IPA may be easily activated and why. She also needs to develop skills for managing conflict in her relationship, and understanding and communicating her emotions effectively. This approach should also assist her to reduce her self-harm/suicidal ideation as well as her aggression. Interpersonal effectiveness skills from DBT may assist with this as well as a cognitive-behavioural or mentalisation-based therapy approach for developing conflict resolution skills. Notably, all these approaches are used in the Positive Futures: Relationships programme.

Shelley should be considered for further specialist psychological intervention to address any clinical levels of post-traumatic stress that may be present.

Conclusion

The Duluth Model has been the first approach to address IPA. On a positive note, it has drawn attention to the plight of victims of IPA. It is an ideological and not a psychological approach, and research has now shown that its core assumptions are not supported empirically. Unlike the Duluth Model, the AP theory has been developed from research into the field of IPA. This is important as forensic psychologists are professionally and legally obligated by the Health and Care Professions Council to critically evaluate research and other evidence to inform their own practice accordingly. Clients then benefit from what research indicates to be the most effective intervention for the time and effort they are investing in addressing their problem behaviour. Effective programmes for people who engage in IPA benefits victims by reducing their likelihood of future victimisation.

The AP theory recognises childhood abuse/trauma experiences as underpinning dysfunction leading to aggression. The AP theory makes a significant contribution to explaining the route for the development of IPA through trauma, attachment insecurity and BP. Understanding emotional reactivity as having a trauma origin not only helps to increase insight but also to promote a more empathic understanding on the part of professionals. This can strengthen the therapeutic alliance between the forensic psychologist and client. Such understanding helps to foster a non-judgemental approach, which is vital for practitioners as it enables difficult behaviours as originating from difficult circumstances. Through understanding the role of attachment in IPA, the AP model helps the forensic psychologist to work collaboratively with the client to understand why jealousy, anger, rejection and abandonment fears are particularly triggering for them. This helps the client to identify that targets for intervention should include emotional regulation.

Prevention approaches for children at risk of developing IPA from exposure to IPA or other ACEs are also necessary. New approaches such as the Positive Futures: Relationships programme, which addresses targets identified as relevant from empirical research and uses relevant evidence-based psychological techniques, may herald a way forward for this significant public health concern.

Learning outcomes

When you have completed this chapter, you should be able to:

1   Identify the core elements of the Duluth Model
2   Identify the core elements of the AP theory
3   Understand how research has supported/not supported the Duluth Model and AP theories
4   Identify threat reactivity as underpinning aggression in the neurocognitive model
5   Understand how the AP theory can be applied to assessment and treatment planning

Key concepts and terms

- Duluth Model
- Feminism
- Borderline personality disorder

- Reactive aggression
- Abusive personality
- Trauma
- Threat activation
- Anxious attachment
- Avoidant attachment
- Developmental trauma
- Fearful attachment
- Power and control

Sample essay questions

- What are the limitations of current approaches to addressing IPA and how could attention to 'What Works' improve approaches?
- Critically analyse two theoretical approaches to understanding IPA making reference to research.
- What does research indicate about the relationship between gender and IPA?
- What does research indicate should be targets for effective interventions for IPA?

Recommended further reading

Dutton, D. G. (2007). *The abusive personality*. Guilford.

Dutton, D. G. (2008). My back pages: Reflections on thirty years of domestic violence research. *Trauma Violence Abuse, 9*, 131–143.

Hines, D. (2008). Borderline personality traits and intimate partner aggression: An international multi-site, cross-gender analysis. *Psychology of Women Quarterly, 32*, 290–302.

References

Andrews, D. A., & Bonta, J. (2010). Rehabilitation through the lens of the riskneeds-responsivity model. In F. McNeil, P. Raynor, & C. Trotter (Eds.), *Offender supervision: New directions in theory, research and practice*. Willan Publishing.

Archer, J. (2000). Sex differences in aggression between heterosexual partners: A meta-analytic review. *Psychological Bulletin, 126*, 651–680.

Blair, J., Mitchell, D., & Blair, K. (2005). *The psychopath: Emotion and the brain*. Blackwell Publishing.

Bowlby, J. (1969). *Attachment and loss: Attachment*. Basic Books.

Brennan, K. A., Clark, C. L., & Shaver, P. R. (1998). Self-report measurement of adult attachment: An integrative approach. In J. A. Simpson & W. S. Rhodes (Eds.), *Attachment theory and close relationships* (pp. 46–76). Guildford Press.

Bushman, B., & Anderson, C. (2001). Is it time to pull the plug on the hostile versus instrumental aggression dichotomy? *Psychological Review, 108*, 273–279.

Cranley, M., Breslin, E., Capers, C., Campbell, J., Quillian, J., & Stanley, J. (2000). Violence as a public health problem. *Journal of Professional Nursing, 16*(1), 63–69.

Capaldi, D. M., Kim, H. K., & Shortt, J. W. (2007). Observed initiation and reciprocity of physical aggression in young, at-risk couples. *Journal of Family Violence, 22*, 101–111.

Corvo, K., Dutton, D., & Chen, W. (2009). Do Duluth model interventions with perpetrators of domestic violence violate mental health professional ethics? *Ethics and Behavior, 19*(4), 323–340.

Critchfield, K., Levy, K., Clarkin, J., & Kernberg, O. (2008). The relational context of aggression in borderline personality disorder: Using adult attachment style to predict forms of hostility. *Journal of Clinical Psychology, 64*(7), 919–919.

Dobash, R. E., & Dobash, R. P. (1977). Love honour and obey: Institutional ideologies and the struggle for battered women. *Contemporary Crises*, *1*, 403–415.

Dutton, D., Ginkel, C., & Landolt, M. (1996). Jealousy, intimate abusiveness, and intrusiveness. *Journal of Family Violence*, *11*(4), 411–423.

Dutton, D. G., Starzomski, A., Saunders, K., & Bartholomew, K. (1994). Intimacy-anger and insecure attachment as precursors of abuse in intimate relationships. *Journal of Applied Social Psychology*, *24*(15), 1367–1386.

Eckhardt, C., & Dye, M. (2000). The cognitive characteristics of maritally violent men: Theory and evidence. *Cognitive Therapy and Research*, *24*(2), 139–158.

Foran, H., & O'Leary, K. (2008). Problem drinking, jealousy, and anger control: Variables predicting physical aggression against a partner. *Journal of Family Violence*, *23*(3), 141–148.

Gardner, F., Moore, Z., & Dettore, M. (2014). The relationship between anger, childhood maltreatment, and emotion regulation difficulties in intimate partner and non-intimate partner violent offenders. *Behavior Modification*, *38*(6), 779–800.

George, C., Kaplan, N., & Main, M. (1985). *Adult attachment interview*. Unpublished manuscript, University of California.

Graham-Kevan, N., & Wilks-Riley, F. R. (2012). *Inner strength*. Unpublished manual, Forensic Psychological Solutions Ltd.

Greenwald, R. (2013). *Progressive counting within a phase model of trauma-informed treatment*. Routledge.

Hambrick, E., Brawner, T., Perry, B., Brandt, K., Hofmeister, C., & Collins, J. (2019). Beyond the ACE score: Examining relationships between timing of developmental adversity, relational health and developmental outcomes in children. *Archives of Psychiatric Nursing*, *33*(3), 238–247.

Hazan, C., & Shaver, P. (1987). Romantic love conceptualized as an attachment process. *Journal of Personality and Social Psychology*, *52*, 511–524.

Holtzworth-Munroe, A., & Stuart, G. L. (1994). Typologies of male batterers: Three subtypes and the differences among them. *Psychological Bulletin*, *116*(3), 476–497.

Home Office. (2019). *The economic and social costs of domestic abuse (Research Report 107)*. Retrieved from https://assets.publishing.service.gov.uk/government/uploads/system/uploads/attachment_data/file/918897/horr107.pdf.

Howe, D. (2011). *Attachment across the lifecourse: A brief introduction*. Palgrave Macmillan.

Howell, K., Barnes, S., Miller, L., & Graham-Bermann, S. (2016). Developmental variations in the impact of intimate partner violence exposure during childhood. *Journal of Injury & Violence Research*, *8*(1), 43–57.

Kimber, M., Adham, S., Gill, S., Mctavish, J., & Macmillan, H. (2018). The association between child exposure to Intimate Partner Violence (IPV) and perpetration of IPV in adulthood: A systematic review. *Child Abuse & Neglect*, *76*, 273–286.

Lie, G., Schilit, R., Bush, J., Montagne, M., & Reyes, L. (1991). Lesbians in currently aggressive relationships: How frequently do they report aggressive past relationships? *Violence and Victims*, *6*(2), 121–135.

Livesley, W. J. (2003). *Practical management of personality disorder*. Guilford Press.

National Office of Statistics. (2019). Domestic abuse prevalence and trends, England and Wales: Year ending March 2019. Published online: *Office for National Statistics*. https://www.ons.gov.uk/people populationandcommunity/crimeandjustice/articles/domesticabuseprevalenceandtrendsenglandan dwales/yearendingmarch2019

Norlander, B., & Eckhardt, C. (2005). Anger, hostility, and male perpetrators of intimate partner violence: A meta-analytic review. *Clinical Psychology Review*, *25*(2), 119–152.

Paymer, M., & Barnes, G. (2007). *Countering confusion about the Duluth model: Battered women's justice project*. Retrieved from www.bwjp.org.

Schrader-McMillan, A., & Raynes, G. (2020). *Inner strength programme evaluation*. Unpublished report, Lancaster Violence Reduction Unit.

Stets, J. E., & Straus, M. A. (1990). Gender differences in reporting marital violence and its medical and psychological consequences. In M. A. Straus & R. J. Gelles (Eds.), *Physical violence in American families: Risk factors and adaptations to violence in 8,145 families* (pp. 151–166). Transaction Publishers.

Simon, T. R., Anderson, M., Thompson, M. P., Crosby, A. E., Shelley, G., & Sacks, J. J. (2001). Attitudinal acceptance of intimate partner violence among U.S. adults. *Victims, 16*(2), 115–126.

Straus, M. A. (1992). Sociological research and social policy: The case of family violence. *Sociological Forum, 7*(2), 211–237.

Straus, M. A., & Gelles, R. J. (1986). Societal change and change in family violence from 1975 to 1985 as revealed by two national surveys. *Journal of Marriage and the Family, 48*, 465–480.

Straus, M. A., Kantor, G. K., & Moore, D. W. (1997). Change in cultural norms approving marital violence. In G. K. Kantor & J. L. Jasinski (Eds.), *Out of the darkness: Contemporary perspective on family violence* (pp. 3–15). Sage.

Velotti, P., Beomonte Zobel, S., Rogier, G., & Tambelli, R. (2018). Exploring relationships: A systematic review on intimate partner violence and attachment. *Frontiers in Psychology, 9*, 1166.

Vigurs, C., Schucan-Bird, K., Quy, K., & Gough, D. (2016). The impact of domestic violence perpetrator programmes on victim and criminal justice outcomes: A systematic review of reviews of research evidence. *What works: Crime reduction systematic review series 5*. College of Policing.

Waterman, C., Dawson, L., & Bologna, M. (1989). Sexual coercion in gay male and lesbian relationships: Predictors and implications for support services. *The Journal of Sex Research, 26*(1), 118–124.

Whitaker, D. J., Haileyesus, T., Swahn, M., & Saltzman, L. S. (2007). Differences in frequency of violence and reported injury between relationships with reciprocal and nonreciprocal intimate partner violence. *American Journal of Public Health, 97*, 941–947.

Wilks-Riley, F. R. (2021). *Positive futures: Relationships programme*. Unpublished manual, Wilks Forensic Psychology Ltd.

Wilks-Riley, F. R., & Graham-Kevan, N. (2017). *Inner strength* (revised). Unpublished manual, Forensic Psychological Solutions Ltd.

World Health Organisation. (2017). *Violence against women* (Factsheet). Retrieved from www.who.int/news-room/fact-sheets/detail/violence-against-women.

10 Deliberate fire-setting

Sally Tilt

Summary

Fires have occurred naturally on earth through human history. Our early ancestors experienced fire through lightning strikes, extreme summer heat and volcanoes. Fires were something to fear. The archaeological record suggests that around 50,000 years ago, humans developed the skill of starting and controlling fire (see Sorenson et al., 2018); this significant event in our history led to an ability to survive in cooler climates, extend the working day and possibly even to increase brain size (Wrangham, 2009).

An interest in and a skill for setting and managing fire therefore may carry a genetic advantage. Indeed, a human interest in fire appears to be a universal human characteristic. One might imagine that there have been points in our history when the ability to deliberately start a fire has been celebrated and these people held in high esteem. However, within a forensic context, we more often find people who have started fires and who are ostracised and stigmatised in society. Instead of being positive and helpful to communities, their fires have been dangerous, fear-invoking and at times catastrophic. This chapter explores why some people start deliberate fires that cause fear and harm, how this risk can be assessed and how this risk might be reduced for the future.

The fear and fascination of fire

Fires are often emotive and memorable events in people's lives. For many reading this chapter, a reference to Grenfell Tower, the Australian fires of 2019/2020 or the fires within the Twin Towers will instantly bring to mind a visual image linked to these events. Further, people may hold strong memories of less well known but locally significant fires that they saw or were aware of during their childhood; with these memories persisting throughout their life. Indeed, in the United Kingdom, the Great Fire of London has retained a place in cultural memory for over 350 years.

In part, the strength of these memories may be explained by an innate fear of fire; since humans learned the skill of controlling fire and using fire for domestic purposes, it has posed a concurrent risk to dwellings and human life. It is protective to be alert to the danger of fire. Alongside, this fear sits an evolutionary advantage to be fascinated by fire. That is, the motivation to master and to control fire enabled our ancestors to heat their homes, cook their food and extend their working days. Later, it allowed the transformation of the properties of materials, for example, through the creation of fired pottery or glass.

Fessler (2006) suggests that fascination with fire provides the drive for humans to learn competence of fire-setting in early life and that fire play is a route to achieve such competence. A difference can be seen between cultures in which fire-setting is

DOI: 10.4324/9781003017103-13

a routine and utilitarian part of life, where mastery of fire competence is achieved in early childhood and those cultures where fire is no longer routinely experienced by humans. Fire interest amongst adults from the former cultures is lower than in Western cultures where children are not required to make and use fire, suggesting that the exposure to opportunities to start fire reduces later fire interest. This exposure theory did not receive support from Murray et al.'s (2015) later study involving adults from two different American states. The studies found no difference between adults with greater childhood exposure to using fires and later fire interest as an adult; although the authors highlight that the amount of fire exposure may not have been sufficient to cross the boundary of exposure.

Who sets fires?

There were 75,558 deliberate fires recorded in England in the year ending September 2019 (Home Office, 2020). This is a decrease of 8% in the previous year, which is consistent with the general downward trend of fire incidents in the United Kingdom more generally. Tyler et al. (2019) highlight the scale of the problem across different countries and call for an adjustment in the focus of attention on deliberate fire-setters to broaden from the current locus in criminal justice, to recognising fire-setting as an international public health issue.

One factor that can cloud the understanding of fire-setting sits in the domain of definition. As outlined in Focus Box 10.1, a number of different descriptors are used when discussing individuals who begin fires; the different definitions leading to a different group of people included. In this chapter, the term fire-setters is used; this has greater relevant inclusivity, including those who do not receive a conviction or a diagnosis relating to their fire-setting behaviour. Whilst the proportion of fire-setters who meet the diagnostic criteria for pyromania is low, it is of note that the perception attached to fire-setters, and their media portrayal is often more aligned to the diagnostic descriptors. Fire-setters in the media are often presented as individuals who repeatedly start fires, driven by a compulsion, and from which pleasure is derived. Research on the characteristics of fire-setters has shown this to be a poor representation of the typical fire-setter, with considerable variability being observed amongst those who deliberately start fires. Despite this, however, the concept of the compulsive fire-setter appears a persistent stereotype.

BOX 10.1   DEFINITIONS RELATING TO PEOPLE WHO SET FIRES

Arson – a crime

In common law, arson is the offence of deliberately setting fire to a property. *(Note: the number of people categorised as arsonists is likely to be significantly less than the number of fire-setters as a conviction for the offence of arson is required. The definition of 'arsonist' also tells us little about a person's motivation for starting a fire. For example, possible motives may include interest in fire, concealing a crime, intent to harm a person or an attempt to claim insurance money amongst many others.)*

Pyromania – a diagnosis

The diagnostic term for a psychiatric disorder involves a compulsion to start fires. In DSM-V, receiving a diagnosis of pyromania requires the presence of a number of specific criteria including an intense desire to start a fire, deriving pleasure from seeing or setting fires, and further that the behaviour is not better explained by another mental disorder such as conduct or antisocial disorder. *(Note: due to the specific descriptors of pyromania, the number of people who meet the criteria for this diagnosis is low. For example, Soltys (1992) summaries three separate studies with groups convicted of arson. Across all these studies (which taken together totalled 331 participants), none of the individuals, all who had a conviction for arson, met the criteria of pyromania.)*

Deliberate fire-setting – a behaviour

Deliberate fire-setting is the most inclusive of these three terms. This describes the behaviour of intentionally starting a fire – when used in the psychology literature, fire-setting (without the 'deliberate' preceding it) most usually describes the behaviour of intentional fire-setting. *(Note: this term is preferred as it is inclusive of all individuals who engage in this behaviour.)*

In answer to the aforementioned question 'who starts fires?' the answer appears to be 'quite a number of us'. Grolnick et al. (1990) explored fire-setting amongst 770 young children (age 6–14). About 38% of participants reported having played with fire at some point in their lives. A correspondingly high level of fire-setting or interest in fire in the non-convicted population has similarly been found in other studies (Kafry, 1980; Block & Block, 1975).

Whilst an interest in fire and a drive to develop mastery may be normative, there remains a need to understand the factors that lead to deliberate fire-setting. According to Dickens et al. (2009), the fire-setter is most likely to be a young man with an early history of offending, instability in childhood, school adjustment problems, a personality disorder or psychosis, a history of drug and alcohol dependency, to have experienced childhood institutionalisation and to have engaged in suicide attempts. These descriptive features are notable, however, by their commonality with those linked to other offence types of behaviour. Gannon et al. (2013) explored whether fire-setters were distinguishable from non-fire-setting offenders. They found overlap between the characteristics of the prisoners convicted of arson and non-arson offences. Yet, they found differences on particular variables namely, anger-related cognition, interest in serious fire, identification with fire, locus of control, self-esteem and fire safety. Ducat et al. (2013) also explored differences between exclusive fire-setters, versatile offenders and non-fire-setting offenders. They found overlap between the groups, with some differences (employment and psychiatric disorders) which distinguished between groups.

Why do people set fires?

Approaches to addressing this question have followed a variety of routes. One of the earlier proposals for a theory was that described by Freud (1932). Making links with Greek philosophers, his theory proposed that the flames of a fire symbolised libido and further that man held a sexualised desire to exercise control over fire through urination. Whilst this theory has been superseded by evidence-based and gender-inclusive approaches, it helps to understand what might be the roots of subsequent explorations of links between fire-setting and both sexual arousal (Quinsey et al., 1989) and enuresis (Slavkin, 2001); neither of which have been found to have a link to fire-setting behaviour.

Subsequent work to understand why people deliberately start fires has explored the motive, as determined by the target of the fire or the approach to the task. Inciardi (1970) examined offence accounts for 138 people who had served sentences in US prisons for arson convictions. Based on the accounts of the offences and subsequent parole records, the offences were categorised by apparent motive, and six categories or typologies of fire-setters proposed are: revenge, excitement, institutionalised (all subjects in this group were held in mental health – or epilepsy – institutions and started fires apparently to be moved from their current setting), insurance claims, vandalism and finally, for the purpose of covering up another crime, such as burglary. By far the largest of the groups in this study was the typology of revenge fire-setter (58%). The sample for this study was those convicted of arson and who had served a custodial sentence. It may be that this represents a subset of those who set fires – a factor which will be discussed further in the following sections.

Attempts to replicate the aforementioned study did not find the same typologies. Typically, they found a greater number of categories (see Prins et al., 1985; Rix, 1994). However, it is of note that each of these studies identified a typology related to 'revenge', and in common with Inciardi's (1970) study, this was the largest group. A helpful model to explain the potential aetiology of this frequently cited motive has been proposed by Barnoux and Gannon (2014). The model suggests three stages: the interpersonal conflict, the emotional or cognitive response to the conflict and the selection of fire-setting as the behaviour response.

BOX 10.2 ETHICS IN RELATION TO SAMPLE TYPE IN FIRE-SETTING RESEARCH

The participant sample used in fire-setting research impacts heavily on findings. This should be an important ethical consideration for practitioners appraising the validity of any research to their client group.

Early fire-setter research explored the characteristics of those convicted of arson offences. Whist the findings of such studies inform on the factors linked to those who are caught, prosecuted and convicted of starting a fire, this likely represents a particular subset of people who start fires. It is likely that this subset is linked to fires which had the most serious outcomes in terms of destruction or injury caused to others. The unpredictability of fire means that the degree of destruction caused by a fire is likely to be a poor indicator of the motivation or the behaviour of the fire-setter (Dickens et al., 2009). That is, the same fire-setting behaviour could lead to a self-extinguishing fire in one context and the destruction of a whole building in another case. The severity of a fire depends on a range of factors additional to the behaviour of the fire-setter, such as the presence of a working smoke alarm, speed of response of fire service and the flammability of surroundings.

Studies have also recruited participants outside of the criminal justice sphere, for example, through social media (Barrowcliffe & Gannon, 2016) and have compared those who self-report having started fires with those who do not. Notably, 18% of the participants who responded to the aforementioned study reported having deliberately set a fire for which they had not been caught. The inclusion of non-apprehended fire-setters allows researchers to begin understanding fire-setting behaviour, which might be more typical of the spectrum of human behaviour.

Other samples include populations which may have specific characteristics. Ducat et al.'s (2015) exploration of factors linked to recidivism in 1,052 people convicted of arson in Australia, included 412 people convicted of arson-related offences. Due to the risk associated with wildfire in Australia this category of offence can include careless use of fire in open areas; however, it is possible that the psychological factors behind this type of fire-setting is distinguishable from other types of fire setting.

Finally, there is little research with those who set fires purely in secure or custodial settings. Without such research, it is not possible to know if this represents a group with different interests and motivation.

Theories of fire-setting

Three multifactorial models have dominated the attention of practitioners working with fire-setters. Jackson et al. (1987) drew on social learning theory to describe the functional analysis model of fire-setting. Fineman (1995) applied dynamic behaviour principles to describe an alternative model (dynamic behaviour model), in which reinforcement contingencies interacted with historical and environmental factors. Building on the aforementioned theories, attempting to address some of the weaknesses and applying the principles advocated by Ward and Hudson (1998), Gannon, Ó Ciardha et al. (2012) developed the multi-trajectory theory of adult fire-setting (M-TTAF). The model consists of two tiers, the first describing the aetiological framework and the second providing proposed subtypes of fire-setting individuals. Figure 10.1 presents the five different trajectories to starting fires as outlined in tier 2. Notably, the framework was developed from literature on both male and female adult fire-setters and therefore is applicable to both genders. An application of this model is made in the case study at the end of this chapter. Increasing the sophistication of theories that explain fire-setting is important for research and practice; there have been positive developments in this direction on which future research can build.

Assessing the risk of fire-setting

Relative to other offence types (such as violent or sexual offending), tools to assist forensic practitioners in understanding an individual's future risk of fire-setting are fewer, and there has been less research into their effectiveness. This section will explore the current tools and the options for practitioners to consider when exploring fire-setting risk.

Structured professional judgement (SPJ) tools for risk assessment, as discussed in chapter four, guide the forensic practitioner to consider and rate factors that the evidence base

Grievance

Individuals on this trajectory typically display difficulties with self-regulation, communication and / or assertiveness. This trajectory describes a pathway to firesetting to resolve interpersonal conflict, fire may be selected out of convenience or due to fire interest.

Fire interest

An interest in fire is the prominent factor for individuals on this trajectory. They may hold fire scripts (learned beliefs) relating to fire and find that the act of setting a fire is rewarded by sensory stimulation.

Emotionally expressive / need for recognition

While considered under the same trajectory – as both are driven by difficulties with communication – this trajectory includes two subtypes that in forensic practice can present quite differently. The first is the individual for whom firesetting is a method to communicate distress. The second is to meet a need for recognition.

Antisocial

The antisocial trajectory describes firesetters for where fire is one among many types of offence on the criminal record. Fire is used as a convenient tool to achieve antisocial goals such as concealing another crime or vandalism.

Multi-faceted

This group present the most complex challenges for forensic practitioners. They are likely to be driven by both anti-social beliefs and fire interest. The multiple goals which may drive their firesetting lead to a complex formulation.

Figure 10.1 Trajectories to fire-setting from tier 2 of the M-TTAF

has shown to be linked to recidivism. They are generally a preferred assessment type, in part, because the items included are empirically supported, and for the standardisation of approach that they offer.

The HCR-20 (v3) (Douglas et al., 2013) is a widely used and researched SPJ for the purpose of assessing risk of violent recidivism. Whilst there may be occasions when fire is used as a weapon of violence towards others, the research referenced previously indicates that there are further motives for fire-setting which would not be described as violent. This limits the scope of the HCR-20 (v3) for use with fire-setters to cases where the practitioner is confident that the fire-setting fits the definition of violence described by the authors. Further, the HCR-20 (v3) is a tool to assess the risk of further violence. This may not be the prominent risk of interest for the practitioner – for example, there are likely to be cases where the risk of further fire setting is of interest as opposed to the risk of violence – the HCR-20 (v3) (and the literature on which it is based) was not designed for this purpose.

A number of checklists and assessment tools have been developed for the purpose of assessing fire-setting risk in adults and juveniles. Respective examples include the Northgate Firesetter Risk Assessment 2.0 (Taylor & Thorne, 2019) and the Firesetting Risk Assessment Tool for Youth (Stadolnik, 2010). To date, the predictive validity of tools in this area is limited and recognised as an area in need of further development (see Tyler et al., 2019).

Psychometric tools to assist in the assessment of specific aspects of fire-setting may also be integrated with the aforementioned approach. The Four Factor Fire Scale (FFFS: Ó Ciardha et al., 2015) is one such measure which has been subject to tests of validation and reliability. Ó Ciardha et al. (2015) found that the FFFS differentiated between fire-setters and non-fire-setters with an offence history on the four factors of: identification with fire, serious fire interest, poor fire safety and fire setting as normal. Notably, in this same study, an everyday interest in fire was not a factor that differentiated between fire-setters and non-fire-setters.

Therefore, the current options available to practitioners for assessing the risk of fire-setting rely on the practitioner maintaining an up-to-date awareness of the developing evidence base for risk and protective factors linked to fire-setting, and the application of this knowledge along with clinical interview and information from a variety of sources. Focus Box 10.3 outlines factors which distinguish between fire-setters and non-fire-setters, and single and repeat fire-setters (Wyatt et al., 2019). Theoretical models, such as those described previously (Jackson et al., 1987; Fineman, 1995; Gannon, Ó Ciardha et al., 2012), can also be valuable in building a formulation of the individual.

BOX 10.3   RISK FACTORS FOR FIRE-SETTING (WYATT ET AL., 2019)

The following factors distinguish between mentally disordered fire-setters and a control group. Fire-setters were more like to have:

- More hospital admissions
- Increased impulsivity
- Premeditated the offence
- Lower substance misuse
- External locus of control
- Lower levels of hostility

The following factors distinguish between single and repeat mentally disordered fire-setters. Repeat fire-setters were more like to have:

- A personality disorder diagnosis
- External locus of control

- Fewer problems with medication non-compliance
- Fewer attempts to extinguish fire

ACTIVITY BOX 10.4

Search for recent news stories that have involved a deliberate fire. Based on the reported information, what would you hypothesise to be the motivation of the person starting the fire? What further information would you like to collect to increase your confidence in your hypothesis?

Interventions with fire-setters

The same general principles for designing interventions to address offending behaviour apply also to fire-setters (Andrews & Bonta, 2014). Practitioners should attempt to understand an individual's needs (supported by the evidence) that relate to the behaviour which is the focus of change and should design or apply interventions which follow risk, need and responsivity principles. Ideally, this approach is then followed by evaluation of such interventions to inform effectiveness and guide future intervention design. Whilst practitioners have worked with fire-setters applying such approaches, evaluations have tended to involve a small sample size and therefore provide little conclusive direction.

As indicated by the title of Gannon et al.'s (2012) paper '*A long time coming? The Firesetting Intervention Programme for Mentally disordered Offenders (FIP-MO)*', prior to the FIP-MO, there was a dearth of intervention provision for fire-setters when compared with those convicted of other offence types. Whilst the FIP-MO and the Firesetting Intervention Programme for Prisoners – FIPP (sister programme for prison settings) were in no way the first interventions targeting deliberate fire-setters, they were the first to provide a standardised training manual and to commit to undertake a large-scale evaluation. Tyler et al. (2017) reported positive indications of change on a study involving 63 participants of the FIP-MO on psychometric measures relevant to deliberate fire-setting. A separate evaluation of the FIPP (Gannon et al., 2015) involving 54 male prisoners completing the programme also showed positive changes on psychometric measures relevant to deliberate fire-setting. Whilst psychometric measures are a positive first step in evaluation, measures of behaviour change to evaluate the impact of the interventions on fire-setting behaviour are not yet available. In addition, evaluation of the interventions with different client subtypes will inform the treatment of specific groups. In the meantime, it appears that there is a need for specific interventions for fire-setters and that a CBT approach to this task appears promising.

Working with fire-setting clients requires the reflective practitioner to be knowledgeable about the science, to consider the available approaches and to agree a plan with the client. The following case study illustrates an example of how this may be done.

Case study

Shane was referred to the psychology department at the prison where he was being held to address his fire-setting behaviour. He had started two fires within prison, both involving setting tissue paper alight in his cell; on each occasion, a member of staff had been close by and had acted to put out the fire before any serious damage occurred.

Shane was serving a sentence for arson. The offence involved starting fires in the toilets of two different pubs on the same evening. One was extinguished quickly, and the second led to significant damage to the building. He had two previous convictions for minor acquisitive crimes as a juvenile.

Initial assessment and formulation of Shane's fire-setting

The psychologist assigned to Shane began by working with him to understand why his fire-setting occurred. They explored his background and his early experiences with fire. Shane described a challenging childhood, with inconsistent parenting and periods when he was looked after in care. He developed strategies to help him to gain the support and attention of adults when he needed help, which included self-harm and antisocial behaviour (including fire-setting). Starting small fires in parks and woodland was a normal part of his childhood, as was calling the fire brigade after setting them. He recalls the kindness of the firefighters, who allowed him to try out their equipment and to sit in their truck.

The psychologist used the M-TTAF to formulate Shane's behaviour. Figure 10.2 describes tier 1 of the M-TTAF for Shane; the model illustrates how his developmental experiences lead to psychological vulnerabilities linked to fire-coping scripts, offence supportive beliefs, communication and emotional regulation difficulties. For much of the time, Shane was able to function well in his life; he had periods of stability when his work and social life ran smoothly. This added to the confusion that both Shane and those around him held towards his fire-setting; it appeared to be untypical of his general behaviour.

Figure 10.2 demonstrates that for the psychological vulnerabilities to be triggered into critical risk factors for starting a fire, proximal factors also needed to be present. For Shane, the triggers were events in his life that he found upsetting (a relationship ending, news of a relative's illness and being threatened by others). When these occurred, he found the resulting emotions difficult to cope with and responded passively. The associated low self-esteem contributed to priming the vulnerabilities, and his response was to start a fire.

On tier 2 of the M-TTAF, his behaviour appeared to fit the emotionally expressive trajectory. His fire-setting appeared to serve the function of communicating his distress or need for help. Shane assisted with the formulation and he stated that it was a relief to see these patterns. He had previously felt confused as to why he started fires, when he was able to manage his life well on other occasions. Shane also completed the Four Factor Fire Scale (Ó Ciardha et al., 2015), which indicated higher than average scores on 'fire safety' and 'fire is normal'.

Intervention

The psychologist identified treatment targets for the intervention, which included sessions targeting: relationships and communication, emotion management, problem-solving, assertiveness, fire safety and fire normalisation. These treatment targets map onto the psychological vulnerabilities and critical risk factors as shown in Figure 10.2.

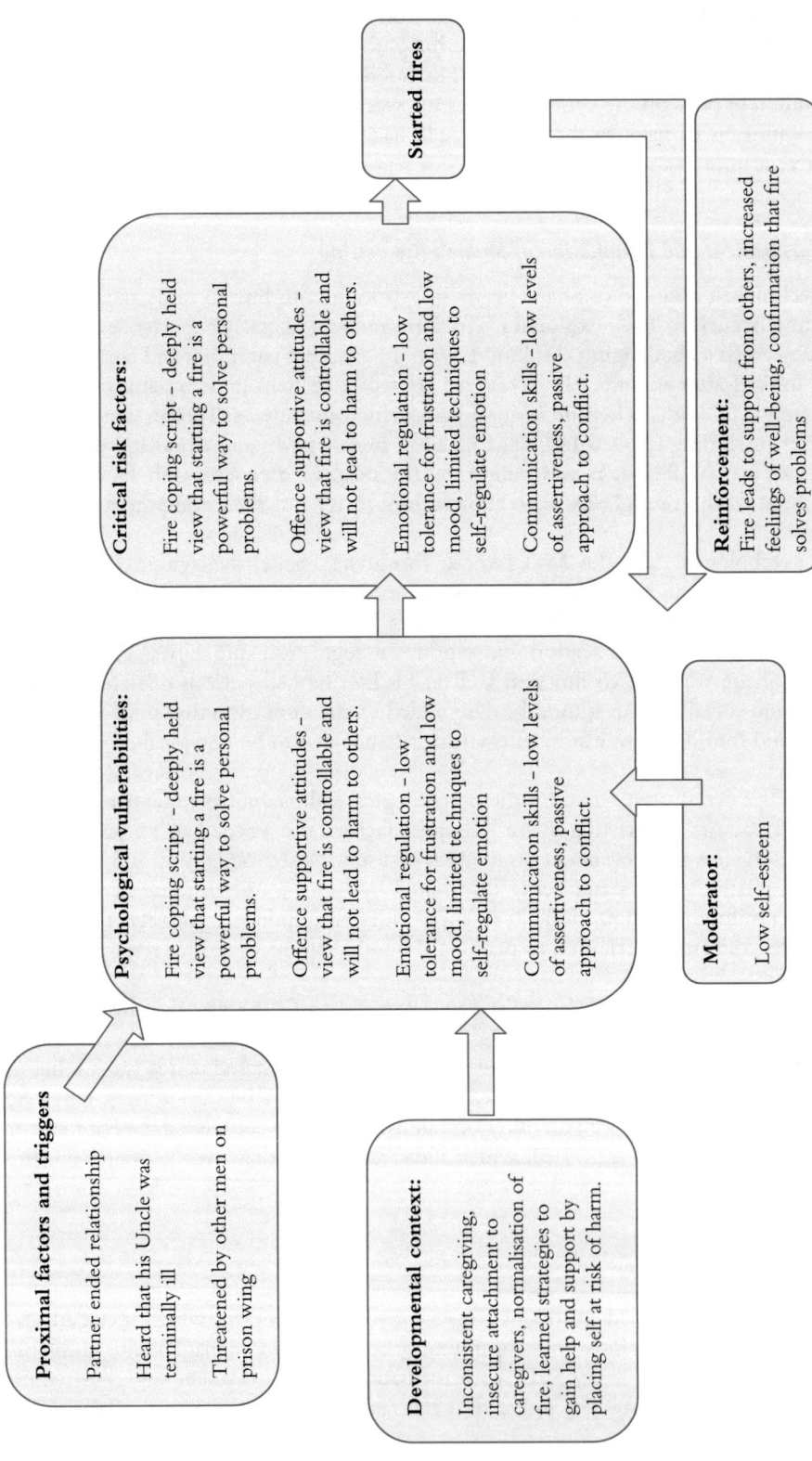

Figure 10.2 Shane's formulation using M-TAFF

Conclusion

Deliberately starting a fire is a skill that has been a great advantage for humans through their history. It is also a cause of great suffering when used without care or to cause harm. Understanding the reasons behind why an important skill becomes a problem for society is of vital importance for forensic psychologists in supporting and changing the behaviour of those with a history of fire-setting. Further attention on this area of behaviour in relation to research and evaluation of interventions will be key to reducing the damage and harm caused.

Learning outcomes

When you have completed this chapter, you should be able to:

1   Know that human interest in fire has an evolutionary history
2   Understand the current research about why people start deliberate fires
3   Know the options available for practitioners to use when assessing the risk of future fire-setting
4   Understand what the evidence suggests is helpful in relation to treatment with fire-setters
5   Have an understanding of how assessment, treatment and intervention may be used in a psychologist's work in a specific case study on fire-setting

Key concepts and terms

- Fire-setting
- Pyromania
- Arson
- Revenge
- Multifactor theory

Sample essay questions

- Why do people deliberately set fires and how has this changed over time?
- In your view, what are the limitations in the current research based on fire-setting behaviour, and what are the priorities for future work?
- Are people convicted of fire-setting offences different to those convicted of other offences? If so, how?

Recommended further reading

Gender differences in fire-setting

Gannon, T. A. (2010). Female arsonists: Key features, psychopathologies and treatment needs. *Psychiatry: Interpersonal and Biological Processes, 73*, 173–189.

Nanayakkara, V., Ogloff, J. R., Davis, M. R., & McEwan, T. E. (2020). Gender-based types of firesetting: Clinical, behavioural and motivational differences among female and male firesetters. *The Journal of Forensic Psychiatry & Psychology, 31*(2), 273–291.

Juvenile fire-setting

Dolan, M., McEwan, T. E., Doley, R., & Fritzon, K. (2011). Risk factors and risk assessment in juvenile fire-setting. *Psychiatry, Psychology and Law*, *18*(3), 378–394.

Johnson, R., Beckenbach, H., & Kilbourne, S. (2013). Forensic psychological public safety risk assessment integrated with culturally responsive treatment for juvenile fire setters: DSM-5 implications. *Journal of Criminal Psychology*, *3*(1), 49–64.

References

Andrews, D. A., & Bonta, J. (2014). *The psychology of criminal conduct* (5th ed.). Routledge.

Barnoux, M., & Gannon, T. A. (2014). A new conceptual framework for revenge firesetting. *Psychology, Crime & Law*, *20*(5), 497–513.

Barrowcliffe, E. R., & Gannon, T. A. (2016). Comparing the psychological characteristics of un-apprehended firesetters and non-firesetters living in the UK. *Psychology, Crime & Law*, *22*(4), 382–404.

Block, J. H., & Block, J. (1975). *Fire and young children: Learning survival skills*. Technical Report for Pacific Southwest Forest and Range.

Dickens, G., Sugarman, P., Edgar, S., Hofberg, K., Tewari, S., & Ahmad, F. (2009). Recidivism and dangerousness in arsonists. *Journal of Forensic Psychiatry & Psychology*, *20*(5), 621–639.

Douglas, K. S., Hart, S. D., Webster, C. D., & Belfrage, H. (2013). *HCR-20V3: Assessing risk of violence: User guide*. Simon Fraser University.

Ducat, L., McEwan, T., & Ogloff, J. R. P. (2013). Comparing the characteristics of firesetting and non-firesetting offenders: Are firesetters a special case? *The Journal of Forensic Psychiatry & Psychology*, *24*(5), 549–569.

Ducat, L., McEwan, T. E., & Ogloff, J. R. (2015). An investigation of firesetting recidivism: Factors related to repeat offending. *Legal and Criminological Psychology*, *20*(1), 1–18.

Fessler, D. (2006). A burning desire: Steps toward an evolutionary psychology of fire learning. *Journal of Cognition and Culture*, *6*(3–4), 429–451.

Fineman, K. R. 1995. A model for the qualitative analysis of child and adult fire deviant behavior. *American Journal of Forensic Psychology*, *13*(1), 31–60.

Freud, S. (1932). The acquisition of power over fire. *The International Journal of Psychoanalysis*, *13*(4), 405–410.

Gannon, T. A., Alleyne, E., Butler, H., Danby, H., Kapoor, A., Lovell, Mozova, K., Spruin, E., Tostevin, T., Tyler, N., & Ó Ciardha, C. (2015). Specialist group therapy for psychological factors associated with firesetting: Evidence of a treatment effect from a non-randomized trial with male prisoners. *Behaviour Research and Therapy*, *73*, 42–51.

Gannon, T. A., Lockerbie, L., & Tyler, N. (2012). A long time coming? The Firesetting Intervention Programme for Mentally disordered Offenders (FIP-MO). *Forensic Update*, *116*, 1–9.

Gannon, T. A., Ó Ciardha, C., Barnoux, M. F. L., Tyler, N., Mozova, K., & Alleyne, E. K. A. (2013). Male imprisoned firesetters have different characteristics than other imprisoned offenders and require specialist treatment. *Psychiatry: Interpersonal and Biological Processes*, *76*(4), 349–364.

Gannon, T., Ó Ciardha, C., Doley, R., & Alleyne, E. (2012). The Multi-Trajectory Theory of Adult Firesetting (M-TTAF). *Aggression and Violent Behavior*, *17*, 107–121.

Grolnick, W. S., Cole, R. E., Laurenitis, L., & Schwartzman, P. (1990). Playing with fire: A development assessment of children's fire understanding and experience. *Journal of Clinical Child Psychology*, *19*(2), 128–135.

Home Office. (2020). Fire and rescue incident statistics: England, year ending September 2019. *Home Office Statistical Bulletin 6/20*. Retrieved from https://assets.publishing.service.gov.uk/government/uploads/system/uploads/attachment_data/file/865256/fire-and-rescue-incident-sep19-hosb0620.pdf.

Inciardi, J. A. (1970). The adult firesetter: A typology. *Criminology*, *8*(2), 145–155.

Jackson, H. F., Glass, C., & Hope, S. (1987). A functional analysis of recidivistic arson. *British Journal of Clinical Psychology*, *26*(3), 175–185.

Kafry, D. (1980). Playing with matches: Children and fire. In D. V. Canter (Ed.), *Fires and human behaviour* (pp. 41–60). Wiley.

Murray, D. R., Fessler, D. M. T., & Lupfer, G. (2015). Young flames: The effects of childhood exposure to fire on adult attitudes. *Evolutionary Behavioral Sciences, 9*(3), 204–213.

Ó Ciardha, C., Tyler, N., & Gannon, T. A. (2015). A practical guide to assessing adult firesetters' fire-Specific treatment needs using the four factor fire scales. *Psychiatry, 78*(4), 293–304.

Prins, H., Tennent, G., & Trick, K. (1985). Motives for arson. *Medicine, Science and Law, 25*, 275–278.

Quinsey, V. L., Chaplin, T. C., & Upfold, D. (1989). Arsonists and sexual arousal to fire setting: Correlation unsupported. *Journal of Behavior Therapy and Experimental Psychiatry, 20*(3), 203–209.

Rix, K. J. B. (1994). A psychiatric study of adult arsonists. *Medicine, Science and the Law, 34*(1), 21–34.

Slavkin, M. L. (2001). Enuresis, firesetting, and cruelty to animals: Does the ego triad show predictive validity? *Adolescence, 36*(143), 461.

Soltys, S. M. (1992). Pyromania and firesetting behaviors. *Psychiatric Annals, 22*(2), 79–83.

Sorensen, A. C., Claud, E., & Soressi, M. (2018). Neandertal fire-making technology inferred from microwear analysis. *Scientific Reports, 8*(1), 10065.

Stadolnik, R. (2010). *Firesetting Risk Assessment Tool for Youth (FRAT-Y): Professional manual.*

Taylor, J. L., & Thorne, I. (2019). Assessing firesetters with intellectual disabilities. *Journal of Intellectual Disabilities and Offending Behaviour, 10*(4), 102–118.

Tyler, N., Gannon, T. A., Ciardha, C. Ó, Ogloff, J. R., & Stadolnik, R. (2019). Deliberate firesetting: An international public health issue. *The Lancet Public Health, 4*(8), e371–e372.

Tyler, N., Gannon, T. A., Lockerbie, L., & Ó Ciardha, C. (2017). An evaluation of a specialist firesetting treatment programme for male and female mentally disordered offenders (the FIP-MO). *Clinical Psychology & Psychotherapy*, 1–13.

Ward, T., & Hudson, S. (1998). The construction and development of theory in the sexual offending area: A metatheoretical framework. *Sexual Abuse: A Journal of Research and Treatment, 10*(1), 47–63.

Wrangham, R. (2009). *Catching fire.* Profile Books Ltd.

Wyatt, B., Gannon, T. A., McEwan, T. E., Lockerbie, L., & O'Connor, A. (2019). Mentally disordered firesetters: An examination of risk factors. *Psychiatry, 82*(1), 27–41.

11 Stalking

Rachael Wheatley

Summary

Stalking is a serious crime that is prevalent and highly destructive and not at all flattering for victims. One in five women and one in ten men will become victims of stalking at some point in their lives in the United Kingdom (ONS, 2019). The unrelenting psychological intrusion conjures an implicit threat of physical harm, and victims suffer emotional, social, financial and vocational problems due to the insidious and persistent nature of stalking. Individuals who stalk are a heterogeneous group, in their behaviours, motivations and psychopathology, and are notoriously difficult to engage in intervention designed to help them. There are no hypotheses to fully explain stalking, no consensus on associated psychopathology, and there is little research exploring components of treatment effectiveness, stalking recidivism or protective factors. This chapter presents a broad overview of aspects for forensic psychologists and students to consider when working with clients who stalk.

What is stalking?

The Protection of Freedoms Act 2012 first introduced the term *stalking* within UK legislation by making amendments to the Protection from Harassment Act 1997. The Stalking Protection Act (2020) makes clear that stalking is a crime of pattern causing physical and/or psychological harm. Stalking is defined by the presence of a fixated and obsessive pattern of unwanted behaviours that cause, or could cause, fear or distress. The notion of fixation is pivotal; the inability of a person to abandon their pursuit is striking. *Normal behaviour* in contrast would feature an ability to give up on the pursuit where there is self-detriment or realisation that the goal is unachievable. Figure 11.1 (McEwan, 2019) illustrates the differences between stalking and 'normal behaviour' in relation to interactions with others.

Stalking consists of offline (such as following and approaching victims, or sending letters) and online behaviours (sending emails or gifts, text messaging, etc.), and often a mixture of both. Stalking differs from harassment in three ways: the context, the motivation of the perpetrator and the impact on the victim. Intrusive behaviours driven by a problem (i.e. a neighbour dispute) that tend to dissipate once a resolution has been reached are best conceptualised as harassment. Stalking is about the person. The perpetrator has formed a fixation on a person for which there is no resolution.

Most individuals who stalk do not use violence. Less than half of stalking victims are assaulted, and it is usually ex-partner stalkers who most readily use violence (McEwan et al., 2017). When they do, it is not usually serious, and only in rare cases, victims will

DOI: 10.4324/9781003017103-14

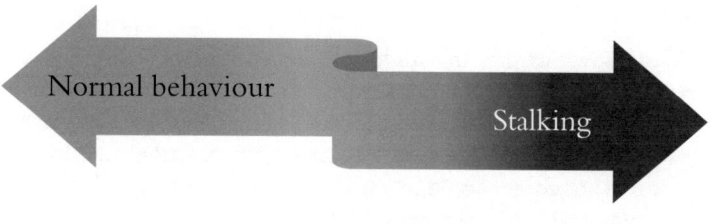

- Desires/goals can be satisfied or abandoned
- Socially appropriate behaviour
- Short-lived attempts to achieve goals

Normal behaviour

Stalking

- Desires/goals cannot be satisfied or abandoned
- Socially inappropriate behaviour
- Persistent attempts to achieve goals

Figure 11.1 Distinguishing stalking from normal behaviour

suffer serious or fatal violence (Wooster et al., 2016). Nonetheless, victims suffer high rates of traumatic stress because even in the absence of violence, fear is central to the victim's experience, exacerbated by persistent (over two weeks of duration) and recurrent stalking. Legal sanctions have little deterrent effect for many and as such reoffending rates are unacceptably high (McEwan et al., 2017).

Understanding stalking

The vast majority of those who stalk are male, and the majority of victims are female. Their average age when presenting to services is mid-30s. According to the National Stalking Helpline survey in 2018, over 50% are an ex-partner, and over 30% an acquaintance; therefore, they are usually known by their victim. The majority do not have a serious mental illness, and reports of psychopathology prevalence will differ between sample settings and typologies – we will explore these later. Personality disorder seems the most common psychopathology feature of individuals who stalk; however, this diagnosis represents vast heterogeneity in itself. As a group, stalkers present with wide-ranging psychopathology features, whilst some individuals do not meet criteria for any diagnoses (Nijdam-Jones et al., 2018). Studies of psychopathology also generally fail to clarify whether the condition under examination is causal, contributory or symptomatic of the toll the episode has taken on the perpetrator.

What takes people towards stalking?

Individuals who stalk do so for a variety of reasons. However, it is usually goal oriented and underpinned by complex psychology. The compelling need for validation from the target(s) and an associated sense of entitlement to this validation is common. Three scenarios precipitate stalking, the ending of a significant relationship, the potential for sex or a sexual relationship or a feeling of being mistreated (Mullen et al., 2009). Whilst no current theory comprehensively explains stalking, two popular theories are attachment theory (Ainsworth & Bowlby, 1991) and relational goal pursuit (RGP) theory (Cupach & Spitzberg, 2004).

Attachment theory

Attachment theory suggests that the underpinning motive of stalking is to restore self-worth. Stalkers more readily recall emotionally neglectful or inconsistent caregiver experiences (MacKenzie et al., 2008), creating an internalised negative self-view such as '*I am not good enough*' and a *preoccupied* survival response towards caregivers. In adulthood, the individual is prone to attachment anxiety and becomes emotionally dependent upon, and psychologically entangled with, significant others. The function is to gain affirmation of one's *self* through the acceptance of another, and achieving this sense of psychological safety is equitable to social survival, a changeable state worth becoming preoccupied with. Hypersensitivity to attachment rupture, however, is thought to contribute to coercive controlling behaviours in relationships, and stalking behaviour post-relationship in order to maintain relationship status. Stalkers typically have an underlying insecure, usually preoccupied, attachment style, and stalking is considered a psychopathology of attachment (Meloy, 2013).

Relational goal pursuit theory

RGP theory similarly asserts that those most likely to stalk will have an insecure, preoccupied attachment style. Within RGP theory, the *relationship* is the desired end goal. Attaining the relationship is linked to higher order meaning, to *life happiness* and *success*; therefore, it is necessary for maintaining one's sense of self-worth. When attainment or maintenance of this goal is thwarted, it is pursued more steadfastly given the linked importance. RGP theory advocates five facets in explaining stalking post-relationship (Brownhalls et al., 2019). *Goal-linking* inflates the importance of re-establishing the relationship, and the person stalking has a belief that the goal is achievable (*self-efficacy*), which influences persistence. Non-attainment causes *rumination* as the person stalking focuses on their distress, commensurate to the higher order goal of self-worth and happiness. Resultant negative feelings, *affective flooding*, further fuel the pursue-rejection cycle. According to RGP theory, it is thought that the preoccupying pursuit in those who stalk is such that the perpetrator does not accept or act upon obvious negative consequences towards themselves, or others. *Rationalisation* of continued pursuits in the face of repeated failure is their psychological mechanism to defend against the reality of rejection, wherein it becomes easier to focus on their own hurt caused by the rejecting partner.

Attachment theory and RGP theory share some similar aspects. Stalking is considered goal directed and functional for the psychological necessity of self-worth and the higher order relational goal of a sense of life happiness. Both theories seek to understand stalking as a symptom of the failure to self-regulate following the loss of an important relationship.

Motivational typologies

There is no such thing as a *typical stalker*. Whilst stalking behaviours can appear similar, the initiating and sustaining motivations, psychopathology features and risk factors of individuals that stalk differ between typologies. Mullen and colleagues (1999) developed a classification system for understanding the heterogeneity amongst stalkers, which intended to account for the initiating motivation, relationship to the victim and psychopathology features and give structure for risk assessment and risk management approaches (see Mullen et al., 2009). Understanding the typology of a client who stalks is crucial in making defensible decisions about risk management, including victim safety planning and formulating treatment approaches. Let's have a look at the five typologies of stalker and some case examples.

The 'rejected' typology

The 'rejected' stalker are the most prevalent, particularly within forensic settings, and are the most likely to use violence. They usually target an ex-partner following the breakdown of a relationship. The stalking becomes the connection substitute for the lost relationship and delays its acceptance, avoiding facing the distress. They seek to re-establish the relationship and can also appear to want revenge to compensate for their experience. They seek to salvage a damaged self-esteem and exude a sense of entitlement to the victim's attention, sometimes complicated by shared children or property. They may display jealousy and believe the relationship is irreplaceable. Research suggests that some post-relationship stalking extends coercive controlling behaviours or intimate partner violence experienced by victims within the former relationship (Senkans et al., 2017). However, post-relationship stalking also commences in the absence of abuse history, with separation being the trigger (McEwan et al., 2017). Rejected typology stalkers often embark on lengthy campaigns of stalking, showing concerning propensity for reoffending against the same or a new victim.

> *Syzmon stalked his ex-partner. For six weeks, he sent daily text messages and left a number of voicemails. The content was either vengeful or distressed, begging for reconciliation, saying he simply could not live without her. Syzmon tracked her movements, then confronted her one day at work demanding answers as to why she had been ignoring him. Frightened, she told him not to contact her anymore and rang the police. Syzmon complied for two days then began sending romantic messages. He sent her flowers at home, apologising and expressing his undying love. Syzmon spiralled negatively in his own distress, began drinking heavily and missing work. Under the influence of alcohol, he went to the victim's house to try one last time to re-establish their relationship. As he arrived, he saw another man leaving her house. Syzmon waited and then knocked the door and then tried to force entry. He was arrested.*

The 'intimacy seeker' typology

The 'intimacy seeker' targets acquaintances or strangers, often driven by fantasy and delusional disorder. The stalking is borne out of loneliness and a lack of intimacy, and they seek a loving and fulfilling relationship with the desired target or indulge the fantasy this relationship exists, to fill the void. Pursuing this fantasised relationship provides hope and gratification from the sense of being *in love*. This typology (along with the 'resentful') is the most likely to present with contributory delusions, thus more prevalent within forensic psychiatry services. They tend to embark on very lengthy stalking campaigns due to their fantasised connection to the victim.

Stephanie's victim was the local bank manager. Stephanie lacked a social network, had never had a lasting intimate relationship and yearned for a family and loving husband. She felt increasingly connected to the male bank manager through her visits. She would loiter and watch him go about his business and build knowledge by asking seemingly innocuous questions. However, this persisted for over three years and caused him and other staff concern. It escalated when she regularly created reasons why she needed the attention of the bank manager. By this point, she was often politely asked to leave the bank. On Valentine's Day, she left him a card and gift referring to their love for one another and their wonderful future together. Stephanie was visited by the police who instructed her not to make any further contact with him. She ignored this and soon noticed the victim's absence at the bank. She approached a new bank clerk and was told he was on paternity leave following the birth of his son. Enraged, Stephanie left a letter for him at the bank accusing him of leading her on, adding that his other girlfriend was not as good as her, and that the baby was probably not his. She suggested that he could come back to her and she would forgive him so they could continue their future together.

The 'resentful' typology

The 'resentful' stalker generally targets a representative of an organisation, an acquaintance or stranger. The stalking is precipitated by a sense of injustice or humiliation, and the behaviours are sustained due to a sense of righteousness. They feel justified in their actions as the perceived victim in the scenario. The stalking is grievance based and fundamental to gaining validation and a sense of power and control in the circumstances. The stalking can be fuelled by a delusional disorder and paranoid traits and can persist for lengthy periods.

When Belinda was made redundant, she struggled to cope. Her mental well-being deteriorated, and she had to sell her car, find cheaper accommodation to rent and her relationship suffered. She had always been socially isolated but enjoyed the routine of work. She always felt undervalued by her manager and they never really got on despite Belinda's efforts to ingratiate herself and do a good job. Belinda became convinced that it would have been the manager who suggested that she be made redundant during the companies downsizing review and felt aggrieved and humiliated that her efforts had not been recognised. She felt justified that someone would need to answer for the deterioration in her life and became fixated on exposing the manager for her unprofessionalism and discrimination. She began a campaign of stalking, relentlessly bombarding the company secretary and director daily with emails. She submitted freedom of information requests about the redundancy review process and any involvement from the manager. She threatened legal action and sought to have the manager fired and herself reinstated in the manager's role as a form of compensation. None of the company responses satisfied Belinda. As the campaign continued, the manager, the company secretary and the director became increasingly concerned by the malicious content and irrational demands, so contacted the police. Belinda was undeterred despite the legal sanctions issued.

The 'incompetent suitor' typology

The 'incompetent suitor' often targets acquaintances, sometimes strangers. The stalking is motivated by the hope of obtaining a date, a sexual encounter or to begin a relationship of some kind, usually in the context of their social isolation and loneliness. The stalker is hampered in their social and courtship skills by global functioning deficits, for example, low IQ, autistic or personality disorder traits. This typology of stalker is often deterred by initial interventions of being told to stop but can be subsequently prone to targeting new victims given their desire for a partner and lack of courtship skills. They are thought to be more common within community rather than forensic or psychiatry settings.

This typology can sometimes appear similar to the intimacy seeker, but they do form completely different subtypes. The intimacy seeker has a far greater level of fantasy-based psychopathology at play. At the core of their pursuit are unfounded beliefs in the existence of the relationship or belief that the relationship will ensue given their stoic belief in the eventual *perfect relationship* with their chosen target. Their use of fantasy is fulfilling in itself, and any counterevidence is swiftly disregarded. The incompetent suitor would like a date or a relationship but employs problematic, clumsy, persistent, intrusive and unskilled behaviours in an attempt to attain that.

> *Danny met the victim at a local community college who was his special educational needs mentor. They became friends and Danny hoped that this meant they could be more than this and eventually get married. Outside of this friendship, Danny had not maintained any other friendships, so this one was important to him. Danny then disclosed his romantic feelings for the victim and asked if they could have a relationship. The victim explained that she just wanted to be his friend. However, Danny thought it would be romantic to pursue her regardless. He would go wherever she would go at college and began showing up at her house and her local gym. He would politely and persistently ask for dates, which she refused. He wrote her a card stating that he wanted to take her for a lovely meal, that she should give him a chance, and said that 'guys are supposed to pursue their gals'. The victim was concerned that he would not take no for an answer and continued to intrude on her daily life so she contacted the police for advice. This had persisted for six weeks until the tutors at college and police met with Danny and told him he could not be friends with the victim anymore. Danny felt confused and upset and stopped contact with the victim. He felt lonely and depressed, but soon after he was assigned a new mentor.*

The 'predatory' typology

The 'predatory' stalker is usually male, targeting females and driven by sexual deviance. The stalking provides voyeuristic gratification. They gain satisfaction from following victims, accessing information about them and feeding fantasies by planning and mentally rehearsing a sexual and/or violent attack. This typology may show psychopathic traits and enjoy the sense of power and domination from the stalking. This typology of stalker is dangerous but thankfully rare.

> *Karl has a previous conviction for rape. His current offence involved identifying a female at the university campus close to his home and spending a number of weeks following her, understanding her movements. He would masturbate to thoughts of the female and started to plan how he could have sex with her and indulge his fantasies of sexual violence. Karl increasingly became more aroused at the prospect of carrying out the attacks as the days wore on. On occasions, he would let the victim know that he was watching, as he enjoyed scaring her. It made him feel powerful as he believed he had total control over what was to happen to her. In the following week, Karl carried out a sexual attack on her.*

Table 11.1 presents proportionate estimates of each typology within a UK stalking sample (Henley et al., 2020). Female clients presenting to this forensic psychiatry service were most likely to be intimacy seekers, whereas males were more commonly rejected types.

Assessment

Robust assessment, involving a bespoke case formulation, is the foundation to understanding stalking behaviour and associated risks. Through these structured and ideally collaborative processes, inferences about effective treatment and risk management strategies can be tailored to the individual. There are two structured professional judgement tools (see Chapter 4) that can be used with men and women who stalk. The first to be published was the **Guidelines for Stalking Assessment and Management** (SAM: Kropp et al., 2008). Factors within domains of 'Nature of Stalking', 'Perpetrator Risk Factors' and 'Victim Vulnerability Factors' are assessed. Evaluation studies suggest moderate-to-strong inter-rater reliability for item scores and risk judgements, good internal consistency and evidence of concurrent validity (Kropp et al., 2008). The only published study of the predictive validity of the SAM risk judgements, however, found that these did not predict stalking recidivism (Foellmi et al., 2016). The **Stalking Risk Profile** (SRP: MacKenzie et al., 2009) also attends to a combination of static and dynamic risk factors related to stalking. Evaluation studies indicate it has good internal consistency, inter-rater reliability (including for typology classification) and predictive validity (McEwan et al., 2018).

The SRP assessment incorporates typology classification, attending to risks for stalking violence (assessed in all cases, including identifying *red flags* which indicate serious and imminent risk), persistence (assessed when stalking is active), recurrence (assessed after a period of cessation of six months, for the same and possible new victim) and risk of psychosocial damage to the stalker (assessed in all cases), which has relevance to increased risk to victims. Stalking is targeted, and as such, unlike many forms of violence, this makes potential victims more identifiable. The risk of persistence is an important domain in stalking assessment given the cumulative impact on victims, and the aim of preventing stalking patterns becoming entrenched. Typologies of stalker most likely to persist with lengthy campaigns are intimacy seeker, resentful and sometimes rejected. Incompetent suitors (with new victims) and rejected (same or new victim) typology stalkers are most likely to reoffend.

In assessing stalkers, it is important to understand the individual's motivations to be able to ascertain ways to deconstruct the *pull* to this behaviour. The risks pertaining to both physical (stalking-related violence) and psychological harms (i.e. through including

Table 11.1 Estimated typology proportion by total sample and gender

Typology	% of total sample	% of males in sample	% of females in sample
Rejected	47	55	25
Intimacy seeker	36	25	50
Resentful	13	14	25
Incompetent suitor	2	4	0
Predatory	2	2	0

assessment of the likelihood of persistent and recurrent stalking episodes) require equal attention to appropriately protect victims. Risk assessments and risk management monitoring will likely be ongoing and dynamic processes. As research advances, SPJ tools will require further evaluation and revision.

ACTIVITY BOX 11.1

Now would be a good point to research these two tools.

- What static and dynamic risk factors do they consist of?
- What research evidence underpins the risk factors?
- Compare and contrast the tools and critically evaluate their application in varied forensic settings (i.e. during police investigations versus assessing clients in prison)

Intervention

Unlike other areas covered in this book, there are no specific interventions for people who stalk. Mullen and colleagues (1999) asserted over two decades ago that abstinence from stalking following prosecution is assisted by a directive therapeutic relationship, yet the issue of successful intervention still remains an emerging field. Given high reoffending rates and the devastation stalking causes, it would be unethical to do nothing other than legally sanction people. To help strengthen the prospect of cessation and future desistance from stalking, forensic psychologists need to make defensible decisions regarding managing risks and proposing treatment intervention. Best practice is to adopt a risk assessment, formulation-led and multidisciplinary approach to treatment intervention and risk management, reflecting the varied needs of those who stalk.

Treatment intervention is likely to warrant psychological input given the predisposing vulnerabilities and psychosocial skills deficits associated with stalking. Forensic psychologists will need to carefully plan bespoke interventions, adapted for any presenting psychopathology, responsivity and psychological vulnerabilities (i.e. emotionally unstable traits, low IQ, autistic spectrum disorder, insecure attachment styles and narcissistic vulnerability). Stalking motivated by major mental illness is believed more treatable (i.e. psychiatric intervention with medication can halt stalking behaviours) than stalking contextual to a personality disorder (Meloy, 2013). Treatment is considered to require long-term and in-depth intervention where stalking is underpinned by personality traits, given their aetiology and longevity (McEwan & Strand, 2013). Table 11.2 provides a suggested structure for the stages of *psychological* assessment and intervention planning which would form part of the multi-agency approach. Within the assessment stage, considerations for motivational typology, psychopathology and responsivity factors are incorporated. Women who stalk have been found not to differ from men in respect of intensity, duration, behaviours, issuance of threats or use of violence; therefore, assessments, interventions, and management strategies will equally apply (Strand & McEwan, 2012).

Table 11.2 Suggested stages for psychological intervention

Stage	Key components
Risk and responsivity assessments	Assessments using appropriate tools to identify levels of risk, static factors, dynamic factors (treatment needs) and responsivity features. Refer to psychiatric assessments if applicable
Risk management planning	Consult on multi-agency risk management strategies, including victim safety planning, as outlined previously
Psycho-education with clients	Provide clear and non-negotiable terms of reference regarding what constitutes stalking, discuss components of stalking legislation and highlight these within the client's own offending
Initial case formulation	Build therapeutic alliance, discuss outcomes of assessments and develop an initial collaborative case formulation (ongoing)
Strengthen willingness for change	Use psycho-education highlighting key aspects of the case formulation that relate to the client and validate their experiences Employ techniques to develop therapeutic alliance and willingness, such as motivational interviewing
Treatment plan	Plan treatment intervention based on identified dynamic risk factors, responsivity features, case formulation and willingness Consider treatment modalities and dose
Deliver treatment intervention	Process-based and skills-focused activity
Review and evaluate	Build in regular reviews of progress against outcome measures and evaluate case formulation. Feed this into the multi-agency team

Practitioner contacts of any kind that adopt compassion-focused and trauma-informed approaches have benefits in nurturing therapeutic alliance. Direct confrontation of the problem and shaming interactions will provoke defensive and possibly offence-supportive responses. However, it is important from the outset to have a clear, shared understanding of what constitutes stalking, what legal sanctions are in place and what the *rules* within the therapeutic engagement are. Being understood and validated in their experiences through relating to or being related to by others is powerful. It allows the practitioner to harness the notion that the offence-driving thoughts and feelings are attributable to their brain development and interpreted life experiences, therefore, not entirely of their own conscious making. Yet, it also makes clear that resultant stalking behaviours are harmful to all and completely in their control, thus their responsibility to change. Collaborative case formulations are encouraged for relating with clients and for them to understand their functioning in this way, identifying that the problematic behaviours are leading them away from achieving their higher order goals. Helping clients learn, practice and hone emotion regulation will improve opportunities for core treatment engagement later on. It is also a crucial personal and interpersonal skill related to the stalking. A formulation-led approach can provide a useful vehicle for agreeing treatment needs to assist stalking-specific goal disengagement, in favour of improving possibilities for achieving higher order goals.

Practitioners will draw on their own skills set as to what treatment modality they will employ for developing willingness to change and delivering core treatment. Although it is expected that psychosocial skills training, for example, would also accompany more process-based intervention to identify, monitor, and address deep rooted inner scripts that predispose the individual to stalking in the first place, improving the stalker's ability to self-regulate their sense of self-worth and emotions is fundamental. Mindful of a lack

Table 11.3 Suggested treatment areas to consider per typology (Purcell & McEwan, 2018)

Typology	Suggested treatment areas
REJECTED	Moving from preoccupation and angry rumination to acceptance of loss, address jealousy
INTIMACY SEEKER	Treat any psychotic illness, cognitive shifting from preoccupation with their love interest
RESENTFUL	Few accept treatment, treat any suspicious/paranoid disorders or related personality traits, look for face-saving withdrawal and focus on personal impact of own behaviour in pursuit of cause
INCOMPETENT SUITOR	Build awareness and empathy, reinforce negative outcomes and improve social skills
PREDATORY	Anti-libidinal medication and psychological therapy

of hypothesis- and empirical-led treatment modalities for intervening with those who stalk, Purcell and McEwan (2018) summarised key components for inclusion in treatment plans. They highlighted some aspects common to all stalkers for consideration plus bespoke approaches with the various typologies as outlined in Table 11.3. The common features to address are (i) emotional dysregulation, (ii) rumination, (iii) attitudes, beliefs and values (e.g. targeting offence-supportive and antisocial attitudes and personality traits maintaining stalking), (iv) interpersonal and self-management skills and (v) contextual, social and practical factors (e.g. shared children, workplace or neighbourhood and developing a new routine and [re-]establishing hobbies).

In the United Kingdom, offending behaviours programmes exist for individuals convicted of violence, intimate partner violence and sexual offences, but they remain largely unsuitable for the majority of stalkers who do not display these behaviours and who may have very different motivations. Whilst such offences can form part of some stalking episodes and those eligible may benefit, successful completion of these programmes is unlikely to address all the drivers of stalking behaviour (Purcell & McEwan, 2018). They could, however, form part of a more holistic treatment intervention. Given the challenges working with, and the huge variation amongst individuals who stalk, it is crucial that practitioners take a risk and formulation-led, multi-agency, collaborative and flexible approach to individual differences in offering treatment. Interventions that aid people in ceasing and desisting will likely take time and patience, given the roots of the behaviours and the complexity of contributory factors. Further, reviewing and evaluating progress against outcome measures within the multi-agency team is important. Peer support, regular information sharing and management of practitioner bias when considering the ongoing risk assessment function can all be upheld in this forum. Resource input and legal sanctioning in its entirety should mirror the risks posed by the individual stalking.

Conclusion

UK legislation is improving, and awareness of stalking as a crime and its devastating impact on victims is slowly increasing. Forensic psychologists and others have a responsibility to continue to educate others, particularly our clients in forensic practice, to ensure they understand their behaviour as stalking and ensure appropriate risk assessments take place swiftly to help protect victims. Treatment and risk management approaches require bespoke development and skilled implementation as part of the wider multi-agency approach, using the legal sanctions at our disposal to manage high reoffending rates. The evidence base needs developing for this client group, and forensic psychologists need to contribute to developing the research that helps us to understand effective approaches to assessment, intervention and risk management.

Recommended further activity

You are encouraged to access the HMPPS Forensic Psychology Podcast (https://pod.link/1533101974) and listen to the following episode which explores concepts discussed in this chapter:

Episode 6: Let's call it stalking [19/11/2020]

Learning outcomes

When you have completed this chapter, you should be able to:

1   Define stalking using key terms (fixated, obsessive, unwanted, repeated, causing alarm or distress)
2   Understand who stalks and why people stalk (demographic and psychopathology features and key theories for stalking)
3   Have an awareness of appropriate risk assessment tools and the domains of risk to consider
4   Describe motivational typologies
5   Have an awareness of current practitioner challenges, ethical issues and research gaps relating to those who stalk
6   Begin to consider appropriate treatment and risk management approaches with those who stalk

Key concepts and terms

*   Stalking
*   Heterogeneity
*   Attachment theory
*   Relational goal pursuit theory
*   Psychopathology
*   Typologies
*   Bespoke treatment approaches

Sample essay questions

*   How well do existing psychological theories explain stalking? What are the similarities, differences, limitations and gaps?
*   What are the motivational typologies proposed by Mullen et al. (1999), and why might it be important for practitioners to apply these when assessing the risk of stalking and planning treatment interventions?

Recommended further reading

Mullen, P. E., Pathé, M., & Purcell, R. (2009). *Stalkers and their victims* (2nd ed.). Cambridge University Press.

Purcell, R., & McEwan, T. (2018). Treatment approaches for stalking. In C. Ireland, J. Ireland, & P. Birch (Eds.), *Violent and sexual offenders: Assessment, treatment and management* (pp. 428–444). Routledge.

References

Ainsworth, M. D. S., & Bowlby, J. (1991). An ethological approach to personality development. *American Psychologist, 46,* 331–341.

Brownhalls, J., Duffy, A., Eriksson, L., & Barlow, F. K. (2019). Reintroducing rationalization: A study of relational goal pursuit theory of intimate partner obsessive relational intrusion. *Journal of Interpersonal Violence,* 886260518822339. Advance online publication.

Cupach, W., & Spitzberg, B. (2004). *The dark side of relationship pursuit: From attraction to obsession and stalking.* Lawrence Erlbaum Associates.

Foellmi, M. C., Rosenfeld, B., & Galietta, M. (2016). Assessing risk for recidivism in individuals convicted of stalking offenses: Predictive validity of the guidelines for stalking assessment and management. *Criminal Justice and Behavior, 43*(5), 600–616.

Henley, S., Underwood, A., & Farnham, F. (2020). National stalking clinic: A UK response to assessing and managing stalking behavior. *Psycho-Criminological Approaches to Stalking Behavior: An International Perspective,* 335.

Kropp, P. R., Hart, S. D., & Lyon, D. R. (2008). *Guidelines for stalking assessment and management (SAM): User manual.* ProActive ReSolutions Incorporated.

MacKenzie, R. D., McEwan, T. E., Pathé, M. T., James, D. V., Ogloff, J. R. P., & Mullen, P. E. (2009). *Stalking risk profile: Guidelines for the assessment and management of stalkers.* Stalkinc Pty Ltd and Monash University.

MacKenzie, R. D., Mullen, P. E., Ogloff, J. R., McEwan, T. E., & James, D. V. (2008). Parental bonding and adult attachment styles in different types of stalker. *Journal of Forensic Sciences, 53*(6), 1443–1449.

McEwan, T. E. (2019). *Resentful stalking: Research update.* XIII International Conference Grudges and Grievances. Cambridge, UK, September 19–20.

McEwan, T. E., Daffern, M., MacKenzie, R. D., & Ogloff, J. R. P. (2017). Risk factors for stalking violence, persistence, and recurrence. *The Journal of Forensic Psychiatry & Psychology, 28*(1), 38–56.

McEwan, T. E., Shea, D. E., Daffern, M., MacKenzie, R. D., Ogloff, J. R., & Mullen, P. E. (2018). The reliability and predictive validity of the Stalking Risk Profile. *Assessment, 25*(2), 259–276.

McEwan, T. E., & Strand, S. (2013). The role of psychopathology in stalking by adult strangers and acquaintances. *Australian and New Zealand Journal of Psychiatry, 47*(6), 546–555.

Meloy, J. R. (2013). Stalking. In J. A. Siegel & P. J. Saukko (Eds.), *Encyclopedia of forensic sciences* (2nd ed., pp. 202–205). Academic Press.

Mullen, P. E., Pathé, M., & Purcell, R. (2009). *Stalkers and their victims* (2nd ed.). Cambridge University Press.

Mullen, P. E., Pathé M., Purcell, R., & Stuart, G. W. (1999). Study of stalkers. *American Journal of Psychiatry, 156*(8), 1244–1249.

Nijdam-Jones, A., Rosenfeld, B., Gerbrandij, J., Quick, E., & Galietta, M. (2018). Psychopathology of stalking offenders: Examining the clinical, demographic, and stalking characteristics of a community-based sample. *Criminal Justice and Behavior, 45*(5), 712–731.

Office for National Statistics. (2019). Crime in England and Wales: Year ending June 2019. Published online: *Office for National Statistics.* https://www.ons.gov.uk/releases/crimeinengland andwalesyearendingjune2019

Purcell, R., & McEwan, T. (2018). Treatment approaches for stalking. In C. Ireland, J. Ireland, & P. Birch (Eds.), *Violent and sexual offenders: Assessment, treatment and management* (pp. 428–444). Routledge.

Senkans, S., McEwan, T. E., & Ogloff, J. R. (2017). Assessing the link between intimate partner violence and post relationship stalking: A gender-inclusive study. *Journal of interpersonal violence*, 0886260517734859.

Strand, S., & McEwan, T. E. (2012). Violence among female stalkers. *Psychological Medicine*, *42*(3), 545–555.

Wooster, L., James, D. V., & Farnham, F. R. (2016). Stalking, harassment and aggressive/intrusive behaviours towards general practitioners:(2) associated factors, motivation, mental illness and effects on GPs. *The Journal of Forensic Psychiatry & Psychology*, *27*(1), 1–20.

12 Terrorism, extremism and radicalisation

Zainab Al-Attar

Summary

The aim of this chapter is to provide a broad synthesis of the existent theory and research that informs our understanding of the psychology of terrorism, extremism and radicalisation, proposing that such theories lead to four types of pathways or motivational trajectories for terrorist offending. Many limitations of the existent research and theory are reviewed, before considering the practice implications of the research and theory.

Introduction

It is hard to think of a crime that is more socially impactful and salient than terrorism, with such salience creating legal, societal and governmental focus on understanding and reducing the threat posed by terrorism. It is therefore not surprising that psychologists have played their role in contributing to analyses of, and responses to, terrorism. As well as being of academic interest, in the United Kingdom, psychologists working in clinical, criminal justice and educational settings are bound by Prevent Duty (HM Government, 2015), at times necessitating their direct contribution to the assessment and reduction of terrorism risk. In most jurisdictions, terrorism is dealt with as a criminal offence, and as a result, terrorist offenders as well as other groups of offenders who raise concerns around potential risk of terrorism may come into contact with forensic psychologists. This complex and often emotionally and politically charged crime demands that psychologists develop the knowledge and expertise to recognise, evaluate and communicate highly complex information, often of a very sensitive nature and which has significant implications for the public. One of the many challenges forensic psychologists face is the acquisition of knowledge in a field that is relatively underdeveloped empirically, when compared to knowledge on other offender groups, their risk and rehabilitation. Nevertheless, psychology, alongside other disciplines such as psychiatry, sociology, criminology and the social, political, behavioural and security sciences has made a contribution to how terrorist behaviour is understood and whilst this has not always been confined to forensic psychology, the contributions clearly have the most significance for forensic psychologists.

Definitions

Whilst the term terrorism conjures up very clear feelings, its actual definition is not as universally clear, due to different states defining terrorism differently, at different times. For forensic psychological purposes, the legal definition adopted by the country in which

DOI: 10.4324/9781003017103-15

the psychologist practices is normally used to base decisions around which behaviour is classified as terrorism. In the United Kingdom, the CPS defines **terrorism** as:

> *The use or threat of action, both in and outside of the UK, designed to influence any international government organisation or to intimidate the public. It must also be for the purpose of advancing a political, religious, racial or ideological cause.*

(CPS, 2020)

Other terms that are often used interchangeably with terrorism, sometimes unhelpfully, are 'extremism' and 'radicalisation'. The UK Government defines **extremism** as the '*vocal or active opposition to fundamental British values, including democracy, the rule of law, individual liberty and mutual respect and tolerance of different faiths and beliefs. Extremism also includes calls for death of members of the armed forces*' (HM Government, 2015). **Radicalisation** is defined as '*the process by which a person comes to support terrorism and extremist ideologies associated with terrorist groups*' (HM Government, 2015). Forensic psychologists may be tasked with understanding and helping to divert the process of radicalisation and/or engagement with extremism and terrorism. Throughout this chapter, the focus will be on terrorism and our psychological understanding of its drivers.

Terrorism research and theories

There are a number of reasons why in spite of significant interest in terrorism from academic psychologists, theories of terrorism remain very limited in scope and empirical testing, leaving us far from a developed psychological science of terrorism. First, terrorism is defined differently across states and times, making a universal, longitudinal measure of terrorist behaviour impractical. Second, terrorist offenders who survive their offences are often inaccessible to researchers. As a result, the field has been at best based on small-scale studies of narrow samples of terrorists (e.g. one ideological group), indirect proxies of terrorism (e.g. attitudes that endorse terrorist acts) or desktop pseudoclinical analyses of hypothesised mind sets of publicly known cases, often using open-source information. Nevertheless, there are some good foundations for theoretically informed hypotheses on why individuals commit terrorism. These theoretical foundations will now be summarised.

Rather than providing a chronological review of the theoretical concepts that shed light on psychological drivers for terrorism, I shall instead break down the theoretical contributions of psychology into the different areas of psychology, including social psychology, moral reasoning and political psychology, cognitive psychology, behavioural psychology, personality and individual differences and abnormal and clinical psychology. Then, I shall attempt to consolidate the different theoretical contributions into a four-pathway model of motivations to engage in terrorism, which lends itself to four distinct practical, rehabilitative approaches. Finally, the methodological limitations of the field will be broadly reviewed, before reflecting on some of the key ethical debates that are raised in this field.

The contributions made by psychology

Each field of psychology has contributed to our understanding of the factors that can contribute to an individual's pathway to terrorism. There is no one theory that purports to explain all levels of terrorism nor should any one field of psychology ever be viewed as explaining all levels of the psychology of terrorism. Instead, each field within psychology contributes to a complex picture of interacting factors that come to shape how and why an individual comes to commit terrorist acts. With this in mind, I will provide some illustrative examples of how each field of psychology has contributed to one or more levels of analysis of terrorist behaviour and comment on how these levels interact and influence each other to move the individual along a pathway to terrorism. Some theories were originally proposed to explain other forms of behaviour but have subsequently been applied to terrorism, whilst other theories were specifically developed to explain terrorism. The current overview is not an exhaustive account of all psychological hypotheses and theories published. Instead, it provides examples of how each area of psychology has begun to contribute to our understanding of terrorism.

Social psychology

Social psychological theories of identity and groups have made an important contribution to our understanding of why individuals may join terrorist groups and how group identity and psychology can shift the individual's worldviews and willingness to carry out acts they would otherwise not carry out without the psychological effect of the group. It is noteworthy that in the modern context, a group may be online as well as offline. In each case, identity needs, such as the need to belong, to have meaning, to be distinct and attain self-worth, are central to a purposeful existence, well-being and psychological survival (Baumeister & Leary, 1995). When such needs are unfulfilled or the individual has a crisis of identity, lowered self-worth or sense of alienation, joining social groups may redress such needs (Tajfel, 1982; Turner et al., 1987). This includes terrorist groups (Silke, 2008). An individual may derive a sense of meaning, belonging, esteem, purpose and distinctiveness from their membership of a terrorist group and their engagement in terrorism on behalf of the group. Identification with a feared, fearless and powerful group or cause can overcome feelings of fear, disempowerment and inferiority and afford a new social image of a hero or warrior (Whitehead, 2005).

Once an individual identifies with a group, they may perceive their ingroup to be more different from outgroups, overestimate the positive qualities of their ingroup and the negative qualities of the outgroup, with such demarcations and generalisations fuelling positive feelings towards the ingroup and negative feelings towards the outgroup. The world comes to be perceived as comprising an ingroup that is morally superior and to whom the individual is bonded and an outgroup to which threat and immorality are attributed, justifying the ingroup's violent defence against the outgroup. The more the individual becomes socially isolated in their group, the more dependent on the group's social support and suspicious of the outgroup they may become, strengthening their defensiveness of the ingroup. Once an individual is strongly bonded with the group and derives a strong sense of identity from it, they may experience 'identity fusion' whereby their identity merges with the group's and they feel a bond akin to a familial bond, the strength of which may facilitate a willingness to sacrifice (Whitehouse et al., 2014). This group's psychological effect may lead to conformity to even the most extreme and violent of group norms and expectations. Schwartz et al. (2009) argued that identity processes that cause the group identity to override the individual's identity operate at the cultural (or religious), social and personal levels and may lead the individual to override their individual identity, self-interest and morality.

Moral reasoning and political psychology

Morality is central to most terrorist narratives and justifications. Typically, at the heart of terrorist causes is the need to redress immoral acts and injustices and to express and bring to light moral outrage, shock or grievance. An injustice may relate to violence and loss of life, loss of land or discrimination and disadvantage whilst threat may be to one's moral values, safety, dignity or identity. In all these instances, terrorism comes to be viewed as a necessary and often the only course of action to redress threat and injustice and to bring about political, social or moral change. Terrorist acts are portrayed as morally necessary, dutiful, courageous and glorious. In order to inhibit any empathy towards the victims or any moral guilt at the harm caused, a process of 'moral disengagement' occurs through attributing blame to the victims, dehumanising them and moving away from one's individual sense of responsibility towards diffusion of responsibility into the wider group. These psychological processes enable individuals who may not otherwise endorse or tolerate violence to commit violent acts against victims without moral deterrents or inhibitions (Bandura, 2004). Other factors that lift inhibitions may include strong moral emotions such as anger, disgust, hatred, indignation, humiliation, fear or insecurity, which may further drive the desire for revenge (Borum, 2004; Silke, 2008).

Some theories shed light on the individual's moral reasoning by examining how they cognitively process information and make decisions, with one theory suggesting that individuals with low levels of 'integrative complexity' (IC) view the world in absolutist black-and-white terms and cannot process and consolidate multiple, complex pieces of information (Guttieri et al., 1995; Suedfeld & Bluck, 1988). This makes them more susceptible to the black-and-white, absolutist, reductionist interpretations of injustices/ threats ('single narratives') used by terrorist groups (Razzaque, 2008). This reduces the blame for injustices/threats to one group/enemy and assigns the solution to one, binary course of action. Narratives used by terrorist groups often portray the enemy in a simplified negative way and the ingroup in a simplified positive way, which reduces the threat to a single source that is then felt to be controllable through a single method. This resonates with individuals who cannot tolerate grey areas and multiple explanations and layers of reasoning for injustices or their solution. This explains why some individuals are more susceptible to extremist moral and political ideologies than others.

It is important to recognise that not all individuals engaging in politically expressed terrorism are themselves driven by moral or political goals. Some may be driven by their need to express their disillusionment with or distinctiveness from the mainstream (Post, 2005). In such cases, moral reasoning may not drive the individual even though they may portray it to do so. Even in such cases, thought processes that incentivise the individual to carry out such acts are clearly important to identify, making cognitive psychology key to understanding all terrorist motives.

Cognitive psychology

As highlighted previously, ideological justifications of terrorist acts may be central in an individual's commitment to terrorism (Sageman, 2004). Internal representations of the self and enemy, the collective positive image of the terrorist group and construal of the terrorist act as heroic, courageous and as part of a grand design, alongside shifting of focus away from the harm to self and victims (Beck, 2002) can all form the basis for cognitive justifications for and positive emotions towards terrorism. In this regard, cognitions, beliefs and attitudes form key drivers for terrorist behaviour (Kruglanski et al., 2009). Cognitive processes can play a key part in lifting moral inhibitions. Maikovich (2005) argued that in order to eliminate any discomfort ('cognitive dissonance') arising from the conflict between terrorism and the individual's moral views, the individual can either lift their behavioural inhibitions through conditioning and repeat training that make the terrorist violence automated (and executed without thinking) or deploy 'cognitive distortions' or cognitive manipulations of reality to reconstrue terrorism as moral. One example of such a cognitive distortion, for example, would be to construe the victims as indirectly culpable in an injustice or to construe violence as a necessary evil that is the moral responsibility of the 'enemy' who is being targeted. Terrorist groups often design propaganda with a 'dominant narrative' that creates such distorted realities, perceptions and beliefs (Canter, 2006).

Group rhetoric can also create 'collective' and 'social' cognitions that may include 'group think', a psychological process that leads group members to underestimate the moral consequences of their actions and which creates an illusion of invincibility (McCormick, 2003). Finally, when one's group endorses immoral acts and distorted beliefs, these can then seem normalised, and hence, distorting one's beliefs into thinking terrorism is normal and acceptable, further diminishing moral inhibitions.

There are psychological factors and processes that can render some individuals more susceptible to terrorist propaganda and ideology and to information on threat. Individuals may become susceptible to ideas around injustice/threat and the necessity of terrorism at times when they are searching for meaning or undergoing changes in their lives that leave them open to new ideas and explanations of the world. This is referred to as 'cognitive openings' and may constitute a transient cognitive susceptibility. Another cognitive susceptibility factor may be immersion in a closed, controlling group alongside isolation from people outside the group. The individual may become increasingly dependent on, uncritical and trusting of the group and mistrustful of people and information from outside the group. This may lead the individual to become more cognitively receptive to the group's beliefs and attitudes (Sageman, 2004). Finally, processing bias and less critical thinking may be associated with threat and the fight-or-flight response in the brain, which means when individuals feel more threatened in their lives, or when threat narratives generate an emotional and neurobiological response in them, they are more likely to remain focused on threat cues (e.g. propaganda) and become less critical in their thinking and less broad in their information processing.

Whilst not always presented as 'cognitive' theories, several psychological theories have been applied to terrorism to explain how beliefs come to drive behaviour. Ajzen and Fishbein's (2005) theory of reasoned action has been used to explain how positive attitudes to terrorism, beliefs that terrorism will be met with social approval and a perception that one can successfully carry out terrorism could shift the individual's subjective norms from mainstream condemnation of terrorism to acceptance of terrorism as socially acceptable, noble and even necessary. It is this shift in beliefs that drives intention and readiness by shaping positive beliefs about terrorism and lifting inhibitions against it. One implication of this theory is that social learning may impact an individual's beliefs and cognitive susceptibility to terrorism.

Behavioural psychology/learning theory

The effect of terrorism on society arises from a learnt association between certain methods of attack and fear that becomes vicariously classically conditioned to it. Such fear is then sustained through the anticipation of future attacks, leading people to experience fear beyond a terrorist event and alter their behavioural routines in order to avoid future threat (Embry, 2007). As well as explaining how society learns to respond to terrorism, learning theories also contribute to explaining why terrorists adopt the methods and ideologies they do. Terrorist methods are often learnt and instrumental, goal-directed behaviours. Technological methods and modus operandi used by terrorists are learnt from past attacks, other groups or instructional materials, explaining why certain methods are used often (Canter, 2006), at times in a copy-cat fashion of successive attacks that use similar methods. These processes of social learning, vicarious learning, conditioning and associations between terrorism and rewards apply to both the methods as well as the values and beliefs of terrorist groups (Saper, 1988). Ideologies and methods that are learnt, reinforced and come to be associated with reward can be strengthened. In summary, behavioural psychology contributes to shedding light on the perpetration of and reaction to terrorism.

Whilst immediate rewards such as social identity, esteem and emotional validation or release may reinforce an individual's engagement in terrorism by generating positive reinforcement or positive feelings and negative reinforcement or removal of negative feelings, Crenshaw (2000) purports that deeper, more abstract and long-term rewards such as personal meaning may be more rewarding than immediate tangible rewards. 'Higher order' rewards as well as social support and positive feelings associated with ideas of nobility and honour all constitute deeper rewards that may be stronger than the punishing effects of terrorism (e.g. injury, prospect of death or imprisonment). The idea of propagating a worthwhile ideology or being part of an act that outlives the individual may act as potent rewards that explain why individuals may sacrifice their immediate personal interest. This is consistent with Bandura's concept of 'intrinsic reward'. However, all individuals don't find the same reward value from such behaviour nor do they all act out their vicarious learning. Clearly, there are many individual factors that determine why some individuals seek and act upon such rewards and others do not.

Personality and individual differences

Some personality traits or types have been argued to be more susceptible to supporting extremist or anti-establishment ideologies, to blindly following group leaders and submitting to group control. Adorno et al. (1950) and Altemeyer (2004) proposed several traits that collectively make up the 'authoritarian' personality, with the latter hypothesising that two subtypes are of relevance, namely authoritarian dominants and submissives. Authoritarians have a preference for absolutist beliefs and strong leaders, with dominants seeking such leadership and fearmongering to sustain their dominance and submissives uncritically following such leaders and being prone to panic and fear. Such personalities have been suggested to be more inclined towards political and religious conservatism whilst authoritarian and foreclosed individuals have been linked with terrorism (Schwartz et al., 2009). This is because such personalities are dogmatic, rigid and unlikely to consider others' views and are less compassionate and less able to maintain their own esteem and regulate their emotions. They prefer, and follow, strong and dictatorial leaders, subscribe to obedience and are driven to prove they are right. These are all traits that may find dogmatic terrorist ideologies and hierarchical terrorist groups that seek to prove their righteousness and disregard others' views, appealing.

Suicide bombers have been reported to exhibit avoidant and dependent personalities that made them more susceptible to social influence (Merari et al., 2009). Terrorist groups and ideologies have also been proposed to appeal to those who view themselves as superior and crave status (Schwartz et al., 2009), namely narcissistic personalities. This trait has been proposed to drive engagement in terrorism when humiliation or rejection causes a narcissistic injury or wound, whereby joining terrorist groups and causes then restores status and redresses such injury (Clark, 1983). Alternatively, an individual may have an inherently heightened need for status, dominance and superiority and terrorist groups or causes fulfil such needs (Silke, 2008). Narcissistic and other personalities may be attracted to specific roles within terrorist groups rather than all aspects of terrorism. Strentz (1988) identified three personality types which he argued are attracted to three types of roles. Narcissistic and paranoid personalities are attracted to 'leader' roles and have vision and intellectual purpose whilst projecting inadequacy onto society. Antisocial personalities, often with criminal histories, are 'opportunist' members who act as the muscle of their group. Finally, inadequate personalities, often young, 'idealistic', with naïve views of social problems, may become ordinary members. The aforementioned personality traits may in some individuals be severe enough to amount to disordered personality, our understanding of which comes from clinical/abnormal psychology.

Abnormal and clinical psychology

The terrorism literature has gone through shifts in focus from terrorists being viewed as mentally disordered, then recognised to have very low levels of psychopathology and to be 'normal' and then in more recent times recognised to be a diverse population in which some subgroups show heightened prevalence of some mental illnesses (Gill & Corner, 2017). Whilst there are many publications that seek to debate prevalence of different diagnoses, there remains limited evidence on any one clinical profile that is associated with susceptibility to terrorism. Overall, the literature converges on two key points, first that many traditional terrorist groups require psychologically healthy, stable, self-disciplined and resilient individuals to carry out their clandestine and well-planned activities, and second, that in some cases, individuals with mental illness may either be recruited if their vulnerability is an asset or at least inconsequential or else self-radicalise. The precise role that different aspects of mental illness may have played in driving pathways to terrorism has not been established by the research. Recent literature has generated hypotheses about the role that may be played by specific symptoms of autism spectrum disorder, personality disorders, mood disorders, psychotic disorders, PTSD and alcohol and drug use (Al-Attar, 2019). It would appear that some subpopulations of terrorists who exhibit mental illness also have histories of criminality, and it is therefore important that theories of general offending are considered when understanding the drivers for such individuals.

Criminological and forensic psychology

Some terrorists may have a juvenile or adult criminal history and problematic behaviour (Weenik, 2015). Terrorism may either afford a replacement identity (as an act of moral redemption or seeking new social groups) or else meet similar needs to general criminality. Like other crimes that afford danger, intensity and risk, terrorism can appeal to individuals due to its sensational, risky or clandestine nature, affording a sense of adventure, excitement, thrill, adrenaline, hedonistic intensity and macho social status amongst peers (Silke, 2008; Bartlett et al., 2010).

In most jurisdictions, terrorism is classified as a crime. The Good Lives Model (Ward & Stewart, 2003) construes any type of criminal offending as a maladaptive means of expressing and meeting adaptive, universal human needs. In this respect, this model can encapsulate elements purported by different fields of psychology to contribute to terrorism, including identity and moral needs. Engagement in terrorist groups or causes may afford a sense of community, companionship, relatedness, inner peace (e.g. alleviation of guilt or distress) and mastery (e.g. feeling skilled or superior).

Finally, some individuals engage in terrorism for purely criminal gains, such as financial or material gains or as part of criminal groups and identities (Post, 2007; Horgan, 2009). In some instances, individuals may seek opportunities to carry out violence and terrorism is opportune (Hoffman, 2006). Prolific violent offenders have been reported to advance attitudes that support crime and are unfavourable to convention (Strand et al., 1999), and these attitudes may extend to terrorism in some instances (e.g. when criminal peers endorse terrorism or it becomes an opportune means to defy convention). In some instances, terrorism and traditional crime may form a reciprocal relationship whereby each group facilitates the other's criminal and practical interests. Narcoterrorism is one such example whereby drug and organised crime groups and terrorist groups facilitate one another's activities in order to survive and succeed operationally, either in the community or in prison. In all the aforementioned cases, traditional theories of criminal behaviour may contribute to explaining involvement in terrorism. Of course, there will always be individuals whose terrorist acts cannot be accounted for by such theories, and it is important to emphasise that there are many other theories and these continue to emerge and develop.

Other theories

There are many more theories of terrorism. These include psychoanalytic, sociocultural, neurocognitive, organisational and political psychological theories. In addition to the drivers for terrorism, psychologists have also actively contributed to understanding the effects of terrorism and informed policy and government messaging and communication about the terrorism threat. Whilst these, and the theories reviewed in this chapter make up a vast array of psychological theories, arising from many thousands of analyses and studies, this ethically complex field remains in its early development and is hindered by many methodological limitations. These limitations will be briefly summarised later in this chapter.

Synthesis of theories – the four pathways

In addition to the aforementioned theories of the drivers to terrorism, there are many theories that seek to explain the 'pathways' that individuals follow as these factors unfold over a period of cognitive and emotional changes, socialisation and operational training. These theories, often labelled radicalisation and pathway theories, are limited in their empirical basis and generalisability to the diverse populations of terrorist offenders. They also rarely consolidate the broad range of psychological concepts and findings in the field of terrorism. A consolidation of the broad range of theories of terrorism reviewed in the current chapter would suggest that there appears to be four different types of motivational trajectories or pathways that could lead individuals to commit acts of terrorism. These four pathways are outlined in Box 12.1.

BOX 12.1　PATHWAYS TO COMMITTING ACTS OF TERRORISM

Ideological/moral-political pathway: Terrorism is driven primarily by moral, political or religious beliefs, goals and emotions.

Psychosocial pathway: Terrorism is driven primarily by social group processes and psychosocial needs such as identity, status, meaning and belonging.

Mental health pathway: Terrorism is driven by an aspect of mental illness or its subjective experience.

Criminal pathway: Terrorism is driven by opportunism, criminal gains, immediate material or hedonistic rewards.

Several of the four pathways may converge and interact for a given individual, with each pathway having primacy at any given point in time. Pathways are neither linear nor only travel in one direction, and individuals may leave a pathway or be diverted. There is a growing literature on desistance and disengagement that identifies factors that may motivate individuals to leave terrorism behind and such factors may include those that motivated terrorist engagement as well as other factors that did not drive entry but may motivate exit.

Implications of theories

Psychological theories of terrorism continue to evolve, and the review in this chapter seeks to organise some of the multitude of theories into the different areas of psychology and to consolidate them into a broad framework for understanding the different pathways to terrorism. Some of the key take-away points from the aforementioned review of theories can be found in Focus Box 12.1, and the applications of such theory can be found in Applications Box 12.1. Of course, the application of theory in this field could have a huge impact for society, and this makes it all the more important for psychologists to consider the limitations of our knowledge as well as the wider ethical considerations that pertain to this sensitive and complex field.

BOX 12.2　KEY TAKE-AWAY POINTS FROM PSYCHOLOGICAL THEORIES OF TERRORISM

1　There is no one profile of a terrorist or homogenous set of factors that explains terrorism. A holistic approach to terrorism that takes into account bio-psychosocial, sociopolitical and environmental factors and their interaction over the course of time is needed.

2   There are at least four types of pathways that can propel an individual to terrorism, and understanding these is important in informing diversion and rehabilitation.

3   Many fields within psychology and other disciplines may add value in explaining the different factors impacting the pathway undertaken by each individual terrorist. There are many limitations to the current research and theory that lead us to exercise caution in our assertions about the drivers for terrorism.

BOX 12.3   APPLICATIONS OF THEORIES OF TERRORISM INTO PRACTICE

Theories of terrorism can inform the way in which offenders who have been convicted of terrorism are risk assessed and rehabilitated. The social, moral/political, cognitive, behavioural learning, personality and clinical needs and criminal tendencies that may have contributed to each offender's pathway to terrorism can be identified and they can be supported to develop legal means to fulfil or manage such needs. Similar approaches can be adopted in preventative measures that support individuals who are deemed to be vulnerable to radicalisation, extremism and terrorist involvement, to divert their risk and prevent them from committing terrorist acts. In terms of risk assessment, Lloyd (2019) provides a summary of some of the current risk assessment methods in use, and most of these build on some of the theories discussed in this chapter. There are many publications on the range of approaches to rehabilitation, with one summary published by Pistonea et al. (2019). Regardless of the theory psychologists use, they must conduct their work in an ethical manner and adhere to their broader ethical code of practice as well as consider the added ethical challenges of working with terrorists. An example of ethical guidelines for practitioner psychologists working with terrorists can be found in Al-Attar et al. (2018).

Methodological limitations and ethical considerations

Researcher access to terrorist samples is very limited due to the sensitive and often dangerous nature of such work and in instances due to the reluctance of some terrorist group members to partake in research. Due to the different definitions of what constitutes terrorism at each time and place, research has included many different types of terrorist behaviours and definitions, making them difficult to compare and contrast and limiting the generalisability of each. Some research studies only focus on very small numbers of subtypes of terrorists (e.g. lone actors), which limits generalisability to other subtypes. Some mix samples of different terrorist roles (e.g. leaders and foot soldiers) without providing analyses of differences across these types of offenders. Most studies focus on male terrorists, which may limit our knowledge of female offenders. Furthermore, some researchers have interviewed small samples whilst most have used open-source information (secondary data) to inform their theories. For offenders who have been interviewed, results may be impacted by social desirability effects, fear or indeed political gains in giving false information, rendering the reliability of even primary data gathered questionable. Finally, many researchers in this field have not worked in practice with terrorist offenders, and many are not psychologists but inform theories that contribute to psychological knowledge.

Other research limitations have been argued to be borne out of cultural and ideological bias. Most terrorism researchers are Western researchers with little in-depth knowledge of the groups and cultural contexts they are researching and whose research is conducted following attacks on the west. Brannan et al. (2001) purport that Westerners studying terrorism have made a number of critical errors that have diminished our understanding of the motivators for terrorism. One example of these errors has been a tendency for Western authors in the terrorism field to approach the analysis from an antagonistic and condescending view of terrorists or at least from an angle that may be based on Western perceptions of the terrorist acts rather than the perpetrators' experiences and subjective psychological and sociopolitical realities. Psychologists have a particular role in delineating the individual's perspective and drivers, remaining objective and independent from their own subjective emotional and social frames of reference in order to counteract researcher and clinician bias. In recent years, many influential terrorism researchers have tried to redress such biases in analysis and emphasised the need for objectivity, an appreciation for subjective and culturally relevant frames of analysis and more nuanced theories that seek to account for different terrorist groups and contexts. This points to a broader fundamental dimension of psychological work with terrorists, namely ethical practice. It is imperative for psychologists to maintain ethical integrity and adhere to their codes of practice when working with any offender group and even more so when working with groups whose offences are emotive and politically impactful.

Conclusion

Forensic psychologists play a critical role in furthering our understanding of the drivers for terrorism and approaches to reducing the threat at the individual level. They adopt theoretically and empirically grounded knowledge to inform their practice with terrorist offenders, whilst adhering to ethical standards. The current chapter reviewed examples of theories from the different areas of psychology, which have informed the work of forensic psychologists working in the field of terrorism. This field is ever-evolving, there is great scope for further research and practice evaluation, and forensic psychology remains at the heart of this, going forward.

Learning outcomes

When you have completed this chapter, you should be able to:

1 Understand the basic psychological theories of terrorism
2 Understand how different psychological factors contribute to different aspects of the process by which an individual may come to be radicalised, engage with extremism and commit terrorist acts
3 Understand the different pathways or motivational trajectories that may lead different individuals to terrorism
4 Identify some of the methodological limitations impacting research and theory in the psychology of terrorism

5   Identify some of the applications of theory to the work that psychologists do with terrorist offenders
6   Identify the ethical considerations that pertain to psychological work with terrorist offenders

Key concepts and terms

- Terrorism
- Extremism
- Radicalisation
- Pathways to terrorism

Sample essay questions

- How do the different fields of psychology contribute to explaining terrorist behaviour?
- Critically review social psychological theories of terrorism.
- 'Psychology cannot inform our response to the terrorism threat'. Critically discuss this statement.

Recommended further reading

Al-Attar, Z., Bates-Gaston, J., Dean, C., & Lloyd, M. (2018). *Ethical Guidelines for Applied Psychological Practice in the Field of Extremism, Violent Extremism and Terrorism*. British Psychological Society.

References

Adorno, T. W., Frenkel-Brunswik, E., Levinson, D. J., & Sanford, R. N. (1950). *The authoritarian personality*. Harper and Row.
Ajzen, I., & Fishbein, M. (2005). The influence of attitudes on behavior. In D. Albarracin, B. T. Johnson, & M. P. Zanna (Eds.), *The handbook of attitudes* (pp. 173–221). Lawrence Erlbaum Associates.
Al-Attar, Z. (2019). *Extremism, radicalisation & mental health: Handbook for practitioners*. Radicalisation Awareness Network (RAN): Health and Social Care, November 2019.
Al-Attar, Z., Bates-Gaston, J., Dean, C., & Lloyd, M. (2018). *Ethical guidelines for applied psychological practice in the field of extremism, violent extremism and terrorism*. British Psychological Society.
Altemeyer, B. (2004). Highly dominating, highly authoritarian personalities. *The Journal of Social Psychology, 144*(4), 421–447.
Bandura, A. (2004). The origins and consequences of moral disengagement: A social learning perspective. In F. M. Moghaddam & A. J. Marcella (Eds.), *Understanding terrorism: Psychosocial roots, consequences and interventions* (pp. 169–185). American Psychological Society.
Bartlett, J., Birdwell, J., & King, M. (2010). *The edge of violence: A radical approach to extremism*. DEMOS.
Baumeister, R. F., & Leary, M. (1995). The need to belong: Desire for Interpersonal attachment as a fundamental human motivation. *Psychological Bulletin, 117*(3), 497–529.
Beck, A. (2002). Prisoners of hate. *Behaviour Research and Therapy, 40*, 209–216.
Borum, R. (2004). *Psychology of terrorism*. University of South Florida.
Brannan, D. W., Esler, P. F., & Strindberg, N. T. A. (2001). Talking to "terrorists": Towards an independent analytical framework for the study of violent substate activism. *Studies in Conflict & Terrorism, 24*(1), 3–24.
Canter, D. (2006). The Samson syndrome: Is there a kamikaze psychology? *21st Century Society, 1*(2), 107–127.

Clark, R. P. (1983). Patterns in the lives of ETA members. *Studies in Conflict and Terrorism, 6*(3), 423–454.

Crenshaw, M. (2000). The psychology of terrorism: An agenda for the 21st century. *Political Psychology, 21*(2), 405–420.

Crown Prosecution Service. (2020). *Terrorism, CPS website*. Retrieved 6 June 2020 from www.cps.gov. uk/terrorism.

Embry, D. D. (2007). Psychological weapons of mass disruption through vicarious classical conditioning. In B. Bongar, L. M. Brown, L. E. Beutler, J. N. Breckenridge, & P. G. Zimbardo (Eds.), *Psychology of terrorism* (pp. 164–174). Oxford University Press.

Gill, P., & Corner, E. (2017). There and back again: The study of mental disorder and terrorist involvement. *American Psychologist, 72*(3), 231–241.

Guttieri, K., Wallace, M. D., & Suedfeld, P. (1995). The integrative complexity of American decision makers in the cuban missile crisis. *Journal of Conflict Resolution, 39*(4), 367–394.

HM Government. (2015). *Counter extremism strategy*. Retrieved 6 June 2020 from https://assets. publishing.service.gov.uk/government/uploads/system/uploads/attachment_data/file/470088/ 51859_Cm9148_Accessible.pdf.

Hoffman, B. (2006). *Inside terrorism*. Columbia University Press.

Horgan, J. (2009). *Walking away from terrorism*. Routledge.

Kruglanski, A. W., Chen, X., Dechesne, M., Fishman, S., & Orehek, E. (2009). Fully committed suicide bombers' motivation and the quest for personal significance. *Political Psychology, 30*, 331–357.

Lloyd, M. (2019). *Extremism risk assessment: A directory*. CREST Full Report, March 2019.

Maikovich, A. K. (2005). A new understanding of terrorism using cognitive dissonance principles. *Journal for the Theory of Social Behaviour, 35*(4), 373–397.

McCormick, G. H. (2003). Terrorist decision making. *Annual Review of Political Sciences, 6*, 473–507.

Merari, A., Diamant, I., Bibi, A., Broshi, Y., & Zakin, G. (2009). Personality characteristics of suicide bombers and organizers of suicide attacks. *Terrorism & Political Violence, 22*(1), 87–101.

Pistonea, I., Erikssona, E., Beckmana, U., Mattsonb, C., & Sagera, M. (2019). A scoping review of interventions for preventing and countering violent extremism: Current status and implications for future research. *Journal of Deradicalization, 19*, 1–84.

Post, J. (2005). The new face of terrorism: Socio-cultural foundations of contemporary terrorism. *Behavioural Sciences and the Law, 23*, 451–465.

Post, J. (2007). *The mind of the terrorist: The psychology of terrorism from the IRA to Al-Qaeda*. Pagrave Macmillan.

Razzaque, R. (2008). *Human being to a human bomb: Inside the mind of a terrorist*. Icon Books.

Sageman, M. (2004). *Understanding terror networks*. University of Pennsylvania Press.

Saper, B. (1988). On learning terrorism. *Studies in Conflict and Terrorism, 11*(1), 13–27.

Schwartz, S. J., Dunkel, C. S., & Waterman, A. S. (2009). Terrorism: An identity theory perspective. *Studies in Conflict & Terrorism, 32*(6), 537–559.

Silke, A. (2008). Holy warriors: Exploring the psychological processes of jihadi radicalisation. *European Journal of Criminology, 5*(1), 99–123.

Strand, S., Belfrage, H., Fransson, G., & Levander, S. (1999). Clinical and risk management factors in risk prediction of mentally disordered offenders: More important than historical data? A retrospective study of 40 mentally disordered offenders assessed with the HCR-20 violence risk assessment scheme. *Legal and Criminological Psychology, 4*, 67–76.

Strentz, T. (1988). A terrorist psychosocial profile: Past and present. *FBI law enforcement bulletin*, April, 13–19.

Suedfeld, P., & Bluck, S. (1988). Changes in integrative complexity prior to surprise attacks. *Journal of Conflict Resolution, 32*(4), 626–635.

Tajfel, H. (1982). *Social identity & intergroup relations*. Cambridge University Press.

Turner, J., Hogg, M. A., Oakes, P. J., Reicher, S. D., & Wetherall, M. S. (1987). *Rediscovering the social group: A self-categorisation theory*. Basil Blackwell.

Ward, T., & Stewart, C. A. (2003). Criminogenic needs and human needs: A theoretical model. *Psychology, Crime & Law, 9*, 125–143.

Weenik, A. (2015). Behavioural problems and disorders among radicals in police files. *Perspectives on Terrorism, 9*(2), 17–33.

Whitehead, A. (2005). Man to man violence: How masculinity may work as a dynamic risk factor. *The Howard Journal, 44*(4), 411–422.

Whitehouse, H., McQuinn, B., Buhrmester, M., & Swan, Jr, W. B. (2014). Brothers in arms: Libyan revolutionaries bond like family. *Proceedings of the National Academy of Sciences of the United States of America, 111,*(50).

13 Working with women in prison

Jude Kelman and Karen Lloyd

Ella's story

Ella was convicted of the murder of a 21-year-old male acquaintance whom she had met through her boyfriend. At the time of the offence, Ella was under the influence of drugs and alcohol. She was convicted alongside her boyfriend and his friend. The offence occurred when Ella was instructed by her boyfriend to lure the victim to their house. Her boyfriend was a drug dealer to whom the victim owed money. Once in the house, the victim was beaten to death by Ella's boyfriend and his friend. Ella was present during the violence and kicked and spat on the victim when he was lying on the floor. She later assisted her co-defendants in concealing the victim's body in nearby woodland.

Summary

Approximately, 5% of individuals in prison within England and Wales are women. Whilst there is some slight variation in this figure; due to a relatively high turnover of individuals moving into or out of the prison system; this gender split has remained similar since 2002. However, proportionally, more women are managed on community sentences, with women constituting around 10% of the probation caseload. This is still far short of the roughly equal gender split within the general population of England and Wales.

Whilst women are under-represented in the criminal justice system (CJS), those women who enter it need to get the right support and access appropriate services to meet their gender-specific needs. The Bangkok Rules (UNODC, 2011) stipulate the requirements for the treatment of women, whether in custody or serving community sentences. These rules supplement the United Nations' standards and norms for the treatment of prisoners and those serving non-custodial sentences (UNODC, 2015), which are not gender sensitive. The starting point therefore – and the reason why this book contains a chapter dedicated to women – is that they should be treated differently (in some ways) to men during their contact with the CJS. Whilst the intention of this chapter is to focus exclusively on women, this should not be taken to indicate that men who come into contact with the CJS do not also face a range of challenges, and neither should it be concluded that other chapters of this book have no relevance to women. Before focusing on the differences in provision and the reasons for those differences, it is first necessary to understand a bit more about the women within the CJS. It should be noted that whilst this chapter focuses on women in prison, similar issues are also faced by women within other parts of the CJS and within the forensic mental health systems in England and Wales.

DOI: 10.4324/9781003017103-16

Women in prison: who are they and what are their needs?

Data published in late 2019 (Prison Reform Trust, 2019) highlight that whilst the number of women in custody remains largely static, there has been an increase in the use of very short prison sentences (i.e. sentences of less than six months) for women over the past two decades, with 62% of the women sentenced between June 2018 and 2019 having received a very short sentence. There is also a high proportion of women who do not receive a custodial sentence having spent a period of time on remand. Whilst at any one time approximately 350 women are serving an indeterminate sentence, the majority of women in prison (80%) have been convicted of non-violent crimes, with the most prevalent offence type being theft. Almost a quarter (23%) of the women receiving prison sentences had no prior convictions or cautions. These figures appear to indicate that many women spend time in prison for relatively minor offences. Short sentences can be disruptive in ways which last far beyond the length of time that they spend in prison (Baldwin & Epstein, 2017). The individual might lose their home and jobs, and those who are primary carers may also have their children taken into care if there are no family members with the capacity to look after them. For forensic psychologists working with women in custody, the short time period that they spend in prison can reduce, or prevent, opportunities for them to engage with psychologists, whether to support them during their sentences, or to work on addressing those aspects of their lives which contributed to them being sent to prison.

Women in prison have consistently been found to be disadvantaged by multiple needs and vulnerabilities (Wright et al., 2012), as well as having experienced social and economic difficulties in their lives prior to imprisonment. This includes poor financial and housing situations and limited employment histories (Gelsthorpe, 2010; McCausland & Baldry, 2017). Many women in custody report mental health issues (Prison Reform Trust, 2019) and women frequently enter the prison system with alcohol or drug addictions (UNODC, 2014) for which they often need immediate support. One or more traumatic experiences have been identified in the lives of many women in prison across many studies (e.g. Messina & Grella, 2006).

BOX 13.1 TRAUMA DEFINITIONS

There is no single agreed definition of what constitutes a traumatic event. For a situation or incident to be considered traumatic, it will usually have been experienced in a strongly negative way.

Trauma is a subjective concept – what one person finds deeply distressing may not be considered so by somebody else.

The extent of the psychological damage caused by the trauma differs depending on a range of factors (e.g. gender, resilience and the availability of support networks) and the prior experiences of the individual(s) experiencing it.

What is post-traumatic stress disorder (PTSD)?

PTSD is the '*exposure to actual or threatened death, serious injury or sexual violence*' (APA, 2013, p. 271) in one or more ways; plus:

- The presence (over at least the past month) of one or more intrusive symptoms (e.g. memories and flashbacks),
- and continued avoidance of things that remind them of the incident
- and substantially negative thoughts and mood which impact negatively on functioning (e.g. anger, hypervigilance and poor sleep).

Whilst trauma histories are also prevalent in the adult male prison, population evidence suggests that the prior trauma experiences of women in custody are more often multiple, and more serious, than those reported to have been experienced by men (Kubiak et al., 2017). Additionally, a large-scale international meta-analysis undertaken by Baranyi et al. (2018) found that the rate of PTSD across many cohorts of women in prison was substantially higher than the rate found amongst male prisoners. It is possible to conclude that there is a consistent pattern, across countries and cultures, of women in custody appearing to have experienced trauma in their lives at higher rates than men. Whilst there is mixed evidence as to the nature of the relationship and extent to which prior victimisation contributes towards female offending (DeHart et al., 2014), women who have experienced trauma prior to their imprisonment may be more vulnerable to mental health difficulties and stress (Anumba et al., 2012). This could impact on their capacity to cope with prison, as well as forming part of the picture of the range of services needed by women in custody.

The impact of imprisonment on women

Prison sentences have been found to have a detrimental effect on women by increasing their likelihood of reoffending (Hedderman & Joliffe, 2015). Additionally, shorter sentences can have a disproportionately negative impact on the lives of individuals, especially mothers (Baldwin & Epstein, 2017; Masson, 2014). Baldwin and Epstein (2017) described the psychological wrench and ongoing anxieties reported by the women, associated with being away from their children during their time in prison, as well as the impact of the separation on their children, which remained for some time after their mother's release from custody. The impact on women of a life sentence was explored by Crewe et al. (2017). Compared with men, women in their study experienced life imprisonment as substantially more psychologically difficult than male participants. Forensic psychologists should consider whether, and how, the experience of imprisonment itself might have impacted the individual's functioning and their presenting behaviour.

The offending-related needs of women within the criminal justice system

In order to reduce the likelihood of women reoffending, evidence (MoJ, 2015) suggests that the following areas should be targeted by the provision of interventions and services designed to support women across the CJS:

- Tackling substance misuse (including binge drinking and chronic alcohol use),
- Addressing mental health needs (including anxiety and depression, as well as personality characteristics which may be problematic, and PTSD and other trauma-related symptoms),
- Building emotion management skills (including temper control and managing the stress associated with parenting),

- The development of a prosocial identity and building social capital and
- Encouraging women to be in control of their daily lives and to set, and strive to achieve, goals, thereby increasing their confidence in the extent to which they can be self-sufficient.

Whilst there are some similarities between men and women within the CJS, the ways in which work is done with men and women may need to be different. This is due to the underlying differences in the personal circumstances of women compared with men. The 'how' is different, even if the 'what' seems the same. Services for women should recognise that women are not a homogenous group and should be gender responsive (i.e. based on evidence about what women need and what works with them). They should also be strength based, trauma informed and trauma responsive. The remainder of this chapter provides practical examples about ways that these goals can be achieved.

Current approaches to working with women in custody

In order to work effectively with women in the CJS, forensic psychologists should focus more broadly on the lives and prior circumstances of the individuals, rather than solely attending to the criminal behaviour. Such a narrow focus potentially misses important aspects of the 'whole story' of that person, including their prior life experiences and the context within which they live. For example, in Ella's case, it is necessary to consider the reasons why she came to use substances in the first place, as well as what contributed to her continued use of drugs or alcohol. This individualised approach enables the psychologist to build the picture of the complex range of factors which are relevant for each woman and which may need to be addressed, in order for them to develop a range of strengths and skills such that they can desist from further offending. This should be done in a trauma-responsive and compassion-focused way (Gilbert, 2013) whereby the resident is invited to better understand her reactions to threats faced in her past and use this as the basis for facilitating self-compassion and change.

Ella's compassion-focused formulation

In trying to understand Ella's whole story, an effective approach might include the forensic psychologist inviting her to complete a collaborative formulation (see Table 13.1) including a life graph of events. This could help Ella's life story to become clearer and the fears and threats to be better understood.

By working collaboratively with Ella, the forensic psychologist would develop a more holistic understanding of Ella and help her to make sense of her experiences. They would use this as a basis to promote feelings of psychological safety, build rapport and sequence treatment needs. This approach enables the client to see themselves as a person, rather than in the narrow focus of being an offender.

Working effectively with women in custody

In order to effectively meet the needs of women during their time in prison, the services provided should be:

- gender responsive
- multi-agency
- trauma informed and trauma responsive.

Table 13.1 Ella's Formulation

Key historical influences	Key fears/threats	Protective/safety strategies	Unintended consequences
• Maternal neglect and drug use • Cycle of being in care from age six • Witnessing domestic violence • Bullied at school and truanted • Moved in with boyfriend age 17 after an argument with mum • Boyfriend lived in a house share with other vulnerable peers and Ella was introduced to drugs	**External** • Mum rejected and abandoned me • Mum put drugs and boyfriends before my needs • Others cannot be trusted; they let you down or use you • It's a dog eat dog world **Internal** • I am unlovable • Others will exploit my feelings if I show them • Everyone looks down on me	• I don't let others get close • I rely on myself rather than others • I keep my head down and try to switch my emotions off • I try to help others so they don't hurt me or reject me	• Avoiding others makes Ella feel unloved and unwanted • Ella blames herself for the bad things that have happened and this is a trigger for self-harm • Ella is ashamed of her cuts and tries to hide them so others do not judge her • Ella's drug use was a means of blotting out her difficult emotions

Gender-responsive services

Whilst the majority of prison residents within Her Majesty's Prison and Probation Service are men, delivering the same services to women as men is not always appropriate. Evidence suggests that services for women are most effective when they are designed specifically for women (Stewart & Gobiel, 2015).

For forensic psychologists undertaking risk assessments with women, there are sometimes additional items or 'risk factors' which need to be considered. An example of this is the Female Additional Manual (FAM: de Vogel et al., 2014) which accompanies the HCR-20 (Douglas et al., 2013) and provides some guidance around how specific items should be considered differently when assessing violence risk with women. The FAM also includes some additional risk factors which research indicates are related to a woman's risk of violence towards others.

In terms of interventions for women in custody, the majority of the core suite of programmes currently available within HMPPS are not suitable for women (in that they were designed for men, and therefore, their likely benefit with women is unknown). Due to the complex range of needs presented by many women in custody, forensic psychologists working in women's prisons are more likely to deliver individually planned interventions. Additionally, it is often the case that women in prison will also be accessing a range of other services to meet their needs (e.g. mental health support or substance misuse services or a more intensive intervention or service to address aspects of their personality which links to their offending).

A multi-agency approach

As stated previously, given the complex range of needs which women in custody can present with, it is usually the case that women will require the input of several different services or agencies during their prison sentence. It is important for therapeutic input to be appropriately sequenced. It is possible that the most pressing needs for the individuals are not necessarily those which might contribute directly to a reduction in reoffending. However, for the person experiencing them, it may not be possible for them to focus on other things until those needs have been met. Attention should therefore be given to those areas of need which impact women in order to support their wider psychological health and functioning. Consequently, this might enable them to feel more psychologically safe and therefore more able to address their offending-related needs. The hierarchy of offending-related or rehabilitative needs is shown in Figure 13.1 and has been adapted from Maslow's hierarchy of needs (Maslow, 1987).

The hierarchy of needs shown in Figure 13.1 is not unique to women. Whilst the main principle is that individuals only progress to the higher order needs once needs at the lower levels have been satisfied, the triangle depicts a complex process, rather than a linear or sequential one. Individuals might move backwards and forwards or overlap through the stages. Forensic psychologists can contribute in different ways to each stage of the hierarchy. The starting point is that individuals need to feel safe and protected from harm and fear. Once individuals feel physically and psychologically safe, then they can progress towards the next stage. This involves the development of positive and rehabilitative relationships with others. Such relationships enable prison residents to begin to believe that they are capable of making changes in their lives, and they can develop hope for a positive future that is offence free.

At the stabilisation stage, individuals can be supported to access a range of services that they need to become and remain drug or alcohol free. They may also receive mental health support. Once the resident is stabilised, they are able to access more intensive services which may be required to enable them to develop the skills and strategies

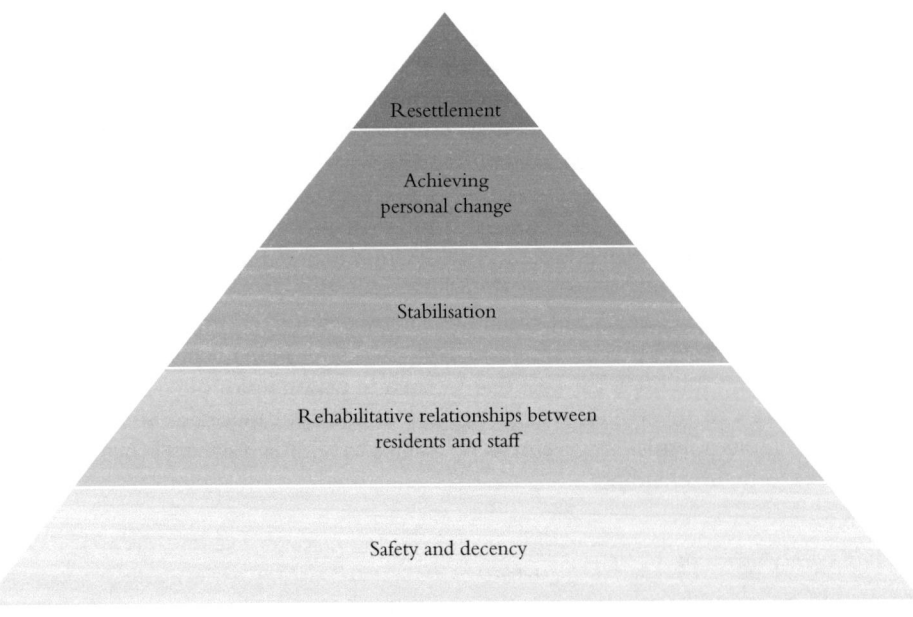

Figure 13.1 The hierarchy of rehabilitative needs

needed to achieve personal change. For some, that might mean undertaking educational or vocational training or learning work skills. For others, that might mean embarking on an intervention through the Offender Personality Disorder Pathway Service (Skett & Lewis, 2019). Within the women's estate, this might be the point at which the resident may engage with a forensic psychologist to complete individual work to address aspects of their offending-related behaviour, attitudes and thinking styles.

The final stage of the hierarchy involves the provision of support for the residents in order that they can become independent and settled as they transition into the community following their prison sentence. This might involve meeting their accommodation needs, supporting them to develop and maintain good family contact, getting suitable employment or accessing education.

A trauma-informed and trauma-responsive service

Across the women's prisons in HMPPS, there is an ongoing programme of staff training to ensure that all staff working in the prisons understand the impact and prevalence of trauma in the lives of women. The goal of this initiative is for all staff to become 'trauma-informed', in order that they can consider the ways in which the trauma histories of the women can shape their responses to stress as well as their prison behaviour. According to Harris and Fallot (2001), a service which is trauma informed, and trauma responsive, is one in which the service users feel physically and emotionally *safe*, as well as one in which they can *trust* the service providers and the system with which they are engaging. Service users should also be able to *collaborate* in key decisions that are made about them and should be able to *choose* where, how and when they access the service. Finally, individuals should be *empowered* by their contact with the service and should be supported to develop skills.

A further objective across the women's prison estate is for prisons to become more 'trauma responsive' in the way they are run. A trauma-responsive service is one in which policies and procedures are adapted to ensure that they do not inadvertently re-traumatise or trigger the women to be reminded of their prior traumatic experiences. This could be both potentially destabilising and psychologically damaging for the residents. One example of a trauma-responsive approach has been the development of supplementary guidance to assist staff when they conduct searches of women. In the additional guidance, staff are encouraged to explain what is about to happen throughout the process. This will help to prepare the residents to anticipate each stage of the search. This aims to minimise the extent to which women are touched without prior warning, which could be triggering for those who have experienced prior physical or sexual abuse.

For forensic psychologists working in women's prisons, working in trauma-informed and trauma-responsive ways has involved engaging with the women in custody to obtain their perspectives and suggestion about ways in which psychologists could adapt their practices to reduce the likelihood that individuals will be further traumatised by their encounters with psychology. Practical guidelines have been developed, in conjunction with the residents, for use by psychologists working across the women's estate. These guidelines include developing procedures with more neutral language to enable clients to agree to participate in assessments or interventions with psychologists without using the term 'consent' or 'consent form'. For example, some residents indicated that this word could be problematic for those individuals who had experienced prior sexual assault or abuse. This was because the word was associated with sexual consent. The word 'agreement' and the term 'agreement form' are now used instead.

Working as a psychologist in a trauma-informed and trauma-responsive manner

Returning to Ella's story and thinking about how a forensic psychologist can apply trauma-informed and trauma-responsive principles in their practice:

> *Ella is in prison and currently works in the textiles workshop. She does not like to speak about her offending, becoming tearful and upset when asked about it. She described it as 'a very traumatic night'. She has been frequently self-harming since coming into prison, a behaviour which she did not engage in prior to custody. She has been cutting her arms and legs with any implements she can find. She has recently started to receive letters from her former boyfriend (the co-defendant), which she said, 'stresses me out'. This is Ella's first conviction and she has found prison quite difficult. Ella is quiet on the wing, largely keeping herself to herself. She speaks to staff when approached but does not seek help. She has twice set fires in the bin in her cell stating that she likes to watch the fire as it calms her down. The manager on Ella's wing has contacted the psychology team to ask whether someone could work with Ella to help address her self-harming behaviour in order to try to reduce the frequency and seriousness of her self-harm.*

ACTIVITY BOX 13.2

Before reading on, think about Ella's current situation and complete the following tasks:

- Considering Figure 13.2, what are Ella's current primary needs (the things we should focus on initially to make her feel safe)?
- Considering Ella's traumatic experiences, think about practical things that a psychologist might do to plan for an initial meeting with Ella to help her feel **safe** about the process and help her to start to develop **trust** in them (e.g. think about things that the psychologist might do before the session to prepare, as well as how they might welcome and introduce themselves to Ella at the start of the session).

This presents an overview of how the psychologist might prepare for, and manage, the initial meeting with Ella by reading about her prison behaviour and experiences, as well as the psychological formulation. Such preparation might help the psychologist understand some of the triggers for Ella's distress, and her self-harm, as well enabling them to identify and examine times in her recent history when she has not self-harmed.

In order to support Ella to feel as physically and psychologically safe as possible, preparation might also involve identifying and arranging a suitable meeting space, within which Ella and the psychologist are not likely to be interrupted or disturbed during the session. This would ideally be one which is away from disruptive noises and activity and where the conversation cannot be overheard. They may also be able to give Ella some choice about when to have the initial meeting.

In order to start to build trust, the psychologist should attend the meeting punctually. They should also be explicit about the length of the meeting and adhere to this. At the outset of the initial meeting, its purpose should be explained, and information should be provided about the likely contents. This might help Ella to feel more prepared to discuss difficult areas. Ella should be given the choice as to whether she wishes to engage with the process at this time and whether she wants to answer each question. The psychologist and Ella may be able to agree which questions will happen earlier in the interview and which will either happen later, or at another time.

The initial meeting should not be rushed, and the psychologist should spend time enabling Ella to relax into the session. It might focus more on the 'meet and greet' aspects rather than discussions about Ella's self-harm, as it may be too soon for Ella to feel safe enough to discuss this. Ella should be given the opportunity to ask questions and should be encouraged to speak freely throughout. The psychologist will also need to explain the limits of confidentiality which will be in place at every meeting (i.e. that if Ella says something which makes the psychologist worried for her safety, the safety of others or the security of the prison they will be obliged to pass that information on).

As the scheduled end time of the meeting draws nearer, the psychologist should try to briefly recap the contents so that Ella is able to see that she has been listened to and heard. The psychologist should explain what will happen next and arrange a further meeting. They should also ask Ella about her current thoughts about self-harm, in order to check how Ella is feeling and whether she has found the session distressing. Such information should then be passed on to the relevant wing staff. Ella should be thanked for her contribution to the meeting and should be praised for any strengths, skills or strategies that she has shown or described during the session. A brief summary of the session should be documented in her prison case record, and a slightly more detailed summary should be entered into her psychology case record.

Working with other professionals to deliver trauma-informed and trauma-responsive services

Forensic psychologists also work with other professionals to enable them to deliver services to residents in trauma-informed and trauma-responsive ways. This is done by first developing a collaborative case formulation with the client to develop understanding. In order to maximise the likelihood that appropriate and effective support and management strategies can be developed and implemented with residents, such work should be underpinned by therapeutic and rehabilitative prison cultures (see Chapter 16) and trauma-responsive environments and systems. Forensic psychologists share the collaborative formulation with operational colleagues (e.g. prison officers) to ensure that it is understood by those staff who come into contact with the resident. This seeks to ensure that the management strategies and therapeutic support being offered are consistently applied. The rationale for this is that responsibilities for case management are shared across professionals, thus providing a supportive and unified approach for those involved in the resident's day-to-day management. This prevents splitting amongst staff and reduces the chance that decisions are made which might undermine the management plan if different staff are on shift.

Supporting staff to work in a trauma-informed and trauma-responsive way with Ella

Thinking about how psychologists may support wing staff to work with Ella in a trauma-informed and trauma-responsive way:

> *Ella is continuing to set fires in the bin in her room. She has been punished each time she sets a fire, as this is against prison rules. She is currently in the care and separation unit (CSU) to temporarily separate her from other residents as punishment following the most recent fire, which was more serious than previous ones. Staff and managers are concerned about her behaviour and her current state of mind as she will not talk to them. She presents as very lethargic and low in mood, showing no interest in engaging in the activities she previously seemed to enjoy such as watching the TV and reading. The CSU manager asks for the psychology team to work with CSU staff to help them understand Ella's current behaviour better so they can support her more effectively.*

The forensic psychologist would ideally work collaboratively with Ella and CSU staff by seeking to share some aspects of the formulation so that the functions of Ella's behaviour in custody can be better understood. The psychologist would be keen to work with Ella to identify distraction methods and self-soothing activities to help reduce her self-harm and fire setting, whilst also building on her strengths and protective factors. This would form part of a wider care plan available to staff supporting Ella. She would be encouraged to take an active and collaborative role in this process. Once staff understand why the distraction methods and self-soothing activities are so important for Ella, they can remind and encourage her to use them at times when it looks like she may find them beneficial.

Conclusion

When forensic psychologists work with residents in women's prisons, their focus is on the whole person and not just the offence(s) that brought them into custody. Ella's story is about more than the offence of murder for which she was convicted. It is about the interconnectedness of her prior life experiences, including her trauma history, and the coping strategies and behaviours that she developed to enable her to feel safer as she grew up. Working in trauma-informed and trauma-responsive ways and using gender-responsive approaches with women in custody can increase the likelihood that the services and interventions provided for them are appropriate and are sequenced most effectively.

Learning outcomes

When you have completed this chapter, you should be able to:

1   Understand how the population differs in women's services and why a holistic approach is needed
2   Understand specific issues faced by women in custody and the impact of imprisonment
3   Identify the offence-related needs of women, know what services are considered effective and understand how to work effectively to be rehabilitative with women
4   Understand the role of trauma and the importance of services being trauma informed and trauma responsive

Key concepts and terms

- Gender sensitive
- Multiple needs
- Trauma
- PTSD
- Trauma informed and trauma responsive
- Compassion-focused formulations
- Effective practice
- Rehabilitative needs

Sample essay questions

- What does it mean to be trauma informed and what are the benefits of working in trauma-responsive ways?
- Why is a gender-sensitive approach important to working with women in prison?

Recommended further reading

McCausland, R., & Baldry, E. (2017). Understanding women offenders in prison. In J. L. Ireland, C. A. Ireland, M. Fisher, & N. Gredecki (Eds.), *The Routledge international handbook of forensic psychology in secure settings* (pp. 25–39). Taylor & Francis Group.

Ministry of Justice. (2015). *Effective interventions for women offenders: A rapid evidence assessment*. National Offender Management Service (NOMS).

References

American Psychiatric Association. (2013). *Diagnostic and statistical manual of mental disorders* (5th ed., DSM-5). American Psychiatric Association.

Anumba, N., DeMatteo, D., & Heilbrun, K. (2012). Social functioning, victimisation, and mental health among female offenders. *Criminal Justice and Behaviour, 39*(9), 1204–1218.

Baldwin, L., & Epstein, R. (2017). *Short but not sweet: A study of the impact of custodial sentences on mothers and their children*. De Montfort University.

Baranyi, G., Cassidy, M., Fazel, S., Priebe, S., & Mundt, A. P. (2018). Prevalence of posttraumatic stress disorder in prisoners. *Epidemiological Reviews, 40*, 134–145.

Crewe, B., Hulley, S., & Wright, S. (2017). The gendered pains of life imprisonment. *British Journal of Criminology, 57*, 1359–1378.

DeHart, D., Lynch, S., Belknap, J., Dass-Brailsford, P., & Green, B. (2014). Life history models of female offending: The roles of serious mental illness and trauma in women's pathways to jail. *Psychology of Women Quarterly, 38*(1), 138–151.

de Vogel, V., de Vries Robbe, M., van Kalmthout, W., & Place, C. (2014). *FAM Female Additional Manual: Additional guidelines to the HCR-20 v3 for assessing risk for violence in women*. Van der Hoeven Kliniek.

Douglas, K. S., Hart, S. D., Webster, C. D., & Belfrage, H. (2013). *HCR-20 V3: Assessing risk for violence*. Simon Fraser University.

Gelsthorpe, L. (2010). Women, crime and control. *Criminology and Criminal Justice, 10*(4), 375–386.

Gilbert, P. (2013). *The compassionate mind*. Robinson.

Harris, M., & Fallot, R. D. (Eds.). (2001). *New directions for mental health services: Using trauma theory to design service systems*. Wiley.

Hedderman, C., & Joliffe, D. (2015). The impact of prison for women on the edge: Paying the price for wrong decisions. *Victims and Offenders, 10*, 152–178.

Kubiak, S. P., Covington, S. S., & Hillier, C. (2017). Trauma-informed corrections. In D. Springer & A. Roberts (Eds.), *Social work in juvenile and criminal justice system* (4th ed., pp. 92–104). Charles C. Thomas.

Maslow, A. H. (1987). *Motivation and personality* (3rd ed.). Pearson Education.

Masson, I. (2014). *The long-term impact of shorter periods of imprisonment on mothers.* Unpublished PhD thesis, King's College, London.

McCausland, R., & Baldry, E. (2017). Understanding women offenders in prison. In J. L. Ireland, C. A. Ireland, M. Fisher, & N. Gredecki (Eds.), *The Routledge international handbook of forensic psychology in secure settings* (pp. 25–39). Taylor & Francis Group.

Messina, N., & Grella, C. (2006). Childhood trauma and women's health outcomes in a California prison population. *American Journal of Public Health, 96*(10), 1842–1848.

Ministry of Justice. (2015). *Effective interventions for women offenders: A rapid evidence assessment.* London: National Offender Management Service (NOMS).

Prison Reform Trust. (2019). *Bromley briefings prison factfile.* Prison Reform Trust.

Skett, S., & Lewis, C. (2019). Development of the offender personality disorder pathway: A summary of the underpinning evidence. *Probation Journal, 66*(2), 167–180.

Stewart, L., & Gobiel, R. (2015). Correctional interventions for women offenders: A rapid evidence assessment. *Journal of Criminological Research, Policy and Practice, 1*(3), 116–130.

United Nations Office on Drugs and Crime (UNODC). (2011). *The Bangkok Rules.* United Nations Rules for the Treatment of Women Prisoners and Non-custodial Measures for Women Offenders with their Commentary. Retrieved 11 March 2020 from www.unodc.org/documents/justice-and-prison-reform/Bangkok_Rules_ENG_22032015.pdf.

UNODC. (2014). *Handbook on women and imprisonment* (2nd ed.). with reference to the United Nations Rules for the Treatment of Women Prisoners and Non-custodial Measures for Women Offenders (the Bangkok Rules). Retrieved 18 April 2020 from www.unodc.org/documents/justice-and-prison-reform/women_and_imprisonment_-_2nd_edition.

UNODC. (2015). *The United Nations standard minimum rules for the treatment of prisoners (the Nelson Mandela Rules).* Retrieved 18 April 2020 from www.unodc.org/documents/justice-and-prison-reform/Nelson_Mandela_Rules-E-ebook.pdf.

Wright, E. M., van Voorhis, P., Salisbury, E. J., & Bauman, A. (2012). Gender-responsive lessons learned and policy implications for women in prison: A review. *Criminal Justice and Behaviour, 39*(12), 1612–1632.

14 Working with young people

Katie Lambert

Summary

Forensic psychologists' work with young people is widely varied dependent on the setting in which they work and on the needs of the young person. They predominately work with young people who have offended or are considered at risk of offending. Due to the nature of the client group, the majority of work occurs within young offender institutions (YOI's), secure children's homes, residential children's homes, secure mental health services or as part of community services. However, it is important to note that not all young people, such as those in residential children's homes, will be involved with the criminal justice system. Forensic psychologists also work with victims, such as those associated with criminal or sexual exploitation or offenders who themselves have been victims. This chapter highlights the theory and evidence that guides the practice of forensic psychologists working with young people in residential and community settings. The application of such theory and approaches in practice will be illustrated with a case example focusing on harmful sexual behaviour (HSB). The role of the forensic psychologist in supporting and educating professionals is also discussed.

Introduction

Forensic psychologists encounter an array of different harmful behaviours in young people, such as HSB, aggression, criminal and sexual exploitation, arson and self-injury. Such young people may also have mental health problems, learning disabilities and/or be neurodiverse, such as ADHD and autism. The task of the forensic psychologist working with these young people is to promote an understanding of the casual factors for their harmful behaviour, or their vulnerability to engage in such behaviours, and to work with the young person to develop alternative behaviours. The main goal is to promote desistance from future offending behaviour and/or to reduce the vulnerability to offending trajectories. This work is challenging, yet very rewarding, and can help to protect against lifelong involvement with criminal justice services. Let's consider how the forensic psychologist contributes to this important area of work.

Key theories that guide practice with young people

Forensic psychologists work on the premise that the problematic or harmful behaviours displayed meet a need for the young person. The behaviours can be a way of coping with intolerable internal states or external circumstances at a family or societal level (Hanson & Holmes, 2014; Case & Haines, 2015). It is important to understand what unmet needs

DOI: 10.4324/9781003017103-17

the behaviour fulfils. To achieve this understanding, the evidence base promotes adopting a holistic and strength-based approach to working with young people. The Good Lives Model of Offender Rehabilitation (GLM: Ward & Stewart, 2003; Fortune, 2018) adopts this approach, arguing that the best way to address harmful behaviour is to balance the management of risk with the development of 'Good Lives'. The model postulates that a sole focus on risk factors, deficits and relapse prevention associated with offending behaviour is not sufficient to effect change and reduce recidivism. It argues that individuals engage in offending or unhelpful patterns of behaviour because they are attempting to meet basic needs, which they cannot meet in healthy ways for particular social or individual reasons. GLM states that effective rehabilitation and intervention requires identification of the needs that were being met through inappropriate means and in turn setting goals and developing skills to allow the individual to meet their needs in more appropriate ways. Thus, the model leads us to target the risks associated with offending, being vulnerable to risky behaviours and/or victimisation, alongside enhancement of the young person's life and well-being.

Adopting a GLM approach helps to understand the young person's needs, goals and functioning in various areas of their life. The necessary areas can then be targeted to develop alternative behaviours to replace the need to engage in risky, problematic and/or harmful behaviours (Purvis et al., 2011; Willis et al., 2012). For example, consider a young person who engages in aggression as a way of feeling 'respected' and liked by peers and in turn reducing their sense of loneliness. Applying the GLM may suggest developing their social skills and self-esteem and promoting their engagement in leisure activities with prosocial peers to make friendships. This would hopefully reduce their sense of loneliness and increase their sense of connection to others, thus, developing a 'Good Life' and reducing the need to engage in offending and/or unhelpful patterns of behaviour.

Whilst the GLM theoretically guides the practice of a forensic psychologist, it can also be used practically with young people, the staff caring for them and with other professionals to create collective goals to develop a 'Good Life'. The approach helps to build skills in young people, develop resilience and instil hope, all of which are known to have a positive impact on self-worth and mental health (Ryan & Deci, 2000). Positive influences of the model on practice with young people have been reported (van Hecke et al., 2019; van Damme et al., 2017), and initial evaluations found that professionals liked the motivational approach. It has helped young people understand their own offending behaviour and feel motivated and hopeful that their situation could get better (Leeson & Adshead, 2013).

In line with providing holistic care, another approach adopted when working with young people is trauma-informed care. The evidence suggests that the majority of young people referred to forensic psychologists have themselves been victims of trauma or adversity. Ford et al. (2019) found, within an adult prison population (n = 468), eight in ten prisoners reported at least one adverse childhood experience (ACE) and nearly half had four or more ACEs. ACEs included verbal, physical and sexual abuse, emotional and physical neglect, parental separation, domestic abuse, parental drug and alcohol misuse, etc. Amongst the prisoners with four or more ACEs, they were four times more likely to have served a sentence in a YOI than those with no ACEs. Similar findings were found in a sample of adult males who had sexual offences (Levenson et al., 2014). The evidence base also indicates that problematic behaviours displayed may be due to earlier trauma or adversities (Hanson & Holmes, 2014; Van der Kolk, 2014; Briere, 2019). Therefore, it is important to recognise the young person's life experiences and any potential trauma or adversity, including any potential contributing role this may in their unhelpful or harmful patterns of behaviour.

BOX 14.1   THE IMPACT OF TRAUMA ON A YOUNG PERSON

Exposure to strong, frequent and/or prolonged adversity or trauma, such as the types of abuse noted in this chapter, can lead to a toxic stress response in the person. The experience of toxic stress impacts on the brain's alarm system that detects threat and places the body and brain into a state of fear. This state of fear activates the young person's 'survival brain' where their response is to fight, flight or freeze. In this state, individuals can act impulsively and on instinct resulting in various different types of behaviour, such as aggression, running away, substance misuse, self-harm and disconnection from others.

A young person's brain that develops in the context of trauma can be more easily triggered into survival mode, even when there is no actual threat. It happens at an unconscious level, so the young person and professionals tend to focus on the behaviour observed rather than the underlying causes of distress. Such circumstances over time can impact upon the individual's relationships (attachment) and the response they receive from others, their emotional regulation, behavioural control, beliefs, cognitions and self-concept (Van der Kolk, 2014). It is, therefore, important when working with those who have experienced trauma that the psychologist acts in a way that helps the client feel safe, secure and avoids triggering their trauma responses. Such responses can make people feel unsafe and impact upon their progress.

A trauma-informed approach to working with young people involves understanding the nature of how trauma works; the affect it can have on their mind, body and behaviour and the optimal ways to work with such presentations. Such models emphasise the importance of establishing and maintaining a safe culture in which individuals can learn adaptive ways of coping with stress (Levenson et al., 2014). Thus, psychologists work collaboratively with the young person to understand 'what happened to you?' rather than 'what's wrong with you?' They encourage professionals supporting the young people to adopt the same mindset and create therapeutic environments and relationships with the young people.

Assessment and formulation of need with young people

Every intervention with a young person is based on an assessment and/or formulation of their needs to ensure the intervention chosen is appropriate for them. In line with the GLM, an assessment should consider their individual life experiences, including the past, present and future, their risk and strengths. For instance, this should involve exploration of their upbringing, current circumstances including functional assessments of presenting problems and their future aspirations. Focusing solely on their offending or the presenting issue would risk a reductionist understanding of their circumstances and potentially miss important vulnerability or contributing factors.

The evidence base indicates that the assessment of risk should generally be based on structured clinical judgement and be balanced in terms of considering both the risk and protective factors (Rogers, 2000). Evidence-based tools such as the Structured Assessment of Violent Risk in Youth (Borum et al., 2006), Juvenile Sexual Offender Assessment Protocol (Prentky & Righthand, 2003) and Structured Assessment of Protective Factors in Youth (de Vries Robbe et al., 2015) enable psychologists to apply structured clinical judgement to determine the level of risk a young person poses. Coupled with a strong formulation, the assessment helps to identify areas to target within intervention and risk management plans.

Considerations for engaging and assessing young people

When working with young people, one of the most important aspects of a psychologists practice is developing and maintaining the therapeutic relationship. Evidence suggests that a strong therapeutic alliance is critical for effective engagement (Ackerman & Hilsenroth, 2003; Kozar & Day, 2012). However, this can sometimes be difficult with young people due to their past experiences of adults and/or limited motivation to explore any areas of concern. Young people in residential/forensic settings generally have limited trust in adults and asking them to engage in an assessment or intervention can be anxiety provoking. Hence, there may be some resistance from young people to build a therapeutic relationship. It is important to adopt a compassionate and reflective view to any resistance, and consider how resistance could be reduced to promote engagement.

Within children's residential settings, assessments are generally completed over a number of weeks, which allows for a rapport to be built. There are also opportunities to interact with the young people outside of formal therapy. For instance, spending time around the home with young people talking, engaging in activities and supporting them with tasks or problems. This informal time with the young person is beneficial to developing and maintaining a relationship, which aids the process of trust, engagement in therapy and can reduce resistance. It is important that this time spent together is genuine and positive.

Psychologically understanding the young person, such as their attachment style (Bowlby, 1973), disclosure styles (Frost et al., 2006) and their level of motivation for changing behaviours (Burrowes & Needs, 2009), can also help guide how to engage with a young person and navigate the dynamics within the therapeutic relationship. The evidence base recommends strategies to help build a strong therapeutic alliance, such as being collaborative, transparent, consistent and flexible to their needs within the premise of professional boundaries, conveying warmth, being non-judgemental, congruent, genuinely interested and empathic (Rogers, 1957; Miller & Rollnick, 2002). Research has found that such approaches have contributed positively to the therapeutic alliance (Ackerman & Hilsenroth, 2003).

Another important aspect is to have an awareness and understanding of adolescent development, typical behaviour and current influences on them, such as puberty, social media and peers. Understanding adolescent trends and current interests can aid rapport-building with the young person but can, also, be areas to consider when exploring their functioning and presenting problems. Internet use, social media and peers can be contributing factors to engaging in risky or offending behaviours and/or be a method by which to offend, such as technology-assisted HSB. It is important to have a working knowledge of these specific adolescence influences to inform practice.

BOX 14.2   IS IT NORMAL BEHAVIOUR?

An important consideration when working with young people is whether the behaviour they are displaying is a normative part of adolescent development or is a problematic or harmful behaviour. It is therefore important to have an understanding of typical adolescent development in the context of social and cultural influences in order to identify any atypical behaviours. Adolescence is a time of change at a physical, emotional and neurobiological level for young people. They become more aligned with their peers, have an increased interest in romantic relationships and sex, can demonstrate more emotional liability and engage in risk-taking behaviours. It is a time when they become more independent, develop their own identity and begin to question the boundaries and expectations that surround them. They also can become challenging and emotionally impulsive (Fahlberg, 2012; Hanson & Holmes, 2014). It is important to encourage healthy development when working with young people and not to label normal adolescent behaviour as problematic. Nevertheless, it is imperative that problematic or harmful behaviours are identified and managed. Thus, a forensic psychologist continually considers whether presenting behaviours are normative and healthy for the young person's age or require attention and management.

For example:

- A 16-year-old is having sexual thoughts about a peer in college. He wants his peer to be his girlfriend and is masturbating to thoughts of consensual sex.
- A 16-year-old is having sexual thoughts about a 13-year old from school who they have noticed in the playground. He is masturbating frequently each day to these thoughts.

The first example would be considered healthy and age appropriate, whereas the latter would be considered inappropriate and requires attention due to the age difference and the frequency of thoughts.

Psychological interventions with young people

Once a collaborative understanding of the young person and their therapeutic needs are established, it is important to develop a therapeutic plan to address their needs, outlining the interventions that will be delivered. The aims of these should be tailored to the individual in line with the risk-need-responsivity principles (Andrews & Bonta, 2014) to promote optimal engagement and learning. All young people present with differing educational needs, levels of functioning and ways of learning; thus, consideration of their cognitive abilities, emotional and social development is needed to inform how to deliver the intervention. All materials and content should be tailored to the young person's needs. Even if the content of the intervention is manualised, this can be adapted to suit the young person's needs (Gannon & Ward, 2014).

Effective communication and creativity are also key to delivering therapeutic work with young people. For some young people, talking will be effective; however, for others, there will be a preference for alternative ways to express themselves, such as through drawing, play and/or worksheets. Creative methods such as making things, playing games, watching videos and practising skills in real-life settings tend to be more appealing and engaging for young people. It can also be helpful to use examples to explore concepts to aid learning in an indirect and less personal manner, such as how a film character dealt with a situation. Once the learning has been achieved, the young person can then apply this to their situation. It is also beneficial to gain an understanding of their likes and interests and incorporate this into the delivery of information where possible as it helps to promote engagement and retain learning. To deliver the creative methods, it is important to find a communication style that fits with the young person in terms of pace and accessible language. The language used needs to be relatable and engaging for the young person; however, the use of their slang is not considered appropriate. The use of appropriate humour and positive language can prove effective. It is, therefore, important for psychologists to understand the young people they are working with and tailor the methods of delivery and communication style.

BOX 14.3   ETHICS AND CONSENT FOR PSYCHOLOGICAL WORK

There are a number of ethical considerations when working with young people such as their ability to consent, safeguarding and disclosure procedures and ensuring professional boundaries are upheld.

In terms of consent, it is essential that consent is obtained from the young person prior to engaging in assessment and intervention work. It is important that they understand the nature of the psychological work being offered, its benefits and the consequences of deciding whether to take part or not. Psychologists need to be transparent about these areas in order for the individual to make an informed decision regarding their engagement. It is particularly important in forensic practice that young people understand the nature of confidentiality, its limits and the potential avenues that may need to be taken if confidentiality needs to be broken, such as reporting information to safeguarding teams, social care and the police (BPS, 2018).

An important reflection point in forensic psychology is the ethical implications surrounding consent when the therapy is contingent on the young person's placement or progression, as this could impact upon the voluntary nature of therapy. There may be a sense of compliance rather than choice in the young person. If individuals feel they do not have a choice in the therapy, then extrinsic motivation can materialise, which can impact negatively on the engagement and outcome of therapy. For forensic psychologists, it is important that a young person understands the nature of consent and the proposed intervention, as outlined previously. If the client is fully informed, then this can help to promote choice.

Flexibility is a further consideration when working with young people. Evidence indicates that a flexible approach is critical for effective engagement (Ackerman & Hilsenroth, 2003; Kozar & Day, 2012) and supporting individuals at a superficial level or being solely focused on the content of sessions can negatively impact upon therapeutic alliance (Marshall, 2009). Thus, the ability to recognise and respond to the evolving needs of the young person in therapy is important, even if it in involves temporarily deviating from the therapeutic aims (Gannon & Ward, 2014). However, young people can sometimes instigate deviation from the content of a session to avoid exploring a topic. It is important to recognise these attempts, respond consistently and continue with the intended content. Thus, in practice, there is a need to recognise when flexibility is genuinely needed and to balance the delivery of the content of therapy with support for the young person.

Supporting multidisciplinary working

Effective and safe work with young people requires good communication and collaboration amongst agencies involved in the young person's life (e.g. those caring for them, school, social services, police and health) in order to inform decisions surrounding their care pathway and risk management. A key part of a forensic psychologist's role is to provide other professionals with a psychological understanding of the young person to inform the care they receive. The psychologist should work closely with the staff teams to promote their understanding of psychological principles and how staff can apply those principles to ensure appropriate and tailored care is provided to the young person. For instance, they may work with staff to increase their understanding of how to build a secure attachment with a young person, provide care that is trauma informed, effectively and appropriately manage risk and ensure they are working within their professional boundaries. This can take place through training and reflective practice.

Staff teams can face a lot of demands each day from the young people they support and often face complex and challenging behaviours. This can sometimes impact upon staff members' resiliency, the team dynamics and care provided. It is, therefore, important for a psychologist to understand the demands on a team, their level of resilience and the culture of the working environment (Johnson & Scholes, 1992) to inform how they can best work with, and support, the team. A good working relationship is also key to enhancing their receptiveness to psychological information and advice. Given the emotive nature of working with young people, it is also important for the forensic psychologist to engage in reflective practice and supervision to ensure their practice remains within professional boundaries and the psychologist's remit.

Conclusion

Working with young people is extremely rewarding and provides the opportunity to intervene and to hopefully prevent further escalation of certain behaviours and future contact with forensic services. Adopting holistic approaches to assessment and intervention are important, and it is fundamental to remember that they are young people. As such, their presenting problems should be contextualised, and the delivery style of the psychologist should recognise this: it is not simply a case of delivering interventions designed for adults in a young person friendly way. Both assessments and interventions should be young person specific and evidence based.

Case study

Luke is a 15-year-old male who is living in a residential children's home in the community which specialises in working with adolescent males who have displayed HSB. Luke was placed in the home due to engagement in sexual behaviour with his two younger siblings.

Assessment and formulation

During the assessment process, Luke discussed how he had experienced physical and emotional abuse in the family home and witnessed domestic violence between his parents, who would drink alcohol regularly. He talked about how he would prepare meals and look after his younger sisters when his parents were intoxicated. He spent a lot of time in his room to stay out of his parent's way, as his sisters did. He saw his maternal grandparents occasionally. He disliked his grandfather as he favoured his sisters but liked his grandmother as he felt that she listened to him. Luke reported having no friends at school and was bullied, which would make him feel angry and resulted in fights. He enjoyed playing computer games and talking to others online. He discussed becoming curious about sex at age 12 when he overheard older peers at school talking about it. This coincided with the start of puberty and him wanting a girlfriend. He started to watch pornography and talk to others online about sex. He gradually began to show his sisters pornography, which led to perpetrating sexual activities against them. When talking about his sexual behaviour with his sisters, Luke became upset as he thought he was a bad person for what he had done.

Through a functional assessment of his HSB, it was established that sexual behaviours helped Luke cope with his feelings of rejection and loneliness, feel connected to others and satisfy his sexual urges and curiosity. It is suggested, from applying social learning theory (Bandura, 1973), that his sexual behaviour was reinforced through feeling positive emotions associated with satisfying his sexual urges, feeling liked and connected to someone and, also, removing negative feelings associated with loneliness and rejection. To understand the casual and risk factors associated with his HSB, his vulnerability factors and situational triggers were considered by applying the Integrated Model of Sexual Offending (Barbaree et al., 1998). Figure 14.1 presents a diagrammatic formulation of Luke's HSB.

Psychological intervention

Luke's HSB helped him to meet his sexual needs, feel better and connected to others. Therefore, to support Luke to live a fulfilled life without acting in a harmful way, it was important for him to learn healthy ways to cope, healthy views associated with sex, increase his self-esteem and develop prosocial ways to feel good and connected to others. The overarching aim was for him to be able to build meaningful and satisfying relationships with others. Therapeutic work, which he consented to, targeted these needs. The intervention, guided by a cognitive behavioural approach, focused on his emotional management, HSB, social skills and developing his strengths and goals for the future. In relation to his HSB, he focused on understanding his triggers and beliefs, reframing such beliefs and developing a safety and management plan to manage triggers and mitigate any further offending. He also focused on understanding appropriate sexual urges and the role of consent to ensure he had the knowledge to engage in healthy sexual relationships. In addition, it was important to help Luke with his unresolved trauma and attachment difficulties, so he engaged

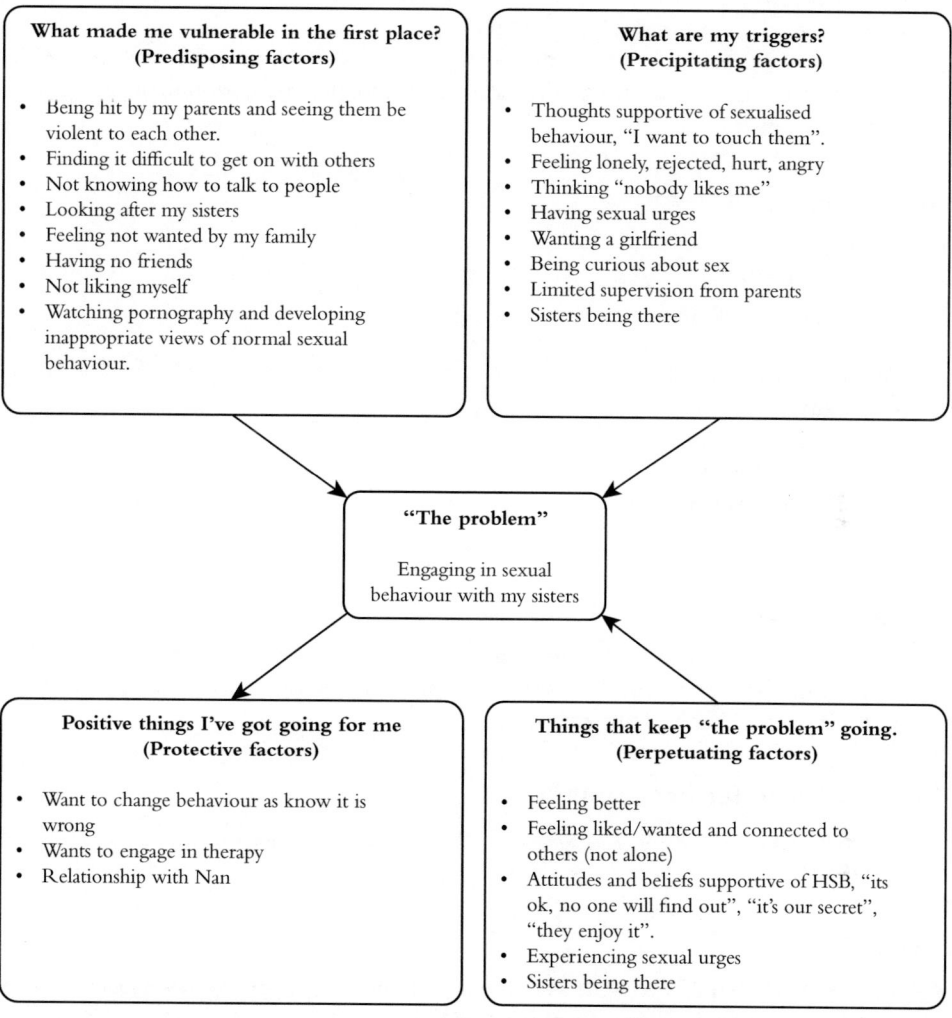

Figure 14.1 Formulation of Luke's engagement in HSB informed by the Integrated Model of Sexual Offending using the 5 P's framework

eye movement desensitisation and reprocessing to target these areas. In conjunction with the therapeutic work, the staff members focused on building therapeutic and trusting relationships with Luke, helping him practice his coping skills learnt in therapy and developing his social skills and prosocial engagement with his peers through leisure activities.

Learning outcomes

When you have completed this chapter, you should be able to:

1   Understand the main approaches to working with young people and the importance of evidence-based practice.

2   Understand the need to work in a holistic manner by attending to both offending behaviour and promotion of a 'good life'.

3   Have an awareness of wider considerations when working with young people, such as multiagency working, the impact of adolescent development and ethical considerations.

Key concepts and terms

- Formulation
- Good Lives Model
- Trauma-informed care
- Consent
- Person-centred practice
- Creativity
- Multi-agency working
- Normative development
- Therapeutic alliance
- Effective communication

Sample essay questions

- Discuss and critically evaluate the main approaches to working with young people.
- Discuss the important considerations a forensic psychologist needs to be mindful of in their practice with young people.

Recommended further reading

Hanson, E., & Holmes, D. (2014). *That difficult age: Developing a more effective response to risks in adolescence.* Research in Practice/ADCS.

References

Ackerman, S., & Hilsenroth, M. (2003). A review of therapist characteristics and techniques positively impacting the therapeutic alliance. *Clinical Psychology Review, 23,* 1–33.

Andrews, D. A., & Bonta, J. L. (2014). *The psychology of criminal conduct* (5th ed.). Anderson.

Bandura, A. (1973). *Aggression: A social learning analysis.* Holt.

Barbaree, H. E., Marshall, W. L., & McCormick, J. (1998). The development of deviant sexual behaviour among adolescents and its implications for prevention and treatment. *The Irish Journal of Psychology, 1,* 1–31.

Borum, R., Bartel, P., & Forth, A. (2006). *Manual for the structured assessment of violence risk in youth.* Psychological Assessment Resources Inc. (PAR).

Bowlby, J. (1973). *Separation, anxiety and anger: Attachment and loss* (Vol. 2). Hogarth Press.

Briere, J. (2019). *Treating risky and compulsive behaviour in trauma aurvivors.* Guildford Press.

British Psychological Society. (2018). *Code of ethics and conduct.* BPS.

Burrowes, N., & Needs, A. (2009). Time to contemplate change? A framework for assessing readiness to change with offenders. *Aggression and Violent Behavior, 14,* 39–49.

Case, S., & Haines, K. (2015). Children first, offenders second: The centrality of engagement in positive youth justice. *The Howard Journal of Crime and Justice, 54*(2), 157–175.

de Vries Robbé, M., Geers, M. C. K., Stapel, M., Hilterman, E. L. B., & de Vogel, V. (2015). SAPROF: Youth version English. In *Guidelines for the assessment of protective factors for violence risk in juveniles.* De Forensische Zorgspecialisten.

Fahlberg, V. (2012). *A child's journey through placement.* Jessica Kingsley Publishers.

Ford, K., Barton, E., Newbury, A., Hughes, K., Bezeczky, Z., Roberick, J., & Bellis, A. (2019). *Understanding the prevalence of adverse childhood experiences (ACEs) in a male offender population in Wales: The prisoner ACE survey.* Bangor University and Public Health Wales NHS Trust.

Fortune, C. (2018). The Good Lives Model: A strengths-based approach for youth offenders. *Aggression and Violent Behavior, 38,* 21–30.

Frost, A., Daniels, K., & Hudson, S. M. (2006). Disclosure strategies among sex offenders: A model for understanding the engagement process in group work. *Journal of Sexual Aggression, 12*(3), 227–244.

Gannon, T., & Ward, T. (2014). Where has all the psychology gone? A critical review of evidence based psychological practice in correctional settings. *Aggression and Violent Behavior, 19*(4), 435–446.

Hanson, E., & Holmes, D. (2014). *That difficult age: Developing a more effective response to risks in adolescence.* Research in Practice/ADCS.

Johnson, G., & Scholes, K. (1992). *Exploring corporate strategy.* Financial Times/Prentice Hall.

Kozar, C., & Day, A. (2012). The therapeutic alliance in offending behaviour programs: A necessary and sufficient condition for change? *Aggression and Violent Behavior, 17,* 482–487.

Leeson, S., & Adshead, M. (2013). The response of adolescents and practitioners to a good lives approach. In B. Print (Ed.), *The Good Lives Model for adolescents who sexually harm.* Safer Society Press.

Levenson, J., Willis, G., & Prescott, D. (2014). Adverse childhood experiences in the lives of male sex offenders: Implications for trauma informed care. *Sexual Abuse: A Journal of Research and Treatment,* 1–20.

Marshall, W. (2009). Manualization: A blessing or a curse? *Journal of Sexual Aggression, 15,* 109–120.

Miller, W. R., & Rollnick, S. (2002). *Motivational interviewing: Preparing people for change* (2nd ed.). Guilford Press.

Prentky, R., & Righthand, S. (2003). *Youth Sex Offender Assessment Protocol-II (J-SOAP II): Manual.* U.S. Department of Justice, Office of Justice Programs, Office of Juvenile Justice and Delinquency Prevention.

Purvis, M., Ward, T., & Willis, G. (2011). The Good Lives Model in practice: Offence pathways and case management. *European Journal of Probation, 3*(2), 4–28.

Rogers, C. R. (1957). The necessary and sufficient conditions of therapeutic personality change. *Consulting Psychology, 21,* 95–103.

Rogers, R. (2000). The uncritical acceptance of risk assessment in forensic practice. *Law and Human Behavior, 24*(5), 595–604.

Ryan, R. M., & Deci, E. L. (2000). Self-determination theory and the facilitation of intrinsic motivation, social development and wellbeing. *American Psychologist, 55,* 68–78.

van Damme, L., Fortune, C., Vandevelde, S., & Vanderplasschen, W. (2017). The Good Lives Model among detained female adolescents. *Aggression and Violent Behavior, 37,* 179–189.

van Der Kolk, B. (2014). *The body keeps the score: Mind, brain and body in the transformation of trauma.* Penguin.

van Hecke, N., Vanderplasschen, W., Van Damme, L., & Vandevelde, S. (2019). The bumpy road to change: A retrospective qualitative study on formerly detained adolescents' trajectories towards better lives. *Child and Adolescent Psychiatry and Mental Health, 13,* 10.

Ward, T., & Stewart, C. A. (2003). The treatment of sex offenders: Risk management and good lives. *Professional Psychology: Research and Practice, 34,* 353–360.

Willis, G. M., Yates, P. M., Gannon, T. A., & Ward, T. (2012). How to integrate the Good Lives Model into treatment programs for sexual offending: An introduction and overview. *Sexual Abuse: A Journal of Research and Treatment, 25*(2), 123–142.

15 Forensic mental health

Emily Glorney and Siobhan Neave

Summary

Forensic mental health broadly refers to people or services that have or address needs relating to both mental disorder and offending behaviour. This chapter will set a context for understanding the relationship between mental disorder and crime, the context of forensic mental health settings in England and Wales, and introduce the Mental Health Act (1983 as amended in 2007). Throughout the chapter, the roles of a forensic psychologist within forensic mental health settings are considered.

Introduction

Across countries of the world, there is a higher prevalence of mental disorder (e.g. mental illness, personality disorders, neurodevelopmental disorders and acquired brain injuries) amongst people in custodial settings such as prisons, in comparison to people living in the community (Brooker et al., 2008; Fazel et al., 2016). People in prisons with mental health problems are likely to have experienced abuse victimisation during their childhood and present with ongoing psychological responses to trauma (Baranyi et al., 2018; Bodkin et al., 2019). What this means for a forensic psychologist is that attention must be paid to the individual beyond their offending behaviour alone. Structured professional judgement approaches to risk assessment include dynamic items on psychosocial functioning, effective coping and communication and healthy stress management (e.g. Douglas et al., 2013), but these factors are also relevant to mental health and well-being. Therefore, forensic psychologists must be aware of, competent to assess and identify appropriate interventions to address mental health need. This chapter sets out some of the considerations for a forensic psychologist about the relationship between mental disorder and offending behaviour, specialist services for people who have dual needs relating to mental health and risk reduction and working in a forensic mental health setting.

Mental disorder and crime

The relationship between mental disorder and crime is complex and cannot be explained through an incorrect assumption that mental disorder causes crime. There are some cases whereby there is a functional link between a person's mental disorder and their offence perpetration; that is, at the specific time at which the crime took place, the person's mental disorder contributed strongly to their behaviour and the offence was unlikely to have happened if mental disorder were not present. Discussions about this functional link typically take place in court trials, and you might be able to think of a number of reasons

DOI: 10.4324/9781003017103-18

why establishing a functional link is tricky. A couple of examples include reliance on retrospective analysis of the circumstances leading up to and at the time of the offence and an absence of a psychological or psychiatric assessment at the time of the offence. There are other cases whereby a person has a mental disorder, but this has no strong contribution to offence perpetration. That is, there is no functional link and the crime would have occurred regardless of the mental disorder. And there are other cases where a person has no experience of mental disorder, commits a crime and receives a custodial sentence and then struggles with the experience of imprisonment (e.g. Crewe, 2011); pre-existing vulnerabilities to mental illness can be triggered by the stress of the environment. The relationship between a person's mental disorder and crime is one factor that can influence the type of forensic setting where treatment can be accessed.

There are, of course, differences in the severity with which people experience mental disorder and the impact that this experience has on their own safety and that of other people. The majority of people with mental disorder are well able to manage activities of daily living, education, employment and relationships, but a minority of people experience substantial problems across these domains. For people with mental disorder who have also committed crimes and are detained in secure services, this has implications for risk reduction and management, as well as rights to care and access to appropriate treatment. The following section provides an overview of specialist services that provide care and treatment for people who have committed crimes and who have mental disorder.

Specialist services that address mental health and criminogenic needs

Prisons are designed to focus on retribution and rehabilitation and are not well equipped to address the mental health and neuropsychological needs with which many people in prison present (Glorney et al., 2020). A National Health Service (NHS) partnership with Her Majesty's Prison and Probation Service (HMPPS) offers mental health in-reach services for the most acutely unwell people in prisons, but there is not an equivalence of service provision to that which would be expected in the community (Forrester et al., 2013). There are dedicated mental healthcare units in prisons, and you can read about Siobhan's reflections on working in this setting in Focus Box 15.1.

BOX 15.1   SIOBHAN'S REFLECTIONS ON WORKING IN A MENTAL HEALTHCARE UNIT IN PRISON

Working in a forensic mental health setting can be very rewarding but the locked environment will impact on patients, staff and the relationship between them. Staff carrying keys and alarms, and having strict security boundaries can hinder therapeutic rapport and trust and restrict the freedom of some conversations. When trying to run therapeutic or psycho-educational groups with patients, I was faced with environmental barriers to therapeutic engagement, mainly relating to the prison regime that was strongly focused on risk and security and seemingly less so on therapeutic engagement and rehabilitation. Despite security processes, some of the patients I worked with witnessed traumatic or violent events, were subjected to bullying or exploitation, and made to feel unsafe in their environment. All these factors (and many more) have an impact on how ready patients feel to engage in therapeutic work with psychologists to address mental health and risk reduction needs. Despite the challenges, through facilitating groups such as the 'Hearing Voices Group' provided by the charity MIND, I was able to provide support and hope in an environment that can feel disempowering and hopeless. I learned a lot about the resilience of patients on healthcare units in prisons and how they conceptualised 'the system' as part of their lives and within the narrative of their journey.

Although prison mental healthcare units can offer care to a small number of people and on a short-term basis, people with severe and enduring mental health difficulties who need an intensive period and/or long-term mental health care and treatment require transfer from the general prison environment to a specialist service.

Provision for personality disorder in the prison and probation services

The Offender Personality Disorder (OPD) Pathway is an NHS-HMPPS partnership in England and Wales designed to address aspects of an individual's interpersonal functioning that are problematic, persistent and pervasive, and designed for people who present with high likelihood and severity of future harm (Skett & Lewis, 2019). The approach sets out sequences of interventions known to be effective in the treatment of personality disorders (such as dialectical behaviour therapy, schema therapy and mentalisation-based therapy) but, crucially, embedded within environments that take account of the difficulties that individuals have experienced in their attachment formations, early life and adolescent experiences and appraisals of events.

The OPD Pathway spans the criminal justice system, across prisons and the community, such that if need is identified within a secure service, a pathway of support and help can be followed through to the community. Change is facilitated through the development and maintenance of positive relationships with specially trained staff but also peers and relationships extending beyond the service to families and other external support. The principles underpinning the OPD Pathway are based on attachment theory and informed by an understanding of trauma (for an overview of the bio-psychosocial model of personality and some of the common presenting needs in forensic services, please see Craissati et al., 2020). In such a Pathway, it is important for all staff to have a psychological understanding of the factors that contribute to social, emotional and behavioural problems and understanding the problematic behaviour. Through this knowledge and ongoing supervision, the whole service and staff group contribute to individual meaningful change and enhanced psychological well-being and risk reduction for people on the OPD Pathway. These are all areas where forensic psychologists can provide input to the effective delivery of the OPD Pathway: training other professionals, providing psychological advice and supervision and conducting psychological assessment and interventions.

ACTIVITY BOX 15.2

We recommend you to read Skett and Lewis (2019) for an overview of the psychological theories and principles that underpin the OPD Pathway, then reflect on how forensic psychologists can contribute to this model of rehabilitation.

For further information about the OPD residential Psychologically Informed Planned Environments (PIPEs) in prisons and approved premises, Enabling Environments across the criminal justice system and Democratic Therapeutic Communities, we recommend you to read Craissati et al. (2020), Kordowicz (2019) and Bennett and Shuker (2017), respectively.

FOCUS BOX 15.3

The term 'personality disorder' is controversial. The label is argued not only to be stigmatising and disempowering but also useful in signposting practitioners to the general needs with which an individual might present. This issue of labelling is highly relevant to forensic settings, where residents and service users are also likely to have a label of 'offender', 'prisoner' or 'ex-prisoner', all of which are stigmatising and disempowering. You can read more about the movement away from the term 'personality disorder' and the importance of psychological formulation of inter-personal functioning in the consensus statement led by Lamb and Sibbold (2018).

Provision for mental disorder in secure hospitals

Secure hospitals provide care and treatment for people who pose a risk of harm to other people (and sometimes themselves) and when that risk is linked to their mental disorder. In England and Wales, secure hospitals are managed by the NHS with an interface to the broader criminal justice system (courts, police, probation, prisons and public protection agencies). Secure hospitals are organised by the level of physical security that they provide: high, medium and low. Patients are admitted to one of the levels of secure hospitals based on the imminence of the risk of harm presented, including whether they are likely to try to escape from their secure care provision. There are also geographical catchment areas based on NHS commissioning, which influence where a patient could be placed.

There are up to 780 beds across three high-secure hospitals in England and Wales (Ashworth, Broadmoor and Rampton), including a small number of beds in specialist services for women, people with learning disabilities and people who are deaf. Patients in high-secure services will have *severe and enduring* mental health difficulties, pose *a serious and immediate risk* of harm to self or others and require a high level of care.

There are up to 5,500 medium- and low-secure beds in England and Wales, providing care for people who present *a risk of harm* to self or others and have *ongoing* mental health-related needs. Quite often, there will be a combination of medium- and low-secure wards on a hospital site, so that patients can move up or down levels of physical security in line with the needs and risks with which they are considered to present.

The Mental Health Act (1983 as amended in 2007)

Due to the nature and degree of mental disorder and the risks posed, patients are typically detained in hospitals under legislation that mandates their detention, provides them with an opportunity to access and engage with treatment relevant to their needs and safeguards the rights of patients whilst their liberty is deprived. Mental health professionals, including forensic psychologists, working in secure hospitals will be working in the context of the Mental Health Act (1983 as amended in 2007; MHA), the legislation that sets out when someone can be sent to hospital and/or receive treatment against their will for the safety of themselves or other people. The MHA offers a framework for the rights of and safeguards for patients across psychiatric and community services, not limited to forensic services. Some of the sections – rules for legal detention – most common in secure hospitals are:

- Section 35 – court direction for assessment/treatment (28 days)
- Section 36 – court direction for treatment (28 days)
- Section 37 – hospital order
- Section 37/41 – hospital order with restrictions
- Section 38 – interim hospital order
- Section 47/49 – transfer to hospital of a sentenced prisoner
- Section 48/49 – transfer to hospital of a prisoner on remand

As you can see from the different sections of the MHA, there are a number of ways in which patients can be referred in to secure hospitals. People who are undergoing court proceedings and for whom there is a concern about their mental health and well-being can be diverted through a liaison and diversion service to mental health care rather than spending time on remand in prison (e.g. Section 35, Section 36). When a court finds that there is a functional link between a person's mental disorder and their offences, then they can be ordered by the court to receive treatment in hospital (Section 37) rather than serve a custodial sentence. For very serious offences, the hospital order is with restrictions (Section 37/41) and the patient can only be discharged from hospital when the Secretary of State for Justice or a Mental Health Review Tribunal is satisfied that the risk with which they present can be managed in the community. People who become acutely unwell in prison can also be transferred to a secure hospital (Section 47/49, Section 48/49), but with restrictions so that their period of detention is not less than the minimum term of the custodial sentence that they received; they can also be returned to prison when they are well enough to do so.

BOX 15.4 SIOBHAN'S REFLECTIONS ON WORKING AS AN ASSISTANT PSYCHOLOGIST IN A SECURE HOSPITAL

After graduating from my undergraduate degree, my goal was to work in a secure unit as an assistant psychologist. When I was given the opportunity to fulfil this dream at a medium-secure hospital, I felt overwhelmed with excitement but also full of anticipation and anxiety about what was to come. It was a long road to becoming an assistant psychologist. I had already worked in a prison mental health team but when I started my new role there was a lot that was unfamiliar to me and a lot to learn, including getting to grips with the Mental Health Act. For my first couple of weeks, I felt like I said everything wrong, focusing too hard on trying to weave psychological jargon into every conversation with my colleagues; I felt intimidated by the knowledge and skills of my colleagues. From my experiences of working in prison, I had developed empathy for the challenges that patients had faced or were part of and, alongside my own experience of entering the secure hospital environment for the first time, I could only imagine how patients must feel having to contend with the fears and anxieties that come with detention in a secure hospital.

In the months following, I found my rhythm and I was learning more about psychology than I had ever thought possible. I was stunned by the breadth of psychological knowledge of my supervisors: one, a clinical psychologist who specialised in mental health and mentored me to work within a CBT framework; the other, a forensic psychologist who specialised in autistic spectrum disorders and mentored me to work within a compassion- and trauma-focused framework. Compassion-focused therapy, in particular, resonated with me and ignited a passion for understanding more about the brain and its relationship with trauma.

It was important to me to understand how the patients I worked with perceived their life beyond the walls of the secure hospital, including the impact of hospital detention on their future well-being and happiness. Working in the secure hospital felt more aligned with my way of working. Although the NHS has its own politics, it felt to me that the primary focus being on healthcare meant I had fewer restrictions to doing my job; there was a strong point of contrast here to my previous role in prison mental health. The working environment felt supportive of therapeutic care, and this was necessary to address the needs of the patients. The psychological work I was doing with the patients in the secure hospital was intense and required me to learn a great deal not only about models of assessment and intervention but also therapeutic and reflective skills. Although I had facilitated therapy groups in prison for nearly three years before, there was still a steep learning curve in the development of my skills. There were days in which I felt a lot of frustration when patients would not 'do what I had taught them'. Finding a balance in the ownership over the responsibility of the patient's behaviour was something that took a while for me to establish within myself. Learning more about the challenging aspects of working with forensic patients, and supervision, helped me to understand and work with my patients in a more therapeutic way. I experienced so many meaningful moments whilst working with the patients, and these memories will never leave me; I will always use these as a reminder of how powerful psychological intervention can be.

Recovery pathways in secure hospitals

The ethos of many secure hospitals in England and Wales is underpinned by the principles of the recovery approach (e.g. Drennan & Alred, 2012). The emphasis in a recovery pathway is to include the patient in the development of a plan that helps the person to move towards what they identify as a meaningful and satisfying life, away from an identity of illness or offending behaviour, and to promote social inclusion. Therefore, recovery is not something that is 'done to' someone or a discrete intervention that is engaged with. Rather, it is an approach to care, assessment and treatment that holds at the core the importance of the patient having control over their life, having opportunities for connection and personal development, and hope for a fulfilling life. There are challenges to this approach within forensic services, where possibilities for hope, control and opportunity are limited, but can be mitigated through the co-production of care plans, collaborative formulation, respect and an environment that promotes agency amongst service users. Thinking broadly about the strengths and identities of patients – such as skills in helping others, being a peer mentor, creative skills, identities relating to family and/or faith groups – strengthen opportunities for therapeutic engagement, respect and positive working relationships (e.g. Glorney et al., 2019; Glorney et al., 2010).

Patients in secure hospitals follow an individualised 'step-down' pathway from admission to discharge (Joint Commissioning Panel for Mental Health, 2013), meaning that they are placed within the least restrictive environment possible to address their needs for care and treatment. Each pathway is based on the specific needs of the individual patient and the level of security required for the safety of themselves and others. There is an expectation that pathways are reviewed regularly because the patient's needs are likely to change over time as their mental health is restored and their risk is reduced (Joint Commissioning Panel for Mental Health, 2013). Regular pathway reviews take place not only through the multidisciplinary team (MDT) responsible for the patient but also through a Mental Health Review Tribunal (MHRT). A role of the MHRT is to ensure that the patient detained under the MHA is not detained in hospital for longer than is necessary, and the care and treatment they receive is appropriate to their needs. A forensic psychologist can be asked to present evidence at a MHRT, to explain the patient's psychological care pathway and comment on risk reduction and mental health restoration.

Multi-disciplinary teams

Working as part of a MDT is a key component in the forensic psychologist role. Some of the skills required for MDT membership are described in Chapter 17, which outlines the stage 2 Core Role of Communicating Psychological Knowledge to Other Professionals. The purpose of a MDT is to take oversight for and action towards a service user's care pathway and recovery and to engage with relevant external stakeholders (e.g. family, probation and social services) as appropriate. MDTs are collaborative and impact greatly on the care provided to forensic mental health patients due to the holistic approach to care and treatment planning and oversight of the recovery pathway by all professionals.

The disciplines that make up the MDT will differ depending on the environment, professional resources and the individual's needs. For example, for a patient with learning disabilities, the MDT might comprise a registered learning disability and mental health nurse, psychiatrist, psychologist, speech and language and occupational therapists and any other professionals specific to the patient's individual needs. All these disciplines contribute to multidisciplinary and multi-agency reviews to shape the sequence of a patient's care pathway. These reviews include the Care Programme Approach, a written document that sets out the coordinated approach to a patient's multidisciplinary care and treatment. This could include the specific medication (mental and/or physical health) that the patient requires, occupational and educational activities that support recovery and personal development, systems and mechanisms for personal support (such as contact with family, faith groups and special interest groups), physical activity, specific dietary needs, plans to address housing and finances, as well as identified risk reduction and mental health needs that might be addressed through psychological intervention and/or further assessment. Psychologists can also be legally responsible for the overall care and treatment of patients detained under the MHA.

As part of an MDT, the forensic psychologist might be asked to be involved in and provide input to multidisciplinary components of the patient's care: for example, attend a ward round to update on psychological assessment and treatment and share psychological formulations of the patient's offending and their behaviour in hospital. The following fictional case study provides a context for the formulation and treatment targets that follow. The formulation-driven summary of the presenting issues would be a typical contribution by a forensic psychologist to an MDT.

Case study

John is a 24-year-old man who grew up with his mother, father and three younger brothers. From a young age, John witnessed his father be violent to his mother and when John tried to intervene he was also assaulted. When John was 12, his father left and broke contact with the family. John's mother started to drink heavily and began to neglect him and his brothers. Sometimes she was verbally and emotionally abusive to the children, blaming them for their father leaving. John's relationship with his mother became strained and he assumed the role of caring for his brothers. As he got older, John found it difficult to manage his thoughts and feelings, particularly related to anger, and his behaviour caused problems for himself and other people. He got involved in petty crime, antisocial behaviour and used alcohol and drugs to try to escape from how he was feeling. On one occasion, the police approached John and his friends – who were drinking alcohol in the local park – following a complaint about the excessive noise they were making. When the male police officer told the young people to go home, John got angry and aggressive and repeatedly complained that the officer was threatening him. The officer attempted to make an arrest and John punched him in the face. John was arrested, entered a guilty plea in court and received a custodial sentence.

John found being in prison very stressful. He was locked in a cell for a long time every day and he began to experience persecutory auditory hallucinations telling him that other people were trying to kill him. This meant that when prison officers opened his cell, John attacked them because he thought they meant him harm. After a serious attempt to take his own life, John told one of the mental healthcare staff about the voices and his suspicions about the intentions of other people. Following an assessment from a psychiatrist, John was diagnosed with a psychotic illness and transferred to a medium-secure unit. A forensic psychologist completed a CBT formulation of John's violent behaviour, using the 'Five-Ps' approach (adapted from Dudley & Kuyken, 2014, p. 21), and this was used to guide treatment.

Presenting issue: what are the key issues for John at the moment?

John's use of violence. John has a diagnosis of mental illness, which is related to his violent behaviour. He feels a lot of anger and confusion. John's coping strategies include taking drugs and alcohol. His personal support is mainly antisocial peers.

Precipitating factors: what are the triggers for the presenting issue?

John's anger and violent behaviour seem to be triggered by the presence of male authority figures whose behaviour John interprets as hostile. Another trigger is feeling trapped or controlled. These triggers might be a trauma response. Alcohol and drugs weaken John's behavioural controls and his ability to manage his emotions and distort his perception of events around him and his thought processes. John's active symptoms of psychosis – specifically his paranoid thinking – further contribute to his violence.

Perpetuating factors: what are the factors that maintain the presenting issue?

John's perception of threat (core belief and paranoid thinking), possible trauma response and active psychosis are likely to maintain his use of violence in response to male authority figures. His difficulties coping with these experiences probably maintain his alcohol and drug use that, in turn, enhances his threat perception and reduces behavioural controls.

Predisposing factors: what are the factors that increase John's vulnerability to the presenting issue?

John's experience of violence victimisation by his father, physical and emotional neglect from his mother and high stress in childhood and adolescence makes him vulnerable to the presenting issue. John's previous alcohol and drug use makes him vulnerable to further substance misuse unless he develops alternative ways to cope with how he feels.

Protective factors: what are the factors that aid John's resilience and strength?

John has a positive relationship with his brothers. John is able to be open about and access support for his mental illness symptoms. Being in an environment that reduces his stress has been protective for John.

Key treatment targets

The key treatment targets were identified as: stabilising John's psychosis through medication, psycho-education and CBT, working through his early-life experiences in individual therapy, developing skills to manage the healthy experience and expression of strong emotions such as anger, engaging in group interventions to address John's use of alcohol and drugs and developing his understanding of his use of violence, including a violence relapse prevention plan. Once John began to feel better within himself, he asked his brothers to start visiting him. Their support was a positive influence in his recovery.

Supervision

Working in a forensic mental health setting can be challenging and emotionally draining but very rewarding. Forensic psychologists need to be prepared for:

- Being faced with unpredictable behaviours.
- Experiencing adversity.
- Having limited control over your own safety and well-being.
- Potentially witnessing or being victim to a traumatic or violent event.
- Engaging in one-to-one or group work with individuals who present with challenging personality traits or mental health symptoms.
- Working with individuals who are not responsive to the therapy provided and finding a way through this.
- Being exposed to upsetting or sensitive information about a patient's offence history, current challenging behaviours and voiced antisocial or harmful thoughts and feelings.

Supervision is critical not only to the health and well-being of psychologists working in forensic mental health settings but also to the patients they work with. Psychologists need to be able to use the supervisory space to reflect on work with their patients, to enhance learning about the needs of their patients and to develop therapeutic skills, so that they can competently and safely provide care and treatment to forensic patients.

Conclusion

In this chapter, we have set out some of the considerations for a forensic psychologist about the relationship between mental disorder and offending behaviour, specialist services for people who have dual needs relating to mental health and risk reduction and working in a forensic mental health setting. The high prevalence of mental disorder in offender populations means that forensic psychologists need to have skills to identify, assess and treat mental health problems and to consider the most appropriate environment within which a person's needs can be addressed. Working with people presenting with dual needs relating to mental health restoration and risk reduction can be very rewarding, and forensic psychologists are well placed to help service users make sense of the relationship between their mental disorder and their offending behaviour, with a view to supporting risk reduction and their pathway to a fulfilling life.

Learning outcomes

When you have completed this chapter, you should be able to:

1   Critically evaluate some of the key issues relating to people who have mental health problems and commit crime/pose a risk to other people or themselves
2   Understand the need for, role and function of forensic mental health settings in prisons and secure hospitals
3   Understand the contribution of psychological knowledge and skills to working with patients in forensic mental health settings
4   Critically evaluate the key issues facing and skills required of forensic psychologists working in forensic mental health settings

Key concepts and terms

• Mental disorder
• Functional link
• Prison healthcare unit
• Secure hospitals
• Mental Health Act
• Multidisciplinary team (MDT)

Sample essay questions

• Critically discuss whether people with mental disorder should be in prison.
• To what extent could the principles of recovery be applied in prisons?

Recommended further reading

Drennan, G., & Alred, D. (2012). *Secure recovery: Approaches to recovery in forensic mental health settings*. Willan.

Vossler, A., Harvard, C., Pike, G., Barker, M. J., Raabe, B., & Walkington, Z. (2017). Therapeutic work in forensic settings. In A. Vossler, C. Harvard, G. Pike, M. Barker, & B. Raabe (Eds.), *Mad or bad? A critical approach to counselling and forensic psychology* (pp. 9–22). Sage.

References

Baranyi, G., Cassidy, M., Fazel, S., Priebe, S., & Mundt, A. P. (2018). Prevalence of posttraumatic stress disorder in prisoners. *Epidemiologic Reviews*, *40*(1), 134–145.

Bennett, J., & Shuker, R. (2017). The potential of prison-based democratic therapeutic communities. *International Journal of Prisoner Health*, *13*(1), 19–24.

Bodkin, C., Pivnick, L., Bondy, S. J., Ziegler, C., Martin, R. E., Jernigan, C., & Kouyoumdjian, F. (2019). History of childhood abuse in populations incarcerated in Canada: A systematic review and meta-analysis. *American Journal of Public Health*, (0), e1–e11.

Brooker, C., Duggan, S., Fox, C., Mills, A., & Parsonage, M. (2008). *Short-changed: Spending on prison mental health care*. Sainsbury Centre for Mental Health.

Craissati, J., Joseph, N., & Skett, S. (2020). *Practitioner guide: Working with people in the criminal justice system showing personality difficulties*. NHS England and Her Majesty's Prison and Probation Service.

Crewe, B. (2011). Depth, weight, tightness: Revisiting the pains of imprisonment. *Punishment & Society*, *13*(5), 509–529.

Douglas, K. S., Hart, S. D., Webster, C. D., & Belfrage, H. (2013). *HCR-20V3: Assessing risk of violence: User guide*. Simon Fraser University.

Drennan, G., & Alred, D. (2012). *Secure recovery: Approaches to recovery in forensic mental health settings*. Willan.

Dudley, R., & Kuyken, W. (2014). Case formulation in cognitive behavioural therapy: A principle-driven approach. In L. Johnstone & R. Dallos (Eds.), *Formulation in psychology and psychotherapy: Making sense of people's problems* (2nd ed., pp. 18–44). Routledge.

Fazel, S., Hayes, A. J., Bartellas, K., CLerici, M., & Trestman, R. (2016). Mental health of prisoners: Prevalence, adverse outcomes, and interventions. *Lancet Psychiatry*, *3*, 871–881.

Forrester, A., Exworthy, T., Olumoroti, O., Sessay, M., Parrott, J., Spencer, S. J., & Whyte, S. (2013). Variations in prison mental health services in England and Wales. *International Journal of Law and Psychiatry*, *36*(3–4), 326–332.

Glorney, E., Perkins, D., Adshead, G., McGauley, G., Murray, K., Noak, J., & Sichau, G. (2010). Domains of need in a high secure hospital setting: A model for streamlining care and reducing length of stay. *International Journal of Forensic Mental Health*, *9*(2), 138–148.

Glorney, E., Raymont, S., Lawson, A., & Allen, J. (2019). Religion, spirituality and personal recovery among forensic patients. *The Journal of Forensic Practice*, *21*(3), 190–200.

Glorney, E., Ullah, H., & Brooker, C. (2020). Standards of mental health care in prisons in England and Wales: A qualitative analysis of reports from Her Majesty's inspectorate of prisons. *International Journal of Forensic Mental Health*, *19*(3), 283–296.

Joint Commissioning Panel for Mental Health. (2013). *Guidance for commissioners of forensic mental health services*. Joint Commissioning Panel for Mental Health.

Kordowicz, M. (2019). *The perceived impact of the Enabling Environments programme within Her Majesty's Prison and Probation Service settings: A qualitative evaluation*. Royal College of Psychiatrists and Her Majesty's Prison and Probation Service.

Lamb, N., & Sibbold, S. (2018). *Shining lights in dark corners of people's lives: The consensus statement for people with complex mental health difficulties who are diagnosed with a personality disorder*. Retrieved from www.mind.org.uk/media/21163353/consensus-statement-final.pdf.

Mental Health Act. Retrieved from www.nhs.uk/using-the-nhs/nhs-services/mental-health-services/mental-health-act.

Skett, S., & Lewis, C. (2019). Development of the offender personality disorder pathway: A summary of the underpinning evidence. *Probation Journal*, *66*(2), 167–180.

Part 4

Forensic settings and professional issues

16 Forensic environments

Jenny Tew and Neil Gredecki

Summary

As has been outlined in this book, forensic psychologists work in a range of settings: prisons, secure hospitals, residential care homes, courts and the list goes on. Forensic psychologists and other professional groups work with clients to support rehabilitation and to support clients to lead productive and offence-free lives in the community as they progress through their individual pathways. Yet, the environments can very much influence the manner in which individual clients engage and the progress they make. It is beyond the scope of this chapter to consider each of these forensic environments and as such, we will consider the prison environment and current approaches to support rehabilitation amongst those within prisons. We will focus on male prisons which represents the largest population and environment for forensic clients in England and Wales. That does not mean, however, that the learning and the psychological theories and concepts cannot be applied in other settings. To the contrary, many of the psychological theories and principles can be applied across various settings. We will also give some consideration as to the impact of the prison setting on culture and experience for prisoners, as well as innovative strategies to reform rehabilitation.

Introduction

Prisons are places of great fascination to many people in terms of what they are like as places in which to live and work, how they operate and what happens on a day-to-day basis. In many ways, prisons are similar to life in society where the day is punctuated by meal times, attending to personal hygiene, engaging in exercise and accessing fresh air, socialisation and work. At the same time, prisons are unique settings. For example, mealtimes are set and access to exercise and socialisation is determined by the regime operating in the prison. They also occur within the physical restrictions of the prison environment (e.g. locked gates and doors and high walls) and the procedural constraints which help to maintain order and control and prevent escape. Thus, prisons remove aspects of choice and autonomy for prisoners who can become reliant on prison officers. Therefore, relationships between the staff and prisoners become very important.

In this chapter, we will consider the prison environment and the prisoner and prison officer roles in the prison context. Considering the prison environment is important in terms of also understanding the other key role of prisons: the rehabilitation of offenders.

DOI: 10.4324/9781003017103-20

Prisons in England and Wales

Within the United Kingdom, prisons are devolved. This means that the responsibility for the running of prisons is different in each of the home nations. Within this chapter, we will focus specifically on the prison system in England and Wales. However, there are perhaps more similarities across the prisons in the home nations than there are differences. If you are interested in knowing more about prison practice in the different home nations, then you can visit the relevant websites to find out more information.

BOX 16.1 PRISON FIGURES AND STATISTICS

According to official statistics, the prison population in England and Wales quadrupled between 1900 and 2019. From the mid-1990s, the prison population saw a high increase in numbers; although this has been more stable from around 2010. Figures at the end of 2019 recorded just under 83,000 people in prison in England and Wales. Up-to-date figures for the prison population in England and Wales can be found on the government website (www.gov.uk). But what does this mean and are these figures high?

A helpful way to think about prison figures is to consider them against the general population. This is usually done by outlining the ratio of people in prison per 100,000 people in the population. In 1900 in England and Wales, there were 86 people in prison for every 100,000 people in the population. In 2018, this figure was 173 prisoners per 100,000 (Sturge, 2020). The most recent complete data set comparing prison numbers across Europe note that England and Wales are ranked as having the 8th highest imprisonment rate across EU countries (see Sturge, 2020).

The Prison Service in England and Wales manages complex and diverse prisoner groups. This includes male and female prisons, as well as young offender institutions (YOIs), the Youth Custody Service and Immigration and Removal Centres, each of which operate slightly differently. Each prisoner group is noted to have different needs in relation to their imprisonment and their offending behaviour more generally. The size of the prison population has implications for how prisons run and what can be achieved with the clients in their care. Prison units are often larger than hospital settings which usually offer more bespoke care for their patients.

Reflecting on the function and purpose of imprisonment, prisons represent the wider society in which they exist and criminal justice policy and practice have been impacted upon by political positions (Cavender, 2004). For example, historical methods of punishment have been strategically and ideologically crucial to the penal system in its modern form (Garland, 1990). Thus, the Prison Service in England and Wales has evolved over the years, and it is necessary to take into account the history and purpose of the Prison Service over previous years in order to understand the 'modern' system (Liebling & Price, 1998). That is to say, it has moved between differing ideals of deterrence, retribution and reform which has had the potential to impact on the culture and climate within prisons.

Culture and climate

As forensic psychologists, we often consider concepts such as the 'therapeutic alliance' (Bordin, 1979) or 'treatment milieu' (Hoffman, 1982) and the impact they can have on our work with clients. The relationships we form with our clients and the environments we create are clearly important for supporting change. However, the wider environment within which we work (the organisation's culture) also impacts on outcomes. Let us consider some of the key terms starting with the term 'Culture'.

Organisational culture is often played out as 'The way we do things around here' (Deal & Kennedy, 1982). It is made up of our attitudes and ideas, our behaviours and the physical things we have around. It has been referred to as the personality of the organisation. Culture has a significant role in influencing all aspects of life within the organisation. The range of factors linked to an organisational culture are vast. As such, an organisation's culture can be difficult to identify and quantify. The **cultural web** (Johnson et al., 2012) provides an approach for examining and looking at an organisation's culture, and we will refer to this later.

If culture is the personality of an organisation, then climate has more to do with its mood or prevailing atmosphere. We may see more fluctuation in the organisation's climate or in different parts of the organisation at different times. Organisational climate could be seen as something more 'surface level' than culture as it relates more to the here and now and in turn it may have more of an impact on how individuals experience being in the particular organisation at a given time. It is more prone to short-term fluctuations. For example, an influx of prisoners with specific offences types may change the climate on a wing for a period of time.

Prison culture and climate

Focusing particularly on prisons, these have been described as distinct societies with their own cultures (Byrne & Stowell, 2007). Whilst the idea of 'culture' often brings positive thoughts about creativity and growth, the idea of a prison culture often brings more negative and hopeless images to mind. There have been different views in the literature about how a prison's culture develops. One view is that it is a result of the criminal culture that individuals bring into prison with them from their life outside. Prisons admit people with violent histories, troubled backgrounds and complex needs, making it likely that a culture including violence will develop (Irwin & Cressey, 1962).

An alternate view is that prison culture develops as a response to the experience of imprisonment (Sekol, 2013; Sykes & Messinger, 1960). Powerlessness, deprivation, stigmatisation, a loss of physical property, disrespect and a fear of violence lead to a need to establish status and increase self-esteem and control, often through violence. Sparks et al. took a holistic view, believing that prison culture was determined by both the experiences of prison and the influences of the outside world, with the additional impact of how the prison was managed (Sparks et al., 1996).

It is not only the subculture of prisoners that shapes a prison but also that of staff alongside the interaction between these two groups. Attitudes and beliefs about why people offend and the purpose of prison shapes behaviours. This is in addition to longstanding expectations of officers as being fearless and resilient authority figures. The result can be a sense of 'us and them' and increased confrontation.

It is important to note that prison culture and climate are not fixed, they can change over time and the relationships between staff and prisoners can impact on these. According to Leibling and Arnold (2004), one of the most important things observed regarding the climate of a prison is the relationship between prison officers and managers, and between staff and prisoners.

Staff–prisoner relationships

Staff–prisoner relationships are said to be at the heart of the prison system in the United Kingdom, and it has long since been recognised that they are fundamental to the effective management of prisons and prisoners (Home Office, 1984; Sparks et al., 1996; Gilbert, 1997). These relationships are central to maintaining decent and stable regimes and in aiding the rehabilitative process (e.g. NOMS, 2008). Therefore, exploring the nature and quality of staff–prisoner relationships can provide insight into prison regimes and prison life.

The roles of staff and prisoners can create a sense of 'us and them'; separate staff and prisoner subcultures can develop which in turn can impact on staff–prisoner relationships. According to Williamson (1990), within the prison system, fundamental roles are assumed. Here, prisoners take on the role of captive and the prison officers, the role of captor which reinforces the 'them and us' mentality. Officers can be a key influence on a prison's culture through their ideas and behaviours. That is, the use of power by officers can be a key source of hope or frustration, especially amongst prisoners serving long sentences (Crewe, 2011). Yet, despite being described as independent groups, they often share similar goals and they demonstrate interdependency in achieving them (Liebling & Arnold, 2004).

Within prisons, expectations around prison officer and prisoner 'roles' can lead to the development of very distinct prisoner and prison officer identities where each group is likely to align themselves with their peers. Where different cultures meet, **acculturation** explains the process of the cultural and psychological change that occurs. Here, individuals adopt the cultural traits or social patterns of another group.

ACTIVITY BOX 16.2

It is well established that *role assignment* (the taking of a specific role within a particular setting) has the potential to impact on interpersonal relationships in forensic settings (see Haney et al., 1973; Haslam & Reicher, 2005; Reicher & Haslam, 2006), particularly where these roles are intrinsically different and reflect varying degrees of power. In turn, these roles assign different rights and responsibilities based on their given label (i.e. prisoner or prison officer) which can impact on prison life.

You are encouraged to further explore the psychology of imprisonment and the notion of role assignment. There have been a number of high-profile studies in this area including the Zimbardo experiment and the rerun of the experiment in 2002 by the BBC. For more information and resources on this topic, visit the following website: www.bbcprisonstudy.org

---

The roles and identities that people adopt within prisons influence their interactions with each other. The prison officer role is diverse and can involve a range of tasks from restraining a prisoner to supporting a prisoner in crisis; they are required to move between security and therapeutic roles. Likewise, prisoners often construct relationships based on the performance of masculinities, conforming to group norms so that they are not treated with suspicion or rejected by their peers. These roles impact relationships which are in turn critical to the type of culture and climate that exists. This means that everyone plays a role in the culture of a prison, and it is something that can be influenced. The recommended reading section provides suggestions for further reading around the construction of the prison officer role. In the next section, we consider the particular prison environments and cultures that can support rehabilitation.

Rehabilitative cultures and environments

Rehabilitative environments

Whilst the aims of the Prison Service include rehabilitation, many of the physical features of prisons and the roles and relationships we have explored here have the potential to be detrimental to rehabilitation (Day & Doyle, 2010). As such, there is a need to explicitly focus on developing environments and cultures that can support individual rehabilitation, and forensic psychologists have a range of roles in helping achieve this. Within prisons, there are specific units and initiatives that pay particular attention to the role the environment and relationships play in supporting rehabilitation. Three examples specific to forensic settings will be outlined including Enabling Environments (EEs), Psychologically Informed Planned Environments (PIPEs) and Therapeutic Communities.

Enabling Environments are environments specifically designed to promote a sense of belonging and to offer opportunities to develop and learn new skills through establishing positive and supportive relationships (HMPPS & NHS England, 2020). There is a recognised need for an increased psychological awareness to be able to achieve this (Johnson & Haigh, 2011). The Royal College of Psychiatrists introduced the Enabling Environment Award as a mark of an organisation that is particularly successful in creating such an environment. The award is made up of a set of ten standards that they identify as necessary, namely: belonging, boundaries, communication, development, involvement, safety, structure, empowerment, leadership and openness. EEs can be created in a wide range of settings, including prisons. Yet, it is perhaps easy to consider potential challenges to achieving the ten standards of an EE where power and authority are open to discussion and spontaneity is encouraged within a prison that, as we have described, has a fixed regime and an inbuilt power imbalance. Despite this, there are numerous such places that have achieved this, for example, the Westgate unit at HMP Frankland (Bennett & Tew, 2018). These environments are psychologically informed rather than psychology led and psychologists play a key role in supporting operational colleagues in implementing the EE standards in practice.

Psychologically Informed Planned Environments is another example of a specialist unit where the environment is key. They are similar to EEs in that they are specifically designed environments where staff have an increased psychological understanding of their work (Turley et al., 2013). These units form part of the OPD Pathway (Joseph & Benefield, 2012) which aims to provide a pathway of psychologically informed services for individuals with highly complex and challenging needs who are likely to have severe personality disorder and who pose a high risk of harm to others (HMPPS & NHS England, 2020). The aim of a PIPE is to ensure that the environment is safe and supportive where everyday interactions can be used as opportunities for development. Staff working in PIPEs support clients to openly explore interpersonal difficulties in a psychologically informed way during daily life on the unit. Again, PIPEs are psychologically informed rather than being psychologically led and so a large part of the psychologist's role within a PIPE is supervision and support of other frontline staff to create the environment and relationships necessary to support progression.

Therapeutic Communities (TCs) are a further example of somewhere where the environment and the relationships that exist are key to supporting change. TCs are holistic treatment approaches that aim to address a range of needs within a living-learning environment using social learning, cognitive behavioural and psychodynamic approaches to treatment within a culture of enquiry (Shuker & Sullivan, 2010). They involve small group therapies and community meetings and make use of everyday interactions and activities to provide opportunity for learning and addressing criminogenic risk factors. TCs exist in custody and community settings and are either residential or operate as day centres. Psychologists are involved in the assessment of individuals, delivery of group-based therapy and in the support of other frontline workers in creating and maintaining the therapeutic environment.

Whilst these units and approaches are clearly helpful in supporting rehabilitation, it remains the case that the wider environment and culture of a prison also plays an important role in its effectiveness as a place of rehabilitation. Rehabilitation is often seen as being supported through structured offending behaviour programmes. However, these programmes are only as good as the environment they are delivered in (Blagden & Thorne, 2013; Woessner & Schwelder, 2014). Culture is important for programme engagement and effectiveness (Lipsey & Cullen, 2007). For example, support from others has been found to be a major factor in the success of treatment; a factor that in prison is provided by staff and peers (Burnett & McNeil, 2005).

A rehabilitative culture

If, as we outlined earlier, culture captures our attitudes and ideas, our behaviours and the physical things around us, then a rehabilitative culture ensures these elements all support people to address the reasons why they might commit crimes: for example, understanding their substance misuse, criminal attitudes or the types of peer and family relationships they have (Bonta & Andrews, 2016). A rehabilitative culture contributes to places being safe, decent, hopeful and optimistic about change and stopping offending. There is also a focus on generating and maintaining hope which is seen as critical for successful change (LeBel et al., 2008; Valle et al., 2006).

BOX 16.3 PRINCIPLES OF A REHABILITATIVE ENVIRONMENT OR CULTURE

The essential qualities of a therapeutic environment have been described by Haigh (2013) as including:

- Attachment (a culture of belonging)
- Containment (a culture of safety)
- Communication (a culture of openness)
- Involvement and inclusion (a culture of participation and citizenship)
- Agency (a culture of empowerment)

Bennett and Shuker (2010) identified five principles of a rehabilitative culture: respect, openness, challenge, trust and responsibility.

A safe and decent environment, positive relationships, good communication and encouraging responsibility are key.

Within prisons a rehabilitative culture can be seen to be made up of the following elements (Mann et al., 2018):

- Relationships that are supportive and collaborative for everyone
- Management and leadership that encourage engagement
- Activities that promote well-being and stopping offending
- Processes and systems that are fair and focus on rehabilitation
- An environment that is normalised and promotes safety, decency and hope

A rehabilitative culture can help reduce reoffending and can help make prisons safer (Byrne & Hummer, 2007; Byrne & Stowell, 2007; Lee & Gilligan, 2006; Ros et al., 2013). Increased support through respectful contact and providing opportunities to learn has been found to reduce aggressive incidents in secure units (Van der Helm et al., 2011). A rehabilitative culture also contributes to safety through addressing areas that contribute to suicide and self-harm, for example, hopelessness, lack of personal control, poor staff–prisoner relationships and poor coping skills (Ludlow et al., 2015). Whilst improvements in safety are clearly of benefit to both staff and prisoners, there are additional benefits of a rehabilitative culture specifically for staff. For prison officers, rehabilitative work has been found to be associated with a source of meaning, lower levels of stress and greater job satisfaction, than a more punitive culture (Dowden & Tellier, 2004; Hepburn & Knepper, 1993; Tait, 2008; Tait, 2011). Rehabilitative cultures can also support the development of staff–prisoner relationships, helping to breakdown 'them and us' barriers.

In the next section, we will consider how a prison's culture can be influenced to be more rehabilitative.

Developing a rehabilitative culture

Understanding the current culture

One of the first steps in trying to influence culture is to understand the current culture. This can then be used to develop a plan for cultural change, identifying positive areas that can be built on and potential barriers to change. One way to get an understanding of the current culture is by using the cultural web (Johnson et al., 2012). The cultural web considers six interrelated areas that the authors consider make up culture namely: stories, symbols, power structures, organisational structures, control systems and rituals and routines. When explored across different groups within an organisation, for example, between prisoners, prison officers, prison managers and visitors, different perspectives can be collated to get as full a picture of the culture as possible.

BOX 16.4   UNDERSTANDING THE CURRENT CULTURE

To be able to influence a culture, it is helpful to first understand the current culture.

You're invited to do consider the current culture of a group or organisation you belong to according to the culture web areas (Johnson et al., 2012).

Example prompts:

- What stories go round about the organisation and what messages do these give?
- Who has power in your organisation and how do they use that power?

- Does your organisation have a hierarchical or flat structure and when are these followed or by-passed?
- What gets rewarded or punished in your organisation and what impact does this have?
- What symbols are important to your organisation?
- What are the habits of your organisation – how do things get done?

To get as complete a picture as possible of the current culture, it is helpful to involve as many people as possible in discussing these areas.

Once the current culture is understood, this can be used to identify ways to influence the relationships, processes and systems, environment, activities and leadership of a prison to be more rehabilitative.

Practical steps towards cultural change

There is not scope in this chapter to cover all the possible ways that aspects of a prisons culture can be rehabilitative. Instead, we will focus on just a couple of examples: the concept of procedural justice and peer worker schemes. Prisons are made up of a multitude of systems and processes that are designed to govern behaviour. How these processes and systems are administered impacts on the prison's culture. An important part of a rehabilitative culture is that everyone feels that they are being treated fairly. Evidence suggests that when people feel they are treated fairly they are more likely to agree with any outcomes and abide by any rules regardless of whether they are in their favour or not (Lind & Tyler, 1988). This can be achieved through processes that are procedurally just.

For people to see things as being procedurally, just, they need to be treated respectfully and have a voice in the process. They also need to see authority figures as acting in a neutral non-biased way, as having trustworthy motives and to care about getting the best outcome for all involved (Tyler, 2008). Procedural justice is relevant to a range of situations in prison, for example, how searches are conducted; how jobs are allocated or how written complaints are responded to. Understanding what is happening and why, being able to ask questions or explain your point of view and being talked to in a respectful way make a big difference to how people feel and consequently how they behave.

For prisoners, procedural justice has been associated with better prison behaviour, increased well-being and lower levels of reoffending (Beijersbergen et al., 2014, 2015, 2016). For prison staff, procedural justice has been associated with reduced stress, improved job satisfaction and greater support for rehabilitation (Fitzalan-Howard & Wakeling, 2019; Lambert, 2003).

BOX 16.5   PROCEDURAL JUSTICE PODCAST EPISODE

To learn more about the concept of procedural justice in secure settings, follow this link (https://pod.link/1533101974) and listen to episode 'Does fairness matter in prison' [12/11/2020]. Flora Fitzalan Howard and Dr Helen Wakeling discuss how concepts such as procedural justice can make a difference.

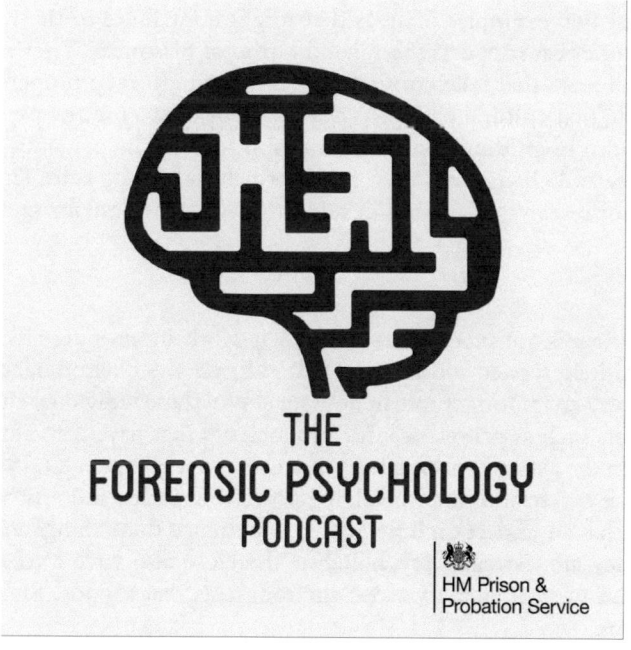

As a very different example, there are lots of activities within a prison that can support or undermine rehabilitation. Opportunities for people to get involved and to help others is one example of this. Peer worker schemes can provide support to people in areas such as improving educational skills or reducing drug use which impacts on the rehabilitation of the person being supported. Peer workers who support others with difficulties they have managed to overcome themselves can have more credibility than staff and are evidence that success is possible, increasing levels of hope. Being a peer worker can also help change how someone sees themselves and how others see them, increasing their confidence and motivation and highlighting their strengths which can help increase their own levels of hope and reduce their own offending (Edgar et al., 2011). There are a wide range of different peer worker schemes in prisons. Some examples include:

- Information and advice sharing roles such as induction or information desk workers
- Support roles such as listeners who are trained by the Samaritans.
- Advocacy roles like being a representative on a council
- Mentoring roles like substance misuse mentors or education mentors.

Whilst the aforementioned examples are focused on peer worker roles for prisoners, there are also similar positions for staff such as mentors for new officers, staff council representatives or care teams who offer confidential support to staff at times of crisis. Whether for staff or prisoners, these roles all encourage empowerment, responsibility and a sense of belonging which contribute to a rehabilitative culture.

These are just two examples of areas that might contribute to the wider culture of a prison being one that supports the rehabilitation of prisoners. They are quite different but are both areas that take considerable time and effort to properly establish and embed, showing that cultural change is not quick or easy. Forensic psychologists have a role to play both in guiding establishments about what the evidence suggests might be helpful to try and change and then in effectively achieving this. They also provide opportunities for research to further develop the evidence base for specific initiatives.

Conclusion

Forensic psychologists are often known for their work in assessing risk and delivering interventions to help reduce and manage that risk, yet the environments within which they work can play an important role in how successful these individual efforts are. Forensics environments such as prisons are discrete societies that have core elements that may seem contrary to the aim of rehabilitation, elements such as the physical security features, the fixed regimes and relationships involving power imbalance and mistrust. The culture within a prison has an impact on how people experience these things and, in turn, how rehabilitative they are. Forensic psychologists therefore also have a role to play in the development and maintenance of wider environments that support their work and the prisons core aims.

Culture is made between people and is changeable over time. As such, everyone involved in a prison plays a part in its culture. Cultural change is not a quick and easy process. It takes time and conscious effort to influence a culture which influences the experiences of the people who live and work there.

Within prisons, there are specialist units that pay particular attention to their environment and the culture they create in order to support effective rehabilitation. There is clear learning from these that can be translated to wider prison settings and whilst not without challenge, this can bring positive impacts for both those living in prison and the staff who work there.

There is evidence that a rehabilitative environment whilst safer is not softer. Trying to build positive supportive relationships and providing opportunities for people to learn and develop can often be mistaken for making life easier for people and not recognising that they are in prison because they have committed serious crimes. On the contrary, creating places where there is an expectation that people engage and make genuine and meaningful changes in their lives and making people accountable for their own choices and actions, rather than taking all the responsibility from them is almost universally described by people involved as being far harder than if they were left alone to survive in a more hostile but more familiar environment.

Recommended further activities

You are encouraged to access the HMPPS Forensic Psychology Podcast (https://pod. link/1533101974) and listen to the following episodes which further explore concepts discussed in this chapter:

Episode 2: What is an ideal environment for change? [22/10/2020]
Episode 7: Is personality disorder a health or justice issue? [26/11/2020]

Learning outcomes

When you have completed this chapter, you should be able to:

1 Define key terms such as organisational culture and climate
2 Consider the impact of the forensic setting and environment on prison culture
3 Outline a number of treatment approaches and places that specifically focus on the environment (e.g. Therapeutic Communities and PIPEs)
4 Understand what is meant by a rehabilitative culture

Key concepts and terms

- Culture
- Climate
- Cultural web
- Acculturation
- Staff–prisoner relationships
- Rehabilitative culture
- Enabling environments
- Therapeutic community

Sample essay questions

- How might staff–prisoner relationships impact on prison climate?
- How might a rehabilitative culture impact on the aims of prisons?

Recommended further reading

Akerman, G., Needs, A., & Bainbridge, C. (Eds.). (2018). *Transforming environments and rehabilitation: A guide for practitioners in forensic settings and criminal justice.* Routledge.

Gredecki, N., & Horrocks, C. (2017). "Crafting identity": Constructions of the prison officer role. In J. L. Ireland, C. A. Ireland, N. Gredecki, & M. Fisher (Eds.), *The Routledge international handbook on forensic psychology in secure settings* (pp. 300–312). Routledge.

Mann, R., Fitzalan Howard, F., & Tew, J. (2018). What is a rehabilitative prison culture. *Prison Service Journal, 235*, 3–9.

Shuker, R. (2010). Forensic therapeutic communities: A critique of treatment model and evidence base. *The Howard Journal, 49*(5), 463–477.

References

Beijersbergen, K. A., Dirkzwager, A. J. E., Eichelsheim, V. I., & Van der Laan, P. H. (2015). Procedural justice, anger, and prisoners' misconduct. *Criminal Justice and Behavior, 42*(2), 196–218.

Beijersbergen, K. A., Dirkzwager, A. J. E., Eichelsheim, V. I., Van der Laan, P. H., & Nieuwbeerta, P. (2014). Procedural justice and prisoners' mental health problems: A longitudinal study. *Criminal Behavior and Mental Health, 24*, 100–112.

Beijersbergen, K. A., Dirkzwager, A. J. E., & Nieuwbeerta, P. (2016). Reoffending after release: Does procedural justice during imprisonment matter? *Criminal Behavior and Mental Health, 43*(1), 63–82.

Bennett, A., & Tew, J. (2018). Creating an enabling environment in high security prison conditions: An impossible task or the start of a revolution? In G. Akerman, A. Needs, & C. Bainbridge (Eds.),

Transforming environments and rehabilitation: A guide for practitioners in forensic settings and criminal justice (pp. 254–270). Routledge.

Bennett, P., & Shuker, R. (2010). Improving prisoner-staff relationships: Exporting Grendon's good practice. *The Howard Journal, 49*, 491–502.

Blagden, N., & Thorne, K. (2013). HMP Whatton: A prison of change. *Prison Service Journal, 208*, 3–9.

Bonta, J., & Andrews, D. A. (2016). *The psychology of criminal conduct* (6th ed.). Routledge.

Bordin, E. S. (1979). The generaliizability of the psychoanalytic concept of the working alliance. *Psychotherapy: Theory, research and practice, 16*, 252–260.

Burnett, R., & McNeil, F. (2005). The place of the officer-offender relationship in assisting offenders to desist from crime. *Probation Journal, 52*, 221–242.

Byrne, J. M., & Hummer, D. (2007). Myths and realities of prison violence: A review of the evidence. *Victims and Offenders: An International Journal of Evidence-Based Research, Policy and Practice, 2*, 77–99.

Byrne, J. M., & Stowell, J. (2007). Examining the link between institutional and community violence: Towards a new cultural paradigm. *Aggression and Violent Behavior, 12*, 552–563.

Cavender, G. (2004). Media and crime policy: A reconsideration of David Garland's the culture of control. *Punishment & Society, 6*(3), 335–348.

Crewe, B. (2011). Soft power in prison: Implications for staff-prisoner relationships, liberty and legitimacy. *European Journal of Criminology, 8*(6), 455–468.

Day, A., & Doyle, P. (2010). Violent offender rehabilitation and the therapeutic community model of treatment: Towards integrated service provision? *Aggression and Violent Behavior, 15*, 380–386.

Deal, T. E., & Kennedy, A. A. (1982). *Corporate cultures: The rites and rituals of corporate life.* Addison Wesley Publishing Company.

Dowden, C., & Tellier, C. (2004). Predicting work related stress in correctional officers: A meta-analysis. *Journal of Criminal Justice, 32*, 31–47.

Edgar, K., Jacobson, J., & Biggar, K. (2011). *Time well spent: A practical guide to active citizenship and volunteering in prison.* Prison Reform Trust. Retrieved from www.prisonreformtrust.org.uk/Projects Research/Citizenship/TimeWellSpent.

Fitzalan-Howard, F., & Wakeling, H. (2019). *Prisoner and staff perceptions of procedural justice in English and Welsh prisons.* HM Prison and Probation Service Analytical Summary 2019.

Garland, D. (1990). *Punishment and modern society.* Clarendon Press.

Gilbert, M. J. (1997). The illusion of structure: A critique of the classical model of organization and the discretionary power of correctional officers. *Criminal Justice Review, 22*, 49–64.

Haigh, R. (2013). The quintessence of a therapeutic environment. *Therapeutic Communities: The International Journal of Therapeutic Communities, 34*, 6–15.

Haney, C., Banks, C., & Zimbardo, R. (1973). Interpersonal dynamics in a simulated prison. *Interpersonal Journal of Criminology and Penology, 1*, 69–72.

Haslam, S. A., & Reicher, S. D. (2005). The psychology of tyranny. *Scientific American Mind, 16*, 44–51.

Hepburn, J. R., & Knepper, P. (1993). Correctional officers as human service workers: The effect on job satisfaction. *Justice Quarterly, 10*, 315–335.

HM Prison and Probation Service & NHS England. (2020). *Practitioners guide: Working with people in the criminal justice system showing personality difficulties* (3rd ed.). Retrieved from https://assets. publishing.service.gov.uk/government/uploads/system/uploads/attachment_data/file/869843/ 6.5151_HMPPS_Working_with_Offenders_with_Personality_Disorder_v17_WEB.pdf.

Hoffman, L. (1982). An historical overview of milieu therapy. In L. Hoffman (Eds.), *The evaluation and care of severely disturbed children and their families.* Springer.

Home Office. (1984). *Managing the long-term prison system: The report of the control review committee.* HMSO.

Irwin, J., & Cressey, D. (1962). Thieves, convicts and the inmate culture. *Social Problems, 10*, 142–155.

Johnson, G., Whittington, R., & Scholes, K. (2012). *Fundamentals of Strategy.* Pearson Education.

Johnson, R., & Haigh, R. (2011). Social psychiatry and social policy for the 21st century: New concepts for new needs-the "Enabling Environments" initiative. *Mental Health and Social Inclusion, 15*, 17–23.

Joseph, N., & Benefield, N. (2012). A joint offender personality disorder pathway strategy: An outline summary. *Criminal Behaviour and Mental Health, 22*, 210–217.

Lambert, E. (2003). The impact of organizational justice on correctional staff. *Journal of criminal Justice*, *31*, 155–168.

LeBel, T. Burentt, R., Maruna, S., & Bushway, S. (2008). The "Chicken and Egg" of subjective and social factors in desistance from crime. *European Journal of Criminology*, *5*, 131–159.

Lee, B., & Gilligan, J. (2006). The resolve to stop prison violence project: Transforming an in-house culture of violence through a jail-based programme. *Journal of Public Health*, *27*, 149–155.

Liebling, A. assisted by Arnold, H. (2004). *Prisons and their moral performance: A study of values, quality, and prison life*. Oxford University Press.

Liebling, A., & Price, D. (1998). *An exploration of staff-prisoner relationships at HMP Whitemoor*. Prison Service Research Report, Institute of Criminology.

Lind, E. A., & Tyler, T. R. (1988). *The social psychology of procedural justice*. Plenum Press.

Lipsey, M. W., & Cullen, F. T. (2007). The effectiveness of correctional rehabilitation: A review of systematic reviews. *Annual: Review of Law and Social Science*, *3*, 297–320.

Ludlow, A., Schmidt, B., Akoensi, T., Liebling, A., Giacomantonio, C., & Sutherland, A. (2015). *Self-inflicted deaths in NOMS' custody amongst 18–24 year olds: Staff experience, knowledge and views*. RAND Europe.

Mann, R., Fitzalan-Howard, F., & Tew, J. (2018). What is a rehabilitative culture? *Prison Service Journal*, *235*, 3–10.

National Offender Management Service. (2008). *Race review 2008: Implementing race equality in prisons: Five years on*. Ministry of Justice.

Reicher, S., & Haslam, S. A. (2006). Rethinking the psychology of tyranny: The BBC prison study. *British Journal of Social Psychology*, *45*, 1–40.

Ros, N., Van der Helm, P., Wissink, I., Stams, J., & Schaftenaar, P. (2013). Institutional climate and aggression in a secure psychiatric setting. *The Journal of Forensic Psychiatry and Psychology*, *24*, 713–727.

Sekol, I. (2013). Peer violence in adolescent residential care: A qualitative examination of contextual and peer factors. *Children and youth services review*, *35*, 1901–1912.

Shuker, R., & Sullivan, E. (2010). *Grendon and the emergence of forensic therapeutic communities: Developments in research and practice*. Wiley-Blackwell.

Sparks, R., Bottoms, A., & Hay, W. (1996). *Prisons and the problem of order*. Oxford University Press.

Sturge, G. (2020). *UK prison population statistics* (Briefing Paper Number CBP-04334). Retrieved from https://commonslibrary.parliament.uk/research-briefings/sn04334/.

Sykes, G., & Messinger, S. (1960). The inmate social system. In R. A. Cloward, D. R. Cressey, G. H. Grosser, R. McCleery, L. E. Ohlin, G. M. Sykes, & S. L. Messinger (Eds.), *Theoretical studies in the social organisation of prison* (pp. 5–19). Social Science Research Council.

Tait, S. (2008). Care and the prison officer: Beyond "turnkeys" and "care bears", *Prison Service Journal*, *180*, 3–11.

Tait, S. (2011). A typology of prison officer approaches to care. *European Journal of Criminology*, *8*, 440–454.

Turley, C., Payne, C., & Webster, S. (2013). *Enabling features of psychologically informed planned environments*. Ministry of Justice Analytical Series.

Tyler, T. R. (2008). Procedural justice and the courts. *Court Review*, *44*, 26–31.

Valle, M. F., Huebner, E. S., & Suldo, S. M. (2006). An analysis of hope as a psychological strength. *Journal of School Psychology*, *44*, 393–406.

Van der Helm, G. H. P., Stams, G. J. J. M., Van Genabeek, M., & Van der Lann, P. H. (2011). Group climate, personality and self-reported aggression in incarcerated male youth. *Journal of Forensic Psychiatry and Psychology*, *1*, 23–39.

Williamson, H. E. (1990). *The corrections profession*. Sage Publications.

Woessner, G., & Schwelder, A. (2014). Correctional treatment of sexual and violent offenders: Therapeutic change, prison climate, and recidivism. *Criminal Justice and Behavior*. Advanced online publication. DOI: 10.1177/00938854813520544.

17 Consultancy in forensic settings

Polly Turner and Amy Freel

Summary

Forensic settings are complex environments in which psychological practice and theoretical models can assist beyond traditional therapeutic work with clients. A core role of the forensic psychologist is to communicate how and when psychology can assist stakeholders and the environment. The forensic psychologist needs to identify opportunities to assist and balance competing demands. This chapter will outline models and frameworks relevant to consultancy and consider the role of forensic psychologists as consultants within the forensic setting. A case study of a psychologist supporting security initiatives in secure settings will be used to bring the evidence to life. This will highlight how forensic psychologists draw upon and share a broad knowledge base of models of human experience in applied practice.

What do we mean by consultancy?

The term 'consultant' is often used to indicate seniority within healthcare settings. For example, 'Consultant Forensic Psychiatrist' denotes successful completion of medical/ psychiatric training and an ability to practice independently. However, this is *not* the meaning of the term consultant or consultancy in the context of this chapter or within forensic psychology (see box 17.1 for an overview of consultancy in the BPS Qualification in Forensic Psychology). Here, we are thinking of the application of knowledge and advice to assist the work of others and/or wider organisations. The use of the term consultancy within the forensic psychology context does not imply 'expert'; in fact, we must ensure we do not fall in to the expert trap (Schein, 2016a; Schwarz, 2006). Paradoxically, it is said that it takes real expertise to avoid being an expert (Wagner, 2016). Yet, this notion will not be new to applied psychologists as focus on respecting the knowledge of others, maintaining clear boundaries and not stepping outside our competence is embodied in our British Psychological Society (BPS) ethical principles. We will consider ethical issues in relation to consultancy throughout the chapter.

BOX 17.1 CONSULTANCY IN THE BPS QUALIFICATION IN FORENSIC PSYCHOLOGY (QFP)

Core Role 3 of the BPS qualification (BPS, 2021) focuses on the forensic psychologist's competence to communicate and consult using psychological knowledge to a range of audiences. It captures the extent to which the psychologist can identify opportunities where offering psychological knowledge can assist others

---

DOI: 10.4324/9781003017103-21

in their job roles and aid wider organisational practices. It includes traditional roles such as feeding back on outcomes of assessment and intervention work in formal settings. It also requires the psychologist to show they can use psychological knowledge and evidence to assist policy development. Ultimately, Core Role 3 aims to ensure all forensic psychologists can adjust and adapt their psychological skills to all stakeholders they work with. It ensures forensic psychologists can, and do, apply psychological knowledge and evidence as broadly as possible to maximise the benefits of applied psychology in forensic services.

Specific competencies developed and demonstrated relating to consultancy and communication during the qualification are as follows:

3.1 Providing psychological advice to aid the formulation of policy and its implementation
3.2 Promoting awareness of the actual and potential contributions of applied psychological services
3.3 Providing psychological advice to assist and inform problem-solving and decision-making
3.4 Preparing and presenting evidence in formal settings
3.5 Responding to informal requests for psychological information
3.6 Providing feedback to clients

Consultancy is best viewed as a collaborative problem-solving endeavour to enhance the functioning of a system (Schein, 2016b; Wagner, 2016). The role of the psychologist here is to work *with* the stakeholders in the system to understand the presenting issue and to *support* the identification of solutions. In consultancy, it is not the role of the psychologist to solve the presenting issue but to support the stakeholders to learn together so that they might resolve future issues themselves (Ireland, 2010a). The aim of a good consultant is to *facilitate* and *encourage* the effective functioning of teams and systems at a broader organisational level. This is achieved by helping and partnering the system to identify how it can adapt to the challenges it faces (Schein, 2016b).

Who is the client in consultancy?

Whilst the psychologist might be approached by one individual for the consultancy task, the 'client' is likely to extend beyond a single person. If we are to help a system function efficiently, then we need to balance and attend to the needs of everyone in the system (Ireland, 2010b). Honkanen and Rus (2017) outline systemic levels in organisations increasing in scope moving from working with the individual, to the group, to the organisation, through to the social and political environment in which the organisation resides. They note the deliberate use of the term systemic, highlighting how change in one level will likely impact other levels. To be effective, the consultant must consider all levels and ensure interventions are targeted appropriately to the different levels. But where do we start when undertaking a piece of consultancy work?

Evidence base for consultancy

The process of a consultancy project should be much the same as how the forensic psychologist might approach an intervention with a client or a research project, by starting with the literature. The psychologist needs to examine what the evidence base advises as to the best way to approach and conduct the work. As outlined in Chapter 1, forensic psychologists learn by drawing on evidence from psychology and other disciplines. This is certainly evident when we consider the consultancy role.

ACTIVITY BOX 17.2

Think about your BSc psychology studies. What models or theories might assist a forensic psychologist in analysing and understanding the functioning of a workplace environment? Perhaps return to this list after you have reviewed this chapter. Reflect on whether your thoughts are similar to the models outlined in the chapter. If not, consider how your ideas might fit with and/or complement the models outlined in the chapter.

In any consultancy task, the psychologist must draw on other areas of applied psychology, particularly occupational and educational psychology but also wider business literature and practices. Whilst the psychologist is seeking to examine a broader system, they are working with people, and therefore, almost all the psychological evidence base will be useful to the consultancy role. Thus, there will likely be a wealth of specific evidence of relevance to each specific consultancy task, though general models and frameworks of consultancy can assist the forensic psychologist in how to approach a consultancy project.

Models of consultancy

The literature presents three models of consultancy, namely, the 'purchase of expertise', the 'doctor–patient' and the process model (Schein, 1999). In each model, the consultant ultimately wants to help the system, although they have different implications for how the consultant approaches the referral. It is suggested that the psychologist might need to utilise all three different approaches according to the referral, at times switching between the three within the same project. Yet, there are important implications if the wrong model is applied.

The **'purchase of expertise' model** is used when the system recruits the consultant as they possess certain knowledge or skills not otherwise available within the system. The system requires the consultant to enact or apply the new knowledge or skill. However, it is reliant on the system correctly identifying the issue that the expert can assist with, communicating this clearly and choosing the right consultant with the right set of skills to match the issue.

The **'doctor–patient' model** places the consultant as the 'doctor' who objectively 'diagnoses' the problem and 'prescribes the cure' to the 'patient' which is the system (Wagner, 2016). The system may request this approach when they are uncertain as to the cause of the presenting issue. A criticism is that this model creates power issues by positioning the consultant in the expert role. It is also dependent on the resulting 'diagnosis' being accepted by the system, which Schein (1999) argues is often a significant challenge.

Process consultation was developed in response to the deficiencies of the former two models. Adopting a process approach, the consultant works with the system to jointly diagnose the presenting issues. Process consultation approaches the referral know-ing the client has the greatest knowledge of their system and culture. The aim is to build skills in the system to address any future issues without the need for a consultant. The model requires strong working relationships to be developed between the consultant and organisation. Some claim the model is too dependent on democratic systems common in Western culture and neglects the diversity seen in modern multicultural workplaces (Kwon et al., 2020). Others suggest the model is poorly understood in practice, yet its strength is the focus on the helping relationship (Lambrechts et al., 2009).

Schein has refined the process model and refers more frequently now to 'humble consulting' and 'humble inquiry' whereby the consultant needs to be curious, caring and committed to being helpful. Consistent with his earlier formulations, the consultant does not have the answer but wishes to support the system to find their own solutions (Schein, 2016b). Where humble consulting differs is in the even greater focus on the relationship with the system. Schein (2016b) describes the need for a personal, trusting and open rela-tionship from the outset. He argues that this requires listening skills and empathy.

This focus on listening and empathy to develop a trusting relationship is no different to our other roles as a psychologist (Llewelyn & Cuthbertson, 2009). The core therapeutic skills of a psychologist are directly transferable to the consultancy process. This includes the ability to show compassion by respecting and hearing the views of all involved. As with therapy, the consultant must be non-judgemental. Clear boundaries must also be maintained with all stakeholders from the outset (Ireland, 2010b). The ethical principles relevant to maintaining equitable and transparent therapy relationships are also critical to consultancy. Further, as with therapy, the relationships will evolve over time. As with ethical dilemmas in therapy, the consultant must attend to any shifts in relationships and adapt where required. We have outlined the wider approach to consultancy; let us now consider the stages involved.

Stages of consultancy

There are various consulting cycles examined in the literature, and whilst there may be subtle differences, the core phases are depicted in Figure 17.1 (see Honkanen & Rus, 2017; Llewelyn & Cuthbertson, 2009; McKavanagh, 2005; Schein, 1999; Vickers et al., 2010).

As can be seen from Figure 17.1, the process is much like other psychological interven-tions. We begin developing rapport for a trusting relationship, we clarify aims and set the parameters of the relationship. Next, we gather data to generate hypotheses which inform formulations to assist us in identifying workable solutions or interventions. Once the solutions are performed, we can conduct a thorough evaluation of the outcomes against initial aims and objectives.

It is the scientist–practitioner skills of the forensic psychologist that add value. For example, they possess analytical skills to synthesise available data to assist the organisation in understanding the issues in greater depth. If adopting a process or humble inquiry approach, the psychologist would ensure collaboration with the organisation at each phase. This would ensure the formulations are informed by valid data and will ensure solutions are workable.

It is important to recognise that cycles and their phases are criticised for being overly simplistic in their attempt to devise discrete phases which may underestimate the com-plexities of organisations and the consultancy task (Bartlett & Francis-Smythe, 2016). Yet

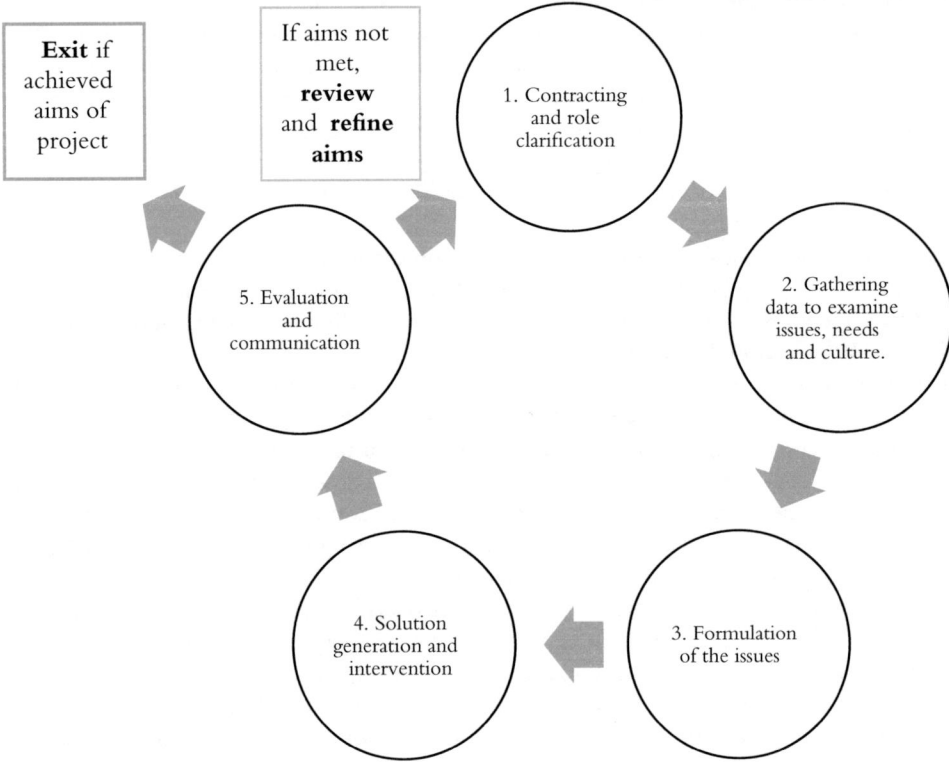

Figure 17.1 Consultancy cycle

for the psychologist new to consultancy, these phases are likely to assist in ensuring the process is approached in a systematic fashion and that all avenues are considered. Equally, it must be remembered that it is the psychologist's ethical duty to ensure they access the evidence base supporting each consultancy project which would always go beyond simple cycles such as those outlined.

What is central to all cycles is the importance of clarifying the presenting issue and developing strong working relationships between the consultant and the organisation. These important first steps will ensure that subsequent phases are effective. In order to do this, the consultant needs to identify and engage with all parties (Ireland, 2010b). This then supports an objective examination of the way in which the organisation functions from all perspectives.

Often in forensic psychology consultation, the psychologist is employed within the organisation and is therefore an internal consultant. Whilst this may offer opportunities in terms of existing working relationships with stakeholders, it may also present challenges in terms of biases or assumptions about the practices and/or culture in the organisation. Adopting the humble inquiry approach would mean the psychologist would need to be curious about their own existing assumptions as well as being curious to the views of all stakeholders. The psychologist needs to ensure they examine the reality of the organisation and not act on their own reality. There are several techniques available to examine the culture and practices of an organisation.

Understanding the system: culture and climate

We saw in Chapter 16 that culture is described as the personality of systems and organisations, whilst climate represents the mood or the prevailing atmosphere of the system or organisation. To understand these factors, the consultant might undertake a culture web as outlined in Chapter 16. They may also adapt models traditionally used for individual level interventions to a wider system. An example of a model that was designed for use within a therapy framework but might be useful at a broader level could be the Social GGRRAAACCEEESSS model, see Focus Box 17.3.

FOCUS BOX 17.3   SOCIAL GGRRAAACCEEESSS MODEL (BURNHAM, 2012)

The following components make up the model and are aspects that position people in society and systems. Each aspect can either enable or disable people, affording or preventing power. Exploring how the aspects impact on people and relationships might open new opportunities within a system. Identifying and overcoming any limiting aspects might offer richer, more meaningful connections within a system. The aspects are judged to be voiced or unvoiced, visible or invisible. This is of great importance in forensic systems where power operates explicitly and implicitly.

Gender
Geography
Race
Religion
Age
Ability
Appearance
Culture
Class/caste
Education
Employment
Ethnicity
Spirituality
Sexuality
Sexual orientation

Social GGRRAAACCEEESSS model (Burnham, 2012)

Burnham's model maps out components of personal and social identity that afford us different experiences of power and privilege. Adopting the model as the consultant would ensure that we are intentionally being aware of, and examining, differences amongst those within the system. This would assist us in examining the power aspects of the culture web in depth. This model could assist in addressing the concerns that process consultation neglects the diversity seen in today's workplaces (Kwon et al., 2020). It could be fruitful to apply the model to consider which of the GRRAAACCEEESSS go voiced versus unvoiced, which are visible or invisible within an organisation.

We learned in Chapter 16 that individual identities, power and privilege can have dramatic influences over a system. The task for the consultant might be to make these aspects visible to the organisation. Indeed, it could be that aspects of the social graces are causing the issues and challenges facing the organisation. It could be that changes are needed to ensure equality and fairness.

Effecting change in systems: interventions

The consultancy process typically arises when a system is faced with a problem or challenge and change is required. The consultancy project might highlight that changes in behaviour or processes are required. Likewise, it might suggest that changes in attitudes and beliefs are needed. As psychologists, we know change can be difficult and threatening, yet we also know the variety of ways in which we can reduce resistance to facilitate change. We know that forcing people to comply with new agendas is likely to be met with resistance and hostility. As a consultant, the psychologist should draw on knowledge from psychological theory and research to assist the functioning of the system.

The psychologist may wish to outline important theories such as self-determination theory (SDT; Deci & Ryan, 2000). SDT tells us that human motivation thrives in the context of autonomy, competence and belonging. Thus, if people within a system are given choice, feel able to perform the required actions and feel part of the community, then they are more likely to be motivated to engage in the process. This knowledge might influence the way in which the consultation process is designed, ensuring all stakeholders are involved and actively engaged. It will likely be critical if an intervention is required to achieve change.

Another concept that can secure active engagement, and be beneficial in effecting change, is compassion. Applying compassion-focused therapy principles to staff support is advocated in forensic settings (Lucre & Taylor, 2020). The business literature has advocated for the benefits of compassion in organisations for some time (see Kanov et al., 2006). Indeed, 'compassionate leadership' is now a well-recognised concept.

Compassionate leadership

Compassionate leadership is embedded within the NHS (NHS England, 2014). The principles of compassionate leadership have particularly come to the fore during the 2020 pandemic, where it was critical that leaders actively turned to the suffering of those in the system, that they listened to the concerns of all stakeholders and responded with kindness and respect. Compassionate leadership has the potential to lead to organisational compassion and contribute to a collaborative culture. Organisational compassion is when all those in the system collectively notice, feel and respond to pain experienced in the system (Kanov et al., 2006). Such a culture would be open to seeing where things can be improved, whilst being supportive of those change affects.

Yet, some leaders and systems may not adopt this compassionate approach and may need support in making change happen. Here, the psychologist can utilise change management models from the business literature, specifically designed to capture issues arising when seeking at a systemic level. Fisher (2012) presents the personal transition curve to highlight the impact of change on individuals. He emphasises the need for consultants and leaders to appreciate varying perceptions of the past, present and future. To reduce conflict and resistance, consultants need to understand the views of those involved and support the organisation to offer education and information about the changes. Fisher's model may seem overly simplistic in capturing the change process for all individuals in an organisation. However, it is not intended to suggest change that occurs in an identical fashion for all individuals; rather, it highlights the importance of acknowledging and supporting all individuals in the system.

ACTIVITY BOX 17.4

Imagine a senior manager approaches you to ask for your assistance with issues regarding high staff turnover in the frontline staff within the establishment (this could be a prison, a forensic hospital or community setting). Think about what you have learned already in this textbook about forensic settings and what you have learned in this chapter about the consultancy process. What might your first steps be? What do you need to know more about? What challenges might you anticipate?

Let us now look at consultancy in practice. The following example will detail a consultancy project which utilised the process consultation model.

Case study: application of process consultation within HMPPS – the security and rehabilitative sourcebook

The following case study describes a consultancy project commissioned and completed within Her Majesty's Prison and Probation Service (HMPPS). Specifically, it will outline the role and key considerations of the forensic psychologist as the consultant.

Relationships within forensic settings are critical to successful organisational outcomes. This includes a broad range of diverse relationships that contribute to the culture within an organisation. Within HMPPS, the relationships between staff and the people in prison are paramount in developing a safe and secure culture that aims to create a firm base for rehabilitation.

A rehabilitative culture is one where all the aspects of our culture support rehabilitation. This includes the prison being safe, decent, hopeful and supportive of change, progression and reducing offending. A rehabilitative culture is not about being soft, passive or always saying yes to people as this would negatively impact safety and security. Instead, it is about adopting ways of working that support the evidence for what can help reduce offending.

Traditional definitions of security have sometimes been limited in depth and breadth and focused on security as a set of practices designed to reduce and manage organisational risks and threats. Whilst this is important, more contemporary and innovative perspectives on prison security take the view that security can and should be more than this (Loader & Walker, 2007; Sparks et al., 1996).

This case study focuses on a project designed to highlight the need for integration between security and rehabilitative culture. The relationship between the two prison approaches was not previously articulated clearly or widely understood. Without this clarity, there was a risk that practices would continue to operate in parallel or even in conflict. The *Security and Rehabilitative Culture Sourcebook* aimed to promote the creation of a prison environment where stronger communities grow and people can thrive alongside continued efforts to address drugs, violence and crime. This broader approach is sometimes referred to as 'human security'. It suggests that people feel secure, not only when they are free from physical threat but also when they can express their rights, are treated fairly and can grow and develop.

The *Security and Rehabilitative Culture Sourcebook* was conceptualised and commissioned by the Deputy Director of the Security Order and Counter Terrorism Directorate within HMPPS. The vision was to support security leaders with the integration of security and rehabilitative cultures by providing information about key areas of work that would be central to everyday security practice. The project would bring together theory, literature and practical working examples within four chapters focusing on:

- staff–prisoner relationships,
- procedural justice,
- promoting diversity and inclusion and
- trauma-informed and trauma-responsive practice.

The consultancy process

As a forensic psychologist working on this project, it was important to start by establishing a rapport with the client and project commissioner. This included making time for initial conversations about the project rationale and purpose. Asking questions and active listening skills were an important part of developing a trusting professional relationship in addition to demonstrating genuine interest and ensuring a clear understanding about expectations and roles. It was important to understand the organisational context for the sourcebook which helped to appreciate the history of the project and how it aimed to influence attitudes and beliefs about security practices along with offering examples of behavioural changes. Further, these initial consultations helped to clarify information about who the target audience was, time frames, purpose, rationale, content, presentational methods and reporting mechanisms between client and consultant.

A period of research and reading was essential for this project. This included a review of relevant literature both from internal organisational searches and external publications to develop an understanding of the depth and breadth of the subject matter evidence base. Examples of these included information about organisational security publications, establishing effective relationships and boundaries, procedural justice, diversity and inclusion, the role of bias in decision-making and trauma-informed practice.

Learning from the review of the evidence led to collaboration with subject matter experts. Chapter authors were approached and invited to contribute to the project, and appropriate objectives and realistic timescales were established. It is a forensic psychologist's ethical responsibility to identify and understand areas of colleagues' expertise. This helps to develop opportunities for joint working and ensures the most reliable and accurate information is communicated effectively. Engagement with colleagues who specialise in certain areas of forensic practice can also include opportunities for continued professional development and for establishing professional working relationships beyond the immediate project.

Once collaboration from a range of experts was secured, opportunities for joint working were identified. This included supporting authors with elements of literature reviewing, providing information about security practice, assisting with visual images for chapters that ensured a broad range of learning styles were included and support with editing. These opportunities were helpful to the project as a means of being able to continuously monitor progress and as a way of being able to provide regular feedback and updates to colleagues. This also had a logistical function in keeping the project running to schedule.

A clear process of regular collaboration and communication with stakeholders helped to develop relationships and anticipate difficulties. These relationships in turn facilitated a more proactive approach to problem-solving. During the editing phase of chapters, there was an unforeseen absence that presented a significant risk to the project. This was sensitively resolved in a timely manner through early identification, collaboration with the client, reallocation of the chapter and a recalculation of time frames. It was important to be transparent about project difficulties with the client. Although difficult at times, it is the responsibility of the forensic psychologist to communicate difficult and sometimes unpopular messages in a clear and transparent way, whilst remaining goal orientated and solution focused. Avoidance of this responsibility may have resulted in the breakdown of trust between the consultant and client and had the potential to cause confusion or mis-communications with other areas of the organisation.

Each of the chapters was sent back to the client of the sourcebook project for review as they were completed. During this process, some chapters were straightforward and accepted quickly, whereas others required some revisions. Having this clear feedback process to check that chapters met the project purpose ensured that any changes were communicated clearly and in a timely manner. Once finalised, all chapters were then edited together in line with the prison service corporate communication standards. This attention to detail with written communication is a key skill for forensic psychologists and ensures that important information is communicated in the most appropriate way to maximise learning potential. The final version was reviewed as a completed project by the client and requested amends made in line with feedback.

As the consultant for this project, it was important to understand the potential for security staff within the organisation to be at different stages of understanding and application of 'human security'. As such, it was necessary to be aware of the stages of individual and organisational change and to work with the client to ensure that a range of communication and dissemination approaches were agreed. This aimed to communicate the learning and final product to as many staff as possible via multiple methods to ensure the learning was embedded within the organisation's security culture. This included the publication of the sourcebook as a stand-alone product alongside the development of a communication plan which provided further opportunities to share and embed learning. Examples included raising awareness of the sourcebook through presentations at a range of organisational forums such as regional security and governors' meetings, publication on the corporate intranet, integration of the chapter material within security capability training and the design of additional products targeting the wider HMPPS workforce.

Applied psychologists are evidence informed in their practice, and so, as a consultancy project ends, they should plan how to evaluate the process and learn about what worked well and what could have been developed. Although the internal publication of the *Security and Rehabilitative Culture Sourcebook* marked the completion of the project, within the organisation, the learning and information from each of the chapters continues to be embedded within security practice. As such, the evaluation process will be measured over time and aims to ensure that attempts are made to capture learning about the process followed and the impact on security practice.

Conclusion

This chapter has highlighted the role of the consultant as the 'helper' and not 'the expert'. The skills that make a good consultant are all those skills that make a good therapist and psychologist. This includes skills such as active listening, empathy and compassion. The relationship is at the heart of both effective therapy and effective consultancy. Forensic psychologists must also ensure that we utilise our skills as scientist–practitioners, drawing on theory and research to analyse the organisational issue and effectively apply the evidence base.

Learning outcomes

When you have completed this chapter, you should be able to:

1   Describe the meaning of consultancy in forensic psychology practice
2   Identify the core skills of a forensic psychologist that are transferrable to consultancy
3   Outline the stages of a consultancy project
4   Critically appraise models of consultancy
5   Identify psychological approaches to examining an organisations culture
6   Identify psychological approaches to achieve change in an organisation

Key concepts and terms

- Consultancy
- The 'purchase of expertise' model
- The 'doctor–patient' model
- Process consultation
- Humble inquiry
- Compassionate leadership

Sample essay questions

- 'The psychologist is best placed to take on the consultancy role'. Discuss the evidence for and against this statement.
- How important is it for psychologists to consider individual needs and views during a consultancy project?
- Compare and contrast the three main models of consultancy.

Recommended further reading

Journal articles

Bartlett, D., & Francis-Smythe, J. (2016). Bridging the divide in work and organizational psychology: Evidence from practice. *European Journal of Work and Organizational Psychology, 25*(5), 615–630.

Kwon, K., Lee, J. Y., Park, J. G., & Zaballero, A. G. (2020). Process consultation within and across cultures. *Journal of Applied Behavioral Science, 56*(3), 322–346.

Books and book chapters

Honkanen, R., & Rus, D. (2017). How do we work with organizations? In N. Chmiel, F. Fraccaroli, & M. Sverke (Eds.), *An introduction to work and organizational psychology* (pp. 469–487). John Wiley & Sons, Ltd.

Ireland, C. A., & Fisher, M. J. (2010). *Consultancy and advising in forensic practice: Empirical and practical guidelines*. BPS Blackwell.

Schein, E. (2016). Taking culture seriously in organisational development. In Rothwell, Stavros, & Sullivan (Eds.), *Practicing organisational development: Leading transformation and change* (4th ed., pp. 233–244). John Wiley & Sons.

References

Bartlett, D., & Francis-Smythe, J. (2016). Bridging the divide in work and organizational psychology: Evidence from practice. *European Journal of Work and Organizational Psychology, 25*(5), 615–630.

British Psychological Society. (2021). *Qualification in forensic psychology (stage 2) candidate handbook*. BPS.

Burnham, J. (2012). Developments in social GRRRAAACCEEESSS: Visible-invisible and voiced-unvoiced. In I. B. Krause (Ed.), *Culture and reflexivity in systemic psychotherapy: Multiple perspectives* (pp. 139–160). Karnac.

Deci, E. L., & Ryan, R. M. (2000). The "what" and "why" of goal pursuits: Human needs and the self-determination of behavior. *Psychological Inquiry, 11*, 227–268.

Fisher, J. (2012). *Process of personal transition* [Online]. Retrieved 17 December 2020 from www.businessballs.com/personalchangeprocess.htm.

Honkanen, R., & Rus, D. (2017). How do we work with organizations? In N. Chmiel, F. Fraccaroli, & M. Sverke (Eds.), *An introduction to work and organizational psychology* (pp. 469–487). John Wiley & Sons, Ltd.

Ireland, C. A. (2010a). The role of a consultant: Function, skills, competences and presentation. In C. A. Ireland & M. J. Fisher (Eds.), *Consultancy and advising in forensic practice: Empirical and practical guidelines* (pp. 3–34). BPS Blackwell.

Ireland, C. A. (2010b). Key stages and factors in the consultancy process and relationship: The importance of stakeholders, organisational boundaries, culture and their management. In C. A. Ireland & M. J. Fisher (Eds.), *Consultancy and advising in forensic practice: Empirical and practical guidelines* (pp. 17–34). BPS Blackwell.

Kanov, J. M., Maitlis, S., Worline, M. C., Dutton, J. E., Frost, P. J., & Lilius, J. M. (2006). Compassion in organizational life. In J. V. Gallos (Ed.), *Organization development* (pp. 793–812). Jossey Bass.

Kwon, K., Lee, J. Y., Park, J. G., & Zaballero, A. G. (2020). Process consultation within and across cultures. *Journal of Applied Behavioral Science, 56*(3), 322–346.

Lambrechts, F., Grieten, S., Bouwen, R., & Corthouts, F. (2009). Process consultation revisited: Taking a relational practice perspective. *Journal of Applied Behavioral Science, 45*(1), 39–58.

Llewelyn, S., & Cuthbertson, A. (2009). Leadership, teamwork and consultancy in clinical psychology. In H. Beinart, P. Kennedy, & S. Lllewelyn (Eds.), *Clinical psychology in practice* (pp. 350–363). John Wiley & Sons.

Loader, I., & Walker, N. (2007). *Civilizing security*. Cambridge University Press.

Lucre, K., & Taylor, J. (2020). Compati | To suffer with: Compassion focused staff support as an antidote to the cost of caring in forensic services. In H. Swaby, B. Winder, R. Lievesley, K. Hocken, N. Blagden, & P. Banyard (Eds.), *Sexual crime and trauma*. Palgrave Macmillan.

McKavanagh, S. (2005). The consulting project lifecycle. In P. Grant, S. Lewis, & D. Thompson (Eds.), *Business psychology in practice* (pp. 22–34). Whurr Publishers Ltd.

NHS England. (2014). *Building and strengthening leadership: Leading with compassion*. NHS England.

Schein, E. H. (1999). *Process consultation revisited: Building the helping relationship.* Addison Wesley.

Schein, E. H. (2016a). Taking culture seriously in organization development. In W. J. Rothwell, J. M. Stavros, & R. L. Sullivan (Eds.), *Practicing organizational development: Leading transformation and change* (4th ed., pp. 233–244). John Wiley & Sons.

Schein, E. H. (2016b). *Humble consulting: How to provide real help faster.* Berrett-Koehler Publishers.

Schwarz, R. (2006). The facilitator and other facilitative roles. In J. V. Gallos (Ed.), *Organization development* (pp. 409–432). Jossey Bass.

Sparks, R., Bottoms, A. E., & Hay, W. (1996). *Prisons and the problem of order.* Clarendon Press.

Vickers, D., Morgan, E., & Moore, A. (2010). Theoretically driven training and consultancy: From design to evaluation. In C. A. Ireland & M. J. Fisher (Eds.), *Consultancy and advising in forensic practice: Empirical and practical guidelines* (pp. 35–50). BPS Blackwell.

Wagner, P. (2016). *Frameworks for practice in educational psychology: A textbook for trainees and practitioners* (2nd ed.). Jessica Kingsley Publishers.

18 Training in forensic settings

Rachel Roper

Summary

Training and developing staff are essential components for any organisation. Indeed, organisations cannot operate effectively without competent staff who have been appropriately trained to perform their role. Training other professionals is one of the core competencies of a forensic psychologist, encapsulating the training journey from identifying the need through to evaluating the outcome. Consequently, they are ideally placed to contribute their expertise to assist organisations in developing the skill set of their staff. Formal training is not always the most appropriate way of resolving organisational issues, and a psychologist has the skills and expertise to determine whether training is relevant or whether other measures would be sufficient to improve the way the organisation functions. This chapter provides a four-step approach on how forensic psychologists create robust and effective training programmes for their organisations. It walks through how to design, develop and evaluate training programmes, provides a case study example and offers some insight into the reasons why people can get it wrong.

Introduction

Forensic settings are complex, dynamic environments within which staff require a range of skills to operate effectively, whilst being resilient in the face of constant challenges in their day-to-day work. The setting itself can contribute to why employees might not be performing their job effectively, alongside personal issues, inadequate policies and procedures, lack of understanding of the role, disinterest or lack of appropriate training. This chapter focuses on the important aspect of training. The role of a forensic psychologist is key in supporting this process and in appropriately advocating when training should be undertaken and how it can be instrumental in enhancing personal and organisational resilience.

Developing a training programme

When we think about training, there is often an assumption that it simply refers to the part that is delivered to learners but it involves a lot more than what goes on in the training room. Goldstein (1993) asserts there is a systematic way of doing this, involving identifying the learner's **need**, **designing**, **implementing** and **evaluating** the programme, as depicted in Figure 18.1. This chapter outlines the suggested approach.

DOI: 10.4324/9781003017103-22

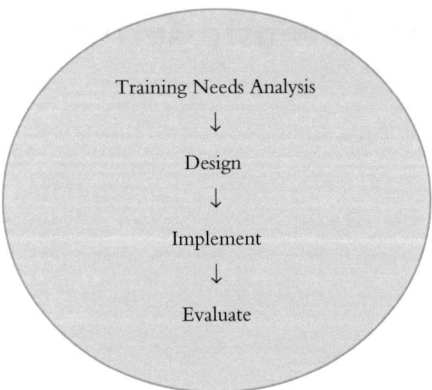

Figure 18.1 Steps to develop a training programme

Step 1: training needs analysis

Training is usually prompted by recognition of a problem in organisational functioning. This means someone (often a manager but sometimes it might be the psychologist) has observed areas of practice where it is thought training might assist. However, before designing a training programme, the psychologist must first understand what has caused the problem. This requires a stakeholder agreement because resources will need to be approved if training is required. Once approved, a Training Needs Analysis (TNA) needs to be undertaken. Ultimately, this will identify if there is a training need amongst staff (Blanchard & Thacker, 2010). A common mistake at this stage is assuming that training is required without adequately exploring whether that is the case as simple guidelines or a change in policy might be sufficient to address the issues that have been identified. If there is a need, the TNA will identify exactly what that is and allow action to be taken to address it. This step alone can save an organisation from significant costs of developing unnecessary training.

Conducting a TNA involves gathering information from a variety of sources. This enables understanding of the existing skill set and needs of the staff involved and the policies in place to support the work being undertaken, as well as a broader awareness of the organisation's overarching aims and mission statement. Questioning staff about their knowledge and skills permits examination of what they do and don't know. Maybe they understand what they should be doing but don't have the necessary skills to do it. Perhaps, they have both the knowledge and the skills, but the organisation's policies and working practices do not allow them to do it properly, or perhaps, there are no consequences for them of not doing their job well. All these need to be explored to determine if training is the right way to address the identified gap that the psychologist has observed or has been asked to fill.

There are various ways in which the required information might be gathered, but it must be done in a structured, consistent way and from as many staff as possible. Questionnaires or interview templates are a good way of asking the questions that need to be answered. To be cost effective, focus groups can be run with relevant staff, which can include possible learners and/or line managers. Directly observing practice can also reveal a lot about what is working and what is not. The questions asked, by whichever means, should relate to the subject matter where the perceived gaps are. Therefore, the psychologist needs to consult the most up-to-date literature to determine if those they are seeking to train are knowledgeable in this or not. A common error is making questions too broad; they need to be specific to the topic area. When collecting data from others, we must be mindful of ethics. Barbazette (2006) reminds us of the importance of confidentiality and to keep information that is used strictly anonymous.

Upon completing the TNA, a report should be produced and the findings fed back to key stakeholders. They need to understand not only the benefits to the organisation if the training goes ahead but also the potential costs if it does not. They must also be aware of the likely requirements involved to deliver it. Stakeholders are often busy but consultation is essential; they must be fully informed of the implications of progressing to step 2. The psychologist should never start the design phase until the outcome of the TNA has been produced and key stakeholders have approved training.

An online resource, hr-guide.com, helpfully covers the areas to consider when conducting a TNA and, importantly, prompts consideration of what the organisation is trying to accomplish, who will receive the training, what their existing knowledge is, why current practices aren't working and if policies and procedures are conducive to the role. This assists in determining if training is the best solution. A case study example highlighting each of the four steps is outlined at the end of this chapter and outlines a TNA in practice.

BOX 18.1   TRAINING NEEDS ANALYSIS – KEY POINTS

- Before embarking on a TNA, consult key stakeholders
- A TNA will identify whether training is required
- The TNA must be specific to the areas staff require development in
- Consult policies and procedures
- A TNA should result in a report that:

    - Reveals the findings of the consultation
    - Outlines how training will benefit staff performance, focusing on what the needs are
    - Generates clear aims and objectives for the training
    - Identifies who needs to be trained and why

- Stakeholders must be informed of the risks if the knowledge and performance of staff is left the way it is and, if there is a training need, commit to providing the time and resources to train staff

---

Step 2: designing the training

Once the needs of the staff are known, the next step is to consider how best to teach them the desired knowledge or skills necessary to successfully, and safely, complete their tasks. In line with the BPS code of ethics and conduct (2018), the psychologist must be mindful of competence. Organisations need the person developing the training to have the relevant competencies to design and deliver training. The trainer must have sufficient experience in the topic area over those they will be training. It is possible for one person to design a training programme and another to deliver it, but the competencies required must be made clear.

The programme must be planned well in advance and should focus on meeting the aims and objectives of learning and job performance outcomes, which are derived from the TNA. At the design stage, the psychologist must also consider how they will evaluate the programme. A number of stages of evaluation (especially assessment) need to be conducted at the time of the training so this must be pre-planned. How learners are selected and prioritised must also be considered, as should planning for the required resources, such as how many learners will attend, the size of room needed, where the training will be delivered and ensuring products, such as handouts and case studies, will be available.

When planning training methods, how attendees learn best should be considered. For years programme designers have drawn upon the literature of Honey and Mumford (1986) whose work was inspired from Kolb's (1984) learning styles model. Honey and Mumford identified four distinct learning styles (or preferences), which advocate that we all learn differently: some of us prefer learning by doing, some like to understand theory, some like to observe and others like experimenting. Despite the learning styles approach receiving criticism (Caple & Martin, 1994; Reynolds, 1997; Willingham et al., 2015), the key, from a design perspective, is to make the training as engaging to learners as possible.

Creating a manual is essential if the training is delivered by someone other than the designer as it helps to clarify exactly what is being taught and how each section addresses the aims and objectives. The actual training methods used should (i) be derived from the literature, (ii) match the type of training being delivered, for example, the approach to knowledge gain compared to skill acquisition will differ and (iii) suit the learner group. Examples include PowerPoint presentation, e-learning, video seminar/webinar, simulator, group discussions, role plays (skills practices) and case studies.

It is often the case that resources are limited. The psychologist needs to be creative. If the TNA allows, e-learning can be useful. Or, if not afforded a sufficient time frame in which to implement training, preparatory work for learners to read beforehand will give them sufficient knowledge on the topic to enable the training to focus on other elements. There will always be ways to work with limited resources; however, cutbacks cannot affect the integrity of the training aims.

It has already been highlighted that stakeholder buy-in is essential. However, stakeholders can put unhelpful restrictions on the trainer. For example, only allowing a certain time frame for training to be done within (e.g. two hours), therefore, it is important to communicate to them the requirements and whether training can be achieved in that time, rather than just accepting it. Refer to the case study for an example of designing a training programme.

BOX 18.2   DESIGNING TRAINING – KEY POINTS

- Ensure there is stakeholder approval identify who is competent to develop the training
- Ensure the design, including the length of the training, is influenced by the aims and objectives identified from the TNA
- Ensure the training is evidence based, and there is a clear link between theory and practice

- Be aware of the different training methods and their strengths and weaknesses: this helps to decide methods most appropriate to content and audience
- Consider how training will be assessed and evaluated. This must form part of the planning
- Ideally, produce a training manual

Step 3: implementation

There are two key elements to implementation: preparation and delivery. Training cannot be implemented well without advance preparation. Preparation involves ensuring that the necessary resources are ready for the start of the event, and all aspects of the proposed venue have been considered to determine its suitability. The training resources must be available – PowerPoint projector, flipchart, pens and learning materials. Appropriate joining instructions must be sent to all those who are attending and any preparatory work has to have been received. Preparation also involves rehearsal of the training material, which is key to effective training delivery (Bolton & Bolton, 2015). It will not be clear beforehand how receptive learners are going to be but knowing the material will not only allow delivery with confidence but also the ability to effectively answer questions as they arise.

When delivering training, it should be within the planned framework but responsive to problems, questions and other issues which might arise (Pont, 1998). The psychologist needs to be sensitive and support the needs of learners, especially when giving feedback. Some learners might be resistant to attending or they might not want to engage, ask questions or share their experiences, which can affect learning (Kauppila, 2018). In these instances, rolling with resistance, an approach adopted by Miller and Rollnick (2012) can be useful where a confrontation is avoided by listening and helping the learner to come up with a solution on how to proceed. It is not the psychologist's role to motivate the learner to do their job, but rather to be a motivating trainer (McLean, 2009). Even when learners are not invested, by understanding their concerns, it is possible to mutually agree goals and how best to teach them (Bolton & Bolton, 2015). Refer to the case study for an example of implementation and how to get learner buy-in.

BOX 18.3   IMPLEMENTING TRAINING – KEY POINTS

- Consider factors which may affect the training, such as the venue, timings and the release of staff
- Prepare all handouts and learning aids in advance
- Rehearse the training, ensuring the content and the timings are clear
- Implement the training so that the aims and objectives are achieved; review this regularly
- Administer the planned assessment procedures during the training in a standardised way
- Be clear, confident and engaging and roll with any resistance
- Be flexible, supportive and listen to the learners

Step 4: evaluation

There are many theories, which can guide an evaluation of training. Kirkpatrick's (1959) four levels of evaluation is probably the most well known. Despite being widely used, Kirkpatrick's work is not without its critics (Reio et al., 2017). Some argue that the framework is too conceptual (Spitzer & Conway, 2002) and makes too many assumptions (Alliger & Janak, 1989). Holton (1996) argues it fails to specify the causal relationships between the four levels. Other evaluation approaches overcoming some of these issues include the CIRO approach developed by Warr et al. (1970) or Phillips' (1995) five-level ROI (Return of Investment) programme.

The evaluative approach selected should be determined by the training programme. Consideration should be given to: (1) the extent to which the training objectives were met, (2) what the learners' learnt, (3) how successful the learners were at implementing the training back in their place of work and (4) whether these changes improved organisational functioning. Given that most training evaluation models utilise the four levels advocated by Kirkpatrick (even if they are called a different name or look at slightly different aspects), they are shown in Figure 18.2 and are explored further here.

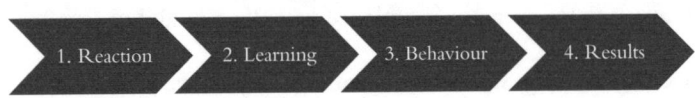

Figure 18.2 Levels of training evaluation

Source: (Kirkpatrick, 1959)

Level 1: reaction to the training

This considers whether the training was pitched at the right level and right pace. Essentially, this evaluates the trainer's style, knowledge and presentation techniques. This is often collected using a questionnaire, which is distributed to learners at the end of the training (this should be anonymous so learners can record their views without fear of upsetting the trainer). This is an important step as even if learners' needs have correctly been identified through an appropriate TNA and the training package adequately addresses these, it still might not obtain the desired results. For example, if the training is too long, too confusing or too boring, this will impact upon learning and stakeholders might conclude that there is little value in rolling out further events. In reality, however, the problem is actually trainer style and how easy the subject material was to follow rather than any flaws with the training design.

Level 2: learning

Learning is a big part of training staff. The only real way of determining learning is through measuring defined learning objectives. The approach chosen will depend on what staff are being trained in (e.g. skills or knowledge). The most commonly used method to assess skills is through observation, whereas knowledge tends to be measured through a test or quiz. The test/quiz needs to consist of the same questions administered immediately before and after the training. During assessment, many make the error of assessing confidence and not actual learning, that is, they measure how confident a learner is at applying their new skills or knowledge, rather than what they have actually learned. Learners should be informed at the start of the training that they will be asked to complete tests at the end, in line with our code of ethics and conduct (e.g. respect: informed consent). Methods used to assess training can include:

- Behavioural observation for skills practices
- Exercises/activities
- Quizzes
- Questionnaires
- Self-assessment

Whatever assessment method is used, it must be administered in a standardised way (Salkind, 2010). It must also have clear scoring criteria to ensure it remains as objective as possible (Andrade & Heritage, 2017). Measures that are not standardised or do not have defined marking criteria are common errors in those new to training delivery. If using a tool that has already been designed, permission must be granted from authors of the tool.

Level 3: behaviour

Training should be evaluated to appraise learners' experiences to see if learning objectives have been attained and to identify whether the training has had the desired effects on job performance. The ways of collecting evaluation data are similar to collecting data for a TNA:

- Questionnaires
- Direct observation
- Consultation with key stakeholders or those with specific knowledge
- Interviews
- Focus groups
- Assessments/surveys

Although the methods might be similar, the questions asked are very different. The TNA seeks gaps in knowledge or skills, whereas the evaluation seeks evidence that the objectives that were derived from the TNA have been met. Following up with staff to see how they are applying their learning and how job performance has improved must be undertaken after a predetermined period of time post-training and not just immediately afterwards.

Level 4: results

Finally, evaluation considers if the training has affected organisational functioning, which is primarily why training is being implemented in the first place. To evaluate level 4, the aims must be considered to determine if they have been met, whilst considering the overarching benefit to the organisation. An evaluation report is a helpful way to compile all the information related to the evaluation to then share with stakeholders. Often, a cost-benefit analysis will be undertaken to reveal if the money has been well spent and if there has been an adequate return on investment.

One of the most significant errors people make is failing to undertake a full evaluation, that is, not reporting on how the training has impacted on job performance and organisational functioning. Many people stop the evaluation process after considering the learners' reaction to the training and their learning. A full evaluation must be undertaken to confidently determine if the training was successful in meeting its aims. Refer to the case study for an example of evaluation.

BOX 18.4   EVALUATING TRAINING – KEY POINTS

- Consider different evaluation models to determine the best method for the training programme
- Evaluate the learner's reaction to the training
- Choose an appropriate assessment method to establish learning (not confidence) as a result of the training
- Ensure fairness by standardising assessments and using/developing scoring criteria, especially if training is a pass/fail event
- Determine whether the aims and objectives have been met
- Post-training, use several sources to determine if the training impacted on job performance (behaviour) and benefitted the organisation
- Produce an evaluation report outlining progress, strengths and weaknesses of the training, with recommendations for improvement
- Ensure the results of the evaluation are shared with stakeholders

---

Conclusion

There is much more to training staff than simply delivering the training to learners. Successful training starts by understanding the problem identified and asking whether training is necessary. A TNA allows those questions about the needs of the staff group – and how to remedy them – to be answered. This directly informs the training design, which should map onto the identified aims and objectives. The design must be guided by the most up-to-date literature on the topic being trained, as well as learning and training methods. Planning and preparation are key to the successful implementation of training. Whilst evaluation is numerical, steps 3 and 4 should not be considered last in the process; identifying the approach to assessment and evaluation should start in the design phase to ensure that both the short- and long-term benefits of the training are adequately explored. Throughout the process, stakeholder engagement and consultation is crucial, as is consideration of ethics, particularly awareness of the sensitivity involved in collecting data on staff. By following the four steps outlined, a robust training programme will be developed, which evaluation can then accurately determine if it did what was intended or not.

Case study: training in a forensic service

Senior Management asked Donna, a forensic psychologist, to help reduce the high levels of absenteeism they had noticed within their administrative team. Donna knew that criminal justice staff can be negatively affected by exposure to vivid and disturbing accounts of crimes (Robertson et al., 2009). Violanti et al. (1996) coined the term 'critical occupation' as a role where there is a frequent risk of contact to potentially traumatic events or material that may impact on the psychological well-being of the individual. The stakeholders were aware of this and presumed that their staff were experiencing negative symptoms from reviewing details of crimes, with the impact being workplace absence. They asked Donna to complete staff training on trauma as a solution.

Step 1: conducting a TNA

Donna had no way of knowing if training was required or if training on trauma would assist the organisation in reducing absenteeism. First, Donna had to confirm the hypothesis that it was the reading material that was affecting staff attendance; whether the staff were experiencing any trauma or difficulty, or if any other reason could be attributed to their absenteeism. Trauma is a vast subject and Donna knew that simply delivering training on trauma was unlikely to address the problem. She needed to be clear about exactly what the issues were.

Donna undertook a TNA, which involved (1) reviewing policies to determine if there was anything in place to support staff and (2) conducting focus groups with staff and requesting line managers complete a questionnaire. Donna asked a variety of specific questions about the staff's role. She ensured that she was familiar with the literature on vicarious trauma so she could ask the staff about the impact that reading violent material might have on them. She also asked what self-care measures they were aware of and what ones, if any, they were using. These activities enabled Donna to determine that:

- Staff did not receive specific training in relation to their role
- Staff knew very little about self-care practices
- Staff had little knowledge regarding how the organisation could support them
- 70% of staff reported they were affected by the material they were reading, and furthermore, they linked this to episodes of sick leave

The outcome of the TNA clarified that there were significant gaps in the staffs' knowledge and that training would be an appropriate method to address the issue. Importantly, the TNA confirmed what the aims of the training should be for staff, which were to: (1) enhance their knowledge of the effects of working with details of crime, (2) increase their understanding of what support was available to them from the organisation and (3) develop their knowledge of self-care and skills in applying self-care methods for themselves. Following approval from stakeholders, Donna then generated objectives to enable her to appropriately assess if learning had taken place. By the end of the training, learners should be able to:

- Display an understanding of the importance of self-care in their role
- Develop a self-care plan, which includes care of psychological, physical, emotional, professional and spiritual needs
- Identify at least five self-care strategies or activities they can use at home
- Identify at least five self-care strategies or activities that could improve workplace/ professional self-care
- Develop awareness of help offered by the organisation

Step 2: Designing the training

Having established the aims and objectives, and receiving stakeholder approval, Donna was able to develop the training programme. She considered the literature on training methodology and decided to use a combination of methods to ensure her training would be focused, interesting and appeal to the different styles within her learner group. She chose PowerPoint slides to communicate information on the effects of reading violent material, as well as slides on how to self-care; exercises to improve learning by engaging in reflection and discussion and having the learners develop their own 'Self-care Pack', which included a self-care assessment that they completed on themselves. This helped them identify how well they took care of their physical, psychological, emotional and spiritual needs.

Donna worked out how long the training would last then advised stakeholders, who agreed to release staff for the amount of time required. Donna also ensured she could access all the materials she needed to deliver the training.

Step 3: Implementing the training

First, Donna ensured the resources required to deliver the training were available and that joining instructions were issued to staff. Donna developed a training plan to ensure that the training was delivered as intended. During the event, Donna was responsive to her learners, regularly checked they understood the material and facilitated the training in an empathic and supportive manner; she was particularly mindful of the sensitive nature of the topic. Whereas most of the learners were receptive, one particular learner was critical and expressed disinterest. Here, Donna rolled with resistance and used a number of strategies such as reflection and reframing to offer a more positive interpretation of the negative information; for example, the learner complained that 'managers didn't care about her mental health and were always nagging her to get the job done'. Donna suggested that the training might help her to speak to managers and 'help them understand what it feels like to read this kind of material, and the pressure you feel'. By listening, empathising and emphasising the potential benefits of the training, Donna was able to motivate the learner who then fully participated in the event.

Step 4: Evaluating the training

After each successful delivery, Donna needed to evaluate the training.

Level 1

Reaction to the training was undertaken using a simple questionnaire, which asked for feedback on aspects such as joining instructions, appropriateness of venue, Donna's style and competence as a trainer and whether the training was pitched at the correct length and level.

Level 2

A test was used to measure learning against the objectives of the training. The same test was administered immediately before and directly after the training so it could be clear whether or not learning had occurred as a result of the training.

Level 3

A focus group was set up with some of the learners at three- and six-month intervals, post-training, which provided data on their view of the impact of the training on job performance. Donna was specifically looking for evidence that the learners were (i) being more open about their experiences with their managers and with colleagues, (ii) seeking more support and (iii) using the self-care measures. Donna found good evidence that the learners were doing all of these. Ultimately, Donna examined how the learners thought their new behaviours affected their job performance and found that there was a significant improvement. Donna also administered a bespoke questionnaire for line managers, which provided a measure of their view of changes in job performance (so the information did not solely come from the learners) and what may have influenced changes (or lack of changes).

The outcome of the evaluation of levels 1, 2 and 3 yielded important findings, and Donna was confident that her training had assisted staff, who thought they were subsequently working more effectively. With these promising results, she then needed to evaluate the impact of her training on the organisation.

Level 4

Donna did this through ongoing monitoring of staff well-being and absenteeism. Staff absenteeism linked with stress was reviewed 12 months after the training to determine the overall impact. Mindful of ethics, Donna did not require the personal details of the staff, rather, the date the individual completed the training and their level of stress-related absenteeism in the 12 months before and after completion of the training.

Learning outcomes

When you have completed this chapter, you should:

1 Understand the importance of gaining key stakeholder approval at every stage of a training project
2 Understand the importance of a TNA and how to conduct one
3 Identify the various methods to design a training programme
4 Understand considerations for how to implement a training programme
5 Understand how assessment fits into the evaluation process and that actual learning must be assessed, not confidence
6 Understand how to conduct the four levels of evaluation and why each level is important

Key concepts and terms

- Training needs analysis
- Evaluation
- Assessment
- Preparation
- Learning styles
- Return of investment

- Key stakeholders
- Focus groups
- Questionnaires
- Standardisation
- Roll with resistance

Sample essay questions

- Describe the importance of conducting a training needs analysis and describe how you would go about undertaking one.
- Why is stakeholder engagement so important to the training process?
- Describe and critique the Kirkpatrick theory of evaluation.
- Discuss how assessment differs from evaluation.

Recommended further reading

Kaufman, P., & Keller, J. M. (1994). Levels of evaluation: Beyond Kirkpatrick, *HRD Quarterly*, *5*(4), 371–380.

Phillips, J. J., & Phillips, P. P. (2016). *Handbook of training evaluation and measurement methods* (4th ed.). Routledge.

www.hr-guide.com.

References

Alliger, G. M., & Janak, E. A. (1989). Kirpatrick's levels of training criteria: Thirty years later. *Personnel Psychology*, *42*(2), 331–342.

Andrade, H., & Heritage, M. (2017). *Using assessment to enhance learning, achievement, and academic self-regulation*. Routledge.

Barbazette, J. (2006). *Training needs assessment: Methods, tools and techniques*. The skilled trainer series. Pfeiffer, A Wiley Imprint.

Blanchard, P. N., & Thacker, J. W. (2010). *Effective training: Systems, strategies and practices* (4th ed.). Pearson, Prentice Hall.

Bolton, R., & Bolton, D. G. (2015). *What great trainers do: The ultimate guide to delivering engaging and effective learning*. Amacon.

British Psychological Society. (2018). *Code of ethics and conduct*. BPS.

Caple, J., & Martin, P. (1994). Reflections of two pragmatists: A critique of honey and Mumford's learning styles. *Industrial and Commercial Training*, *26*(1), 16–20.

Goldstein, I. L. (1993). *Training in organisations: Needs assessment, development and evaluation* (3rd ed.). Pacific Grove.

Holton. E. F. (1996). The flawed four-level evaluation model. *Human Resource Development Quarterly*, *7*(1), 5–21.

Honey, P., & Mumford, A. (1986). *Manual of learning styles*. P Honey.

Kauppila, O. P. (2018). How does it feel and how does it look? The role of employee motivation in organizational learning type. *Journal of Organizational Behavior*, *39*(8), 911–1043.

Kirkpatrick, D. L. (1959). Techniques for evaluation training programs. *Journal of the American Society of Training Directors*, *13*, 21–26.

Kolb, D. A. (1984). *Experiential learning: Experience as the source of learning and development*. Prentice Hall.

McLean, A. (2009). *Motivating every learner*. Sage.

Miller, R. W., & Rollnick, S. (2012). *Motivational interviewing: Helping people change (Applications of motivational interviewing)* (3rd ed.). Guilford Press.

Phillips, J. (1995). *Return on investment: Beyond the four levels.* Academy of HRD 1995 Conference Proceedings.

Pont, T. (1998). *Developing effective training skills* (2nd ed.). McGraw-Hill.

Reio, G., Tonette, J. R., Rocco, S. S., & Chang, E. (2017). Critique of Kirkpatrick's evaluation model. *New Horizon in Adult Education and Human Resource Development, 292*(2), 35–53.

Reynolds, M. (1997). Learning styles: A critique. *Management Learning, 28*(2), 115–133.

Robertson, N., Davies, G., & Nettleingham, B. (2009). Vicarious traumatisation as a consequence of jury service. *The Howard Journal, 48*(1), 1–12.

Salkind, N. J. (2010). *Encyclopaedia of research design.* Sage Publications.

Spitzer, D., & Conway, M. (2002). *Link training to your bottom line.* American Society for Training and Development.

Violanti, J. M., Vena, J. E., Marshall, J. R., & Petralia, M. S. (1996). A comparative evaluation of police suicide rate validity. *Suicide and Life-Threatening Behavior, 26*(1).

Warr, P., Bird, M., & Rackham, N. (1970). *Evaluation of management training.* Gower Press.

Willingham, D. T., Hughes, E. M., Dobolyi, & David, G. (2015). The scientific status of learning styles theories. *Teaching of Psychology, 42*(3), 266–271.

Index